Breast Diseases

This comprehensive textbook incorporates all aspects of breast disease, including basic science, benign breast diseases, malignant neoplasms, diagnostics, multidisciplinary therapeutic options, and molecular biology research. It focuses on information useful for trainees, medical students, and practicing breast surgeons and oncologists. The highlight of the book is to present the controversies and arrive at a consensus in an evidence-based narrative. It aims to be useful not only for daily practice but also to establish a firm knowledge platform for clinicians and research scientists by outlining the guidelines for the treatment plan.

Key Features

- Has a global perspective and encourages implementation of the guidelines for management in daily practice
- Enriched with high-quality illustrations and flowcharts for easy understanding of trainees, fellows, and breast surgeons
- Covers the latest innovations and research in breast disease management

Breast Diseases
Guidelines for Management

Edited by
Diptendra Kumar Sarkar

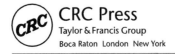

CRC Press
Taylor & Francis Group
Boca Raton London New York

CRC Press is an imprint of the
Taylor & Francis Group, an **informa** business

Designed cover image: Shutterstock
First edition published 2024
by CRC Press
2385 NW Executive Center Drive, Suite 320, Boca Raton, FL 33431

and by CRC Press
4 Park Square, Milton Park, Abingdon, Oxon, OX14 4RN

CRC Press is an imprint of Taylor & Francis Group, LLC

© 2024 Taylor & Francis Group, LLC

ISBN: 9780367421281 (hbk)
ISBN: 9780367609696 (pbk)
ISBN: 9780367821982 (ebk)

DOI: 10.1201/9780367821982

Typeset in Times
by KnowledgeWorks Global Ltd.

Contents

Editor

Diptendra Kumar Sarkar is a Professor of Surgery and Chief of the Breast Surgery and Research Unit at the Institute of Post Graduate Medical Education and Research, Kolkata, India. He was awarded the prestigious GB Ong award by the Royal College of Surgeons of Edinburgh for securing the highest position in the FRCS exam in 2000. He is currently the President of the Association of Breast Surgeons of India and the Honorary Secretary of the Asian Society of Mastology. He is the Associate Editor of the *Indian Journal of Surgery* and the *Journal of Indian Medical Association*. He is an international tutor-examiner with the Royal College of Surgeons of Edinburgh. He was awarded the prestigious Hauck Visiting Professorship in May 2019 by the Mayo Clinic, Rochester, Minnesota. He is a member of the Working Group Committee on Breast Cancer Screening in India and has been the international resource person for early diagnosis of breast cancer in Bangladesh. He is presently a member of the Governing Council of Association of Surgeons of India. His areas of interest include research in prognostic markers and locally advanced breast cancer. He has written more than 40 peer-reviewed articles and contributed to three book chapters.

Contributors

Sanjit Agarwal
Department of Breast Oncosurgery
Tata Medical Center
Kolkata, India

Rosina Ahmed
Department of Breast Oncosurgery
Tata Medical Center
Kolkata, India

Amanda L. Amin
Department of Surgery
University Hospitals
Cleveland, Ohio

Rudradeep Banerjee
Department of General Surgery
IPGME&R and SSKM Hospital
Kolkata, India

Srija Basu
Department of General Surgery
IPGME&R and SSKM Hospital
Kolkata, India

Ashok BC
Department of Plastic & Cosmetic Surgery
Manipal Hospital
Bengaluru, India

Saurabh Bharadwaj
Department of General Surgery
IPGME&R and SSKM Hospital
Kolkata, India

Hannah L. Bromley
Department of Clinical Oncology
The Christie NHS Foundation Trust
and
Division of Cancer Sciences
University of Manchester
Manchester, UK

Leena S. Chagla
Mersey and West Lancashire Teaching Hospitals
    NHS Trust
Merseyside, England

Suma Chakrabarthi
Department of Radiology and Imaging
Peerless Hospitex Hospital and Research Center
    Limited
Kolkata, India

Sumohan Chatterjee
University Hospital of South Manchester NHS
    Foundation Trust
Manchester, UK

Sharat Chopra
Cardiff University
Health Education and Improvement Wales (HEIW)
Aneurin Bevan University Health Board
Royal Glamorgan and Nevill Hospital
Newport, Wales

Kakali Choudhury
Department of Radiation Oncology
Murshidabad Medical College
Murshidabad, India

Soumen Das
Department of Surgical Oncology
Netaji Subhas Chandra Bose Cancer Hospital
Kolkata, India

Amy C. Degnim
Department of Surgery
Mayo Clinic Comprehensive Cancer Center
Rochester, Minnesota

SVS Deo
Department of Surgical Oncology
BRA–IRCH
All India Institute of Medical Sciences
New Delhi, India

Debashis Ghosh
Surgical Oncology
Royal Free London NHS Foundation Trust
London, UK

Joydeep Ghosh
Department of Medical Oncology
Tata Medical Center
Kolkata, India

Matt Green
The Royal Wolverhampton NHS Trust
West Midlands, UK

Ismail Jatoi
Division of Surgical Oncology and Endocrine
    Surgery
University of Texas Health Science Center
San Antonio, Texas

Heba Khanfar
Surgical Oncology
Royal Free London NHS Foundation Trust
London, UK

Ashutosh Mishra
Department of Surgical Oncology
BRA–IRCH
All India Institute of Medical Sciences
New Delhi, India

Afshin Mosahebi
Royal Free Hospital & University College
London, UK

Amitabh Ray
Chittaranjan National Cancer Institute–New Town
    Campus
Kolkata, India

Bahaty Riogi
Kisii Teaching and Referral Hospital
Kisii, Kenya

Ronit Roy
Department of General Surgery
IPGME&R and SSKM Hospital
Kolkata, India

Agnimita Giri
Paediatric and Adolescent Breast Clinic
Institute of Child Health
Kolkata, India

Nikita Shorokhov
Eurasian Federation of Oncology
Russian Federation
Moscow, Russia

Ayush Keshav Singhal
Department of General Surgery
IPGME&R and SSKM Hospital
Kolkata, India

Somasundaram Subramanian
Eurasian Cancer Research Council
Mumbai, India

Saima Taj
Surgical Oncology
Royal Free London NHS Foundation Trust
London, UK

Jajini Susan Varghese
Royal Free Hospital & University College
London, UK

Raghavan Vidya
The Royal Wolverhampton NHS Trust
West Midlands, UK

CORE AREA I: EPIDEMIOLOGY

Epidemiology of Breast Cancer

1

Saurabh Bhardwaj and Diptendra Kumar Sarkar

INTRODUCTION

Cancer is the leading cause of death and an important deterrent to increasing life expectancy in every country of the world (1). According to estimates of the World Health Organization (WHO) in 2019 (2), cancer is the first or second leading cause of death before 70 years in 112 of 183 countries.

According to GLOBOCAN 2020, there were an estimated 19.3 million new cases and 10 million cancer deaths worldwide in 2020 (3).

Female breast cancer is the most commonly diagnosed cancer (11.7% of total cases). In women, breast cancer is the leading cause of cancer death.

INCIDENCE AND POPULATION TRENDS

Female breast cancer has an estimated 2.3 million new cases. It is the fifth highest cause of cancer mortality worldwide, with 685,000 deaths. In women, breast cancer represents one in four cancer cases and accounts for one in six cancer deaths. It tops the incidence rate and mortality rate in 159 out of 185 countries and 110 out of 185 countries.

Incidence rates are 88% higher among transitioned countries than in transitioning countries (55.9 and 29.7 per 100,000, respectively). The highest incidence rates are found in Australia/New Zealand, Western Europe (Belgium has the world's highest incidence), North America, and Northern Europe and the lowest rates are found in Central America, Eastern and Middle Africa, and South Central Asia.

The higher incidence rates in higher Human Development Index (HDI) countries reflect a long-standing higher prevalence of reproductive as well as hormonal risk factors (early age of menarche, later age of menopause, higher age at first birth, fewer children, less breastfeeding, menopausal hormone therapy)

DOI: 10.1201/9780367821982-1

1

and lifestyle factors (alcohol intake, obesity, physical inactivity), as well as increased detection through screening.

Incidence rates of breast cancer are rising fast in transitioning countries in South America, Africa (4), and Asia (5), as well as in high-income Asian countries (Japan and the Republic of Korea) (6), where rates have historically been low. Changes in lifestyle and sociocultural environments brought about by growing economies with an increase in the proportion of working women have had an impact on the prevalence of breast cancer risk factors—the postponement of childbirth and having fewer children, excess body weight, and physical inactivity—have in turn resulted in a convergence toward the risk factor profile of Western countries, causing a narrowing of international gaps in breast cancer morbidity.

DISTRIBUTION ACCORDING TO TYPE

Histological Classification

The WHO describes at least 18 different histological breast cancer types. Invasive breast cancer of no special type (NST), also known as invasive ductal carcinoma, is the most frequent subgroup (40%–80%). About 25% of invasive breast cancers show distinctive growth patterns and cytological features; hence, they are recognized as specific subtypes (invasive lobular carcinoma, tubular, mucinous A, mucinous B, neuroendocrine) (7).

Molecular Classification

The breast cancer subtype of hormone receptor positive/human epidermal growth factor receptor 2 negative (HR+/HER2–) is the most common subtype, with an age-adjusted rate of 88.1 new cases per 100,000 women, based on 2014–2018 Surveillance, Epidemiology, and End Results Program (SEER) data. This is a rate more than six times higher than the triple-negative breast cancer rate of 13.1 and the HR+/HER2+ breast cancer rate of 13.4, and over 16 times higher than the HR–/HER2+ breast cancer rate of 5.5 (8).

The best survival pattern was seen among women with the HR+/HER2– subtype, followed by HR+/HER2+ subtype and then the HR–/HER2+ subtype. The HR–/HER2– subtype, also known as the triple-negative subtype, had the worst survival (9).

The distribution of breast cancer subtypes varies by age, race, ethnicity, stage, and other factors. Compared with women with the HR+/HER2– subtype (the most common subtype), those diagnosed with the other three subtypes were more likely to be younger, belong to minority groups, and diagnosed with cancer at a later stage.

MORTALITY TRENDS

Breast cancer was the leading cause of cancer deaths among women in the world in 2020 (GLOBOCAN 2020). Mortality in low-income countries such as Fiji, Jamaica, Samoa, Nigeria, and Cameroon were higher than that in high-income countries (South Korea, Australia, the United States, and the United Kingdom). The geographic variations in breast cancer mortality indicated a disparity in access to early screening and treatment. In highly developed countries in Europe and America, there was a downward mortality trend, which started in 1988–1996, and the highest decrease was 39% between 1989 and 2015, which probably was a result of early detection by mammography screening and improvements in treatment. Limited financial support given to health in low-income countries led to a majority of breast cancer patients diagnosed with advanced-stage disease being unable to receive timely treatment, which was also the reason for the poor prognosis in these countries The trends of breast cancer mortality decreased in the United States, Australia, and the United Kingdom between 2000 and 2015 (10). The decline of breast cancer mortality in these countries owed to early detection by mammography and improvements in medical treatment. "Delay" is the key factor for poorer survival in low- and middle-income countries. Delay can be in the pre-diagnostic phase (lesser access of rural populations to modern health care), diagnostic phase (lack of one-stop clinics and trained manpower), and treatment delay (delay in initiation of treatment due to various factors).

CONCLUSION

Despite a decline in mortality rates in breast cancer, the prevalence of the disease is on a steady rise. As of the end of 2020, there were 7.8 million women alive with breast cancer in the past 5 years, making it the world's most prevalent cancer. There are more lost disability-adjusted life years (DALYs) by women to breast cancer worldwide than any other type of cancer. Hence, several attempts have to be made globally to decrease the morbidity of the disease and to offer a better standard of living for the survivors.

REFERENCES

1. Bray F, Laversanne M, Weiderpass E, Soerjomataram I. The ever-increasing importance of cancer as a leading cause of premature death worldwide. *Cancer*. 2021 Aug 15;127(16):3029–30.
2. Global health estimates: Leading causes of death [Internet]. [cited 2022 Apr 13]. Available from: https://www.who.int/data/gho/data/themes/mortality-and-global-health-estimates/ghe-leading-causes-of-death
3. Sung H, Ferlay J, Siegel RL, Laversanne M, Soerjomataram I, Jemal A, et al. Global Cancer Statistics 2020: GLOBOCAN estimates of incidence and mortality worldwide for 36 cancers in 185 countries. *Cancer Journal for Clinicians*. 2021 May;71(3):209–49.
4. Joko-Fru WY, Jedy-Agba E, Korir A, Ogunbiyi O, Dzamalala CP, Chokunonga E, et al. The evolving epidemic of breast cancer in sub-Saharan Africa: Results from the African Cancer Registry Network. *International Journal of Cancer [Internet]*. 2020 [cited 2022 Apr 13];147(8):2131–41. Available from: https://onlinelibrary.wiley.com/doi/abs/10.1002/ijc.33014
5. Bray F, McCarron P, Parkin DM. The changing global patterns of female breast cancer incidence and mortality. *Breast Cancer Research [Internet]*. 2004 Aug 26 [cited 2022 Apr 13];6(6):229. Available from: https://doi.org/10.1186/bcr932
6. Heer E, Harper A, Escandor N, Sung H, McCormack V, Fidler-Benaoudia MM. Global burden and trends in premenopausal and postmenopausal breast cancer: A population-based study. *Lancet Global Health [Internet]*. 2020 Aug 1 [cited 2022 Apr 13];8(8):e1027–e37. Available from: https://www.sciencedirect.com/science/article/pii/S2214109X20302151
7. Łukasiewicz S, Czeczelewski M, Forma A, Baj J, Sitarz R, Stanisławek A. Breast cancer—Epidemiology, risk factors, classification, prognostic markers, and current treatment strategies—An updated review. *Cancers (Basel) [Internet]*. 2021 Aug 25 [cited 2022 Apr 13];13(17):4287. Available from: https://www.ncbi.nlm.nih.gov/pmc/articles/PMC8428369/
8. Female breast cancer subtypes—Cancer stat facts [Internet]. SEER. [cited 2022 Apr 13]. Available from: https://seer.cancer.gov/statfacts/html/breast-subtypes.html

9. Howlader N, Cronin KA, Kurian AW, Andridge R. Differences in breast cancer survival by molecular sub-types in the United States. *Cancer Epidemiology, Biomarkers & Prevention*. 2018 Jun;27(6):619–26.

10. Lei S, Zheng R, Zhang S, Wang S, Chen R, Sun K, et al. Global patterns of breast cancer incidence and mortality: A population-based cancer registry data analysis from 2000 to 2020. *Cancer Communications (Lond) [Internet]*. 2021 Aug 16 [cited 2022 Apr 13];41(11):1183–94. Available from: https://www.ncbi.nlm.nih.gov/pmc/articles/PMC8626596/

CORE AREA II: RADIOLOGY

Breast Imaging for the Surgeon

2

Suma Chakrabarthi

INTRODUCTION

Looking through the eyes of the radiologist, the myriad gray dots fashion themselves into the colorful kaleidoscope of information! Imaging is the science and art of discovering information that is not visible to the naked eye or clinically palpable. It is important for the clinician to understand the role, advantages, indications, and contraindications of various imaging modalities that are available. It is equally important to utilize radiological tests intelligently in a resource-constrained environment, and a good understanding of the radiological investigations helps achieve optimal results. This chapter will hopefully equip you to image your patient in the most favorable way irrespective of where you practice in the world.

THE PILLARS OF BREAST IMAGING – MAMMOGRAPHY AND ULTRASOUND

Choosing the Right Modality – Basic Principles

Mammography and ultrasound studies complement each other. While most abnormalities are demonstrated on both modalities, some features are specifically better visualized on only one of these modalities. Small grouped microcalcifications are not usually visualized on ultrasound, but are distinctly seen on mammograms (1). Ultrasound is an excellent modality to differentiate a solid mass from a cyst, although on mammograms both are visualized as masses. Hence, any significant abnormality demonstrated on one modality should ideally be correlated with the other to get the whole picture. (Figure 2.1). An algorithm to help decide which modality to choose as the starting point of imaging investigations is useful (Flowchart in page 11).

DOI: 10.1201/9780367821982-2

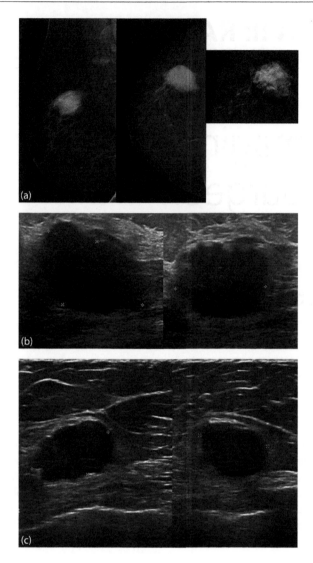

FIGURE 2.1 A 56-year-old woman presented with a palpable mass in the right upper outer breast. (a) Right MLO, CC, and CC spot compressions views *(left to right)* demonstrate the palpable right upper outer breast dense, irregular-shaped mass with indistinct margin. (b) Ultrasound demonstrates the corresponding hypoechoic 3.9 cm × 2.3 cm × 3 cm (outlined by the small cursors in the image) irregular-shaped mass with indistinct margin in the right upper outer breast at the 10 o'clock position, 2 cm from the nipple. Core biopsy confirmed this to be an invasive ductal carcinoma. (c) Ultrasound also demonstrates a posteriorly situated smaller mass in the right lower inner breast at the 5 o'clock position. It measures 1.8 cm × 1.1 cm × 1.5 cm (outlined by the small cursors in the image) and is about 3 cm from the nipple. This demonstrates the importance of performing both mammography and ultrasound.

In the presence of breast symptoms such as a palpable lump, clinically significant nipple discharge, or breast pain, mammography is used as the first investigation for women aged 40 years or more, with the addition of ultrasound when indicated (2). Any suspicious abnormality demonstrated on mammography must be investigated with breast ultrasound. Ultrasound is recommended in certain situations even if the mammograms are normal. For example, if a woman presents with a palpable breast lump or blood-stained nipple discharge, breast ultrasound must be performed even if the mammography images are normal.

Small intraductal masses are better appreciated on ultrasound, and the ability to palpate the mass as one scans the breast cannot be underestimated in diagnosing the palpable lump.

The theoretically increased radiation risk of mammography, low incidence of breast cancer, and relatively denser breast tissue which reduces mammographic sensitivity in the less-than-30-years age group, make ultrasound the imaging method of choice in this age group. This is also the modality of choice during pregnancy and lactation (3, 4). However, mammography should be performed if there is a suspicious finding on ultrasound in these groups.

In the 30–39 years age group, both ultrasound and mammography may be good options. Clinical correlation is advised before requesting/performing a mammogram in this age group. For example, a 34-year-old woman with a clinically obvious palpable fibroadenoma may only need a ultrasound to confirm the same. However, a woman presenting with a suspicious hard palpable mass would benefit from both mammography and ultrasound at the outset.

Mammograms performed to investigate women presenting with breast symptoms are called diagnostic mammograms. Screening mammography refers to mammograms in women who do not have breast symptoms or obvious clinical signs of breast cancer. The aim of this is to detect breast cancer early, thereby reducing the morbidity and mortality from the disease (5). Many countries have population-based breast screening programs and start screening women periodically from an age that the program deems apt for their population. Some examples of breast screening programs/guidelines are the National Health Service Breast Screening Programme (UK) and American College of Radiology Guidelines (6, 7). Whereas the former recommends screening women every 3 years from the age of 50–70 years, the latter advises annual screening from the age of 40 years to an age at which life expectancy is less than 5–7 years due to age or comorbid conditions. Ultrasound may be used as an adjunct to screening mammography in women with dense breasts, but it needs to be kept in mind that this increases false-positive examinations (8, 9). Early screening with mammograms at less than 40 years is appropriate in high-risk groups. These include women with a lifetime risk of breast cancer of ≥ 20% according to risk assessment tools, women with known *BRCA1* or *BRCA2* gene mutations, their untested first-degree relatives, and women who have had radiation therapy to the chest between 10 years and 30 years of age (6, 7, 9). Screening with annual mammography is recommended from the age of 30 years or 10 years before the age of diagnosis of a first-degree relative with breast cancer, whichever is later. With a history of mantle radiotherapy, annual mammography should be started 8 years after radiation therapy. However, screening mammography is not to be started for any woman before the age of 25 years, irrespective of the cause of the high risk. Annual breast MRI is recommended as an adjunct to mammography-based screening for these high-risk women. Only breast MRI for screening is advised for women with TP53 (Li–Fraumeni) syndrome and A-T homozygotes (7, 9). If MRI is contraindicated or if the woman cannot tolerate an MRI study, breast ultrasound should be used instead (9).

Many countries have established national guidelines for mammography and ultrasound, both for the choice of the appropriate first investigation for breast symptoms (2–4) and for screening. In a country that does not have such guidelines, the options include following one of the established guidelines or to develop one's own guidelines based on the available local data of the prevalence and incidence of breast cancer in different age groups in the country (10).

Technique – Mammography

Mammography is the process of using low-energy X-rays to acquire radiographs of the breast. Standard mammography images include mediolateral oblique (MLO) and craniocaudal (CC) views of each breast. Bilateral mammograms are advised even if symptoms are unilateral, as otherwise subtle asymmetric abnormalities may be missed. Digital mammography (DM) is preferred over conventional film screen mammography, particularly in women < 50 years of age and with dense breast tissue (11). If a suspicious abnormality is detected, additional views such as lateral, spot compression, and magnification views, are acquired. The lateral view helps confirm whether a lesion that is approximately in the line of the nipple on the MLO view is actually in the upper or lower half of the breast. Magnification views are for further assessment of microcalcifications, while spot compression views are for further assessment of masses, architectural distortions, and asymmetries. Other views, such as the laterally/medially extended CC views and the valley view, help visualize areas of the breast that are not well visualized on the standard views. For women with implants, special views with the implants displaced are also acquired for better visualization of breast parenchyma. The dose of radiation must be kept to the minimum without reducing the image quality. Automated Exposure Control (AEC) system which is inbuilt in most modern mammography machines helps minimize radiation for the given breast thickness and composition. Optimal compression must be applied during acquisition of images. Exposure time must be as low as possible to reduce the dose, to avoid motion artifact, and to minimize discomfort to the woman being imaged.

Digital breast tomosynthesis (DBT)

DBT is a quasi-3D imaging technique in which several low-dose images are acquired as the X-ray tube rotates along an arc around the breast. A 3D dataset is reconstructed from these projection images and viewed as thin slices. The main advantage is that it removes the superimposition of tissues, thereby helping the radiologist identify a true abnormality rather than an apparent abnormality caused by the overlap of normal tissues. It is especially helpful in young women with dense breasts (12). The indications for diagnostic DBT and screening DBT are the same as for 2D DM (13). Synthesized 2D mammography (SM) images, which are maximum-intensity projections, can be created from the DBT dataset. If DM and DBT are used together, the radiation dose to the patient increases by a factor of 2.25 when compared to the dose for DM alone. However, if DM is replaced by SM, the radiation dose can be reduced by 45% (14). There are multiple studies that demonstrate that the combination of SM and DBT is as good as the combination of DM and DBT (15–17). DBT should be used only for implant-displaced views for imaging breasts with implants (13).

Contrast-enhanced spectral mammography (CESM)

CESM is a mammographic method of assessing tumoral angiogenesis, thereby acquiring physiological information about the mass along with the morphological information acquired on DM. Nonionic, low-osmolar contrast medium is injected intravenously, and two sets of images are acquired, one at low energy and another at high energy. Thus, CESM is a dual-energy technique. The low-energy images are subtracted from the corresponding high-energy images, giving an image that demonstrates areas of contrast uptake in areas of tumoral angiogenesis. The low-energy images are interpreted as routine DM images. This is not, however, a kinetic study, and time-intensity curves cannot be acquired, as is possible in contrast-enhanced (CE) MRI. It has better diagnostic accuracy than DM, especially in dense breasts (18, 19). It is capable of accurate assessment of tumor size (20). It is also an effective tool for the assessment of response to neoadjuvant chemotherapy (21) and in the postoperative breast for assessment of recurrence (22). It may a good screening test for intermediate-risk women with dense breasts (23). As there are two exposures involved, the radiation dose may be up to 81% higher upon comparison with standard DM (24).

Technique – Ultrasound

Ultrasonography is a imaging technique that uses high-frequency sound waves produced from a probe to interrogate tissues. Based on the echoes that are reflected from the tissues back to the probe, as well as the time taken for return of echoes, an image is created which is analyzed by the operator. A high-resolution probe (12–5 MHz, 18–6 MHz) with a center frequency of at least 10 MHz is required to perform breast ultrasound (25).

Patient positioning is vital for optimal visualization of breast tissue. The woman lies in the supine position with arms placed above the head. To assess the lateral aspect of the breast, the woman turns to the opposite side and lies in a semi-lateral decubitus position with the arm placed above her head to ensure that the lateral part of the breast is flattened over the chest wall while scanning. Application of gel on the skin is mandatory to perform ultrasound studies. This is because the gel acts as a lubricant for easy movement of the probe over the skin and also obliterates the air between the probe and the skin, which impedes transmission of sound waves through the skin. Gentle pressure is applied over the breast while performing ultrasound. The gray-scale settings should be optimized for the study. The focal zone is set at the level of the abnormality that is being assessed. To get a cutaneous or a superficial lesion into the focal zone, a thick layer of gel can be applied on the skin. The gain setting is said to be optimal when subcutaneous fat appears medium gray (26). Color flow imaging is very useful in certain situations, such as confirming vascularity within small intraductal lesions for the diagnosis of papillomas.

Elastography is a new adjunct in breast ultrasound which assesses the elasticity of tissues and classifies lesions as soft, intermediate, and hard. There are two types of elastography: Strain elastography and shear wave elastography. Although elastography findings may aid in diagnosis, they must not be used in isolation to evaluate a lesion. In strain elastography, size ratio and strain ratio values are obtained. Elasticity values are documented in kilopascals (kPa) or meters/second (m/s) in shear wave elastography (27).

Automated breast volume scan (ABVS) is a special type of breast ultrasound which uses a mechanically driven wide linear array transducer that can image whole breast volumes in three dimensions. The data are sent to a separate workstation to be analyzed by the radiologist (28). ABVS is less operator dependent, more reproducible, and is being explored as a potential tool for breast cancer screening in women with dense breasts (29). Lesions detected on ABVS need further evaluation with handheld ultrasound. Suboptimal visualization of the axillary tail and axilla, as well as artifacts in the nipple area, are some of the limitations of ABVS.

BREAST MRI

The minimum requirement to provide a breast MRI service is a 1.5 tesla magnet with dedicated breast surface coils capable of simultaneous bilateral imaging. The equipment must be able to provide high spatial and temporal resolution for morphologic and kinetic assessment, respectively, of the lesion. Kinetic assessment is performed by acquisition of a series of images after injecting gadolinium contrast intravenously at a dose of 0.1 mmol/kg and drawing a time-intensity curve of contrast uptake (30). Typically, a malignant mass demonstrates fast uptake in the initial phase and a washout pattern in the delayed phase. In contrast, a typically benign curve shows slow uptake in the initial phase and persistent enhancement in the delayed phase (31). The morphology of the lesion and its kinetics are both taken into account to characterize it.

MRI is an excellent modality for assessing the extent of disease in newly diagnosed breast cancer. It demonstrates multifocality and multicentricity better than mammography and ultrasound, especially in dense breasts (Figure 2.2). Posterior breast tumors are also better assessed on MRI. As it has high sensitivity, MRI may demonstrate suspicious lesions not initially shown on mammography and ultrasound. Of these MRI-only lesions, masses are more likely to have a sonographic correlate than non-mass-like lesions, 65% and 12%, respectively, on second-look ultrasound. Malignant mass lesions are more likely to be demonstrated on second-look ultrasound correlation, with 85% seen sonographically (32). MRI is the examination of choice for assessing response to neoadjuvant chemotherapy. It is important to perform a baseline MR study prior to starting neoadjuvant chemotherapy in order to be able to assess response to treatment. MRI accurately detects occult primary breast lesions in 62%–86% of cases that present as unilateral metastatic axillary lymphadenopathy with unknown primary malignancy (33). It is very useful in differentiating a postoperative scar from local recurrence. It is the modality of choice for the assessment of the integrity of breast implants, which is very well facilitated by silicone selective sequences.

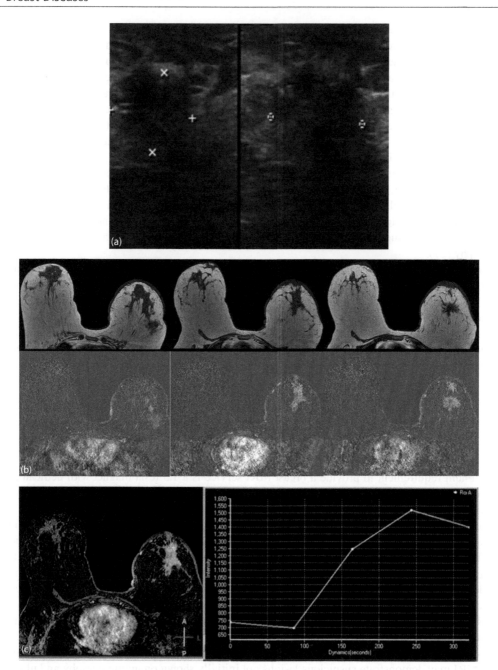

FIGURE 2.2   (a) Ultrasound image of a 50-year-old woman who presented with a palpable mass in the left upper breast at the 12 o'clock position. The 1.6 cm × 1.8 cm × 1.9 cm (delineated by cursors in longitudinal and transverse section) mass at 12 o'clock is irregular shaped, has indistinct margins, and is nonparallel to the skin. Core biopsy demonstrated invasive ductal carcinoma. (b) *Top row:* Precontrast axial T1-weighted representative images of breasts below the level of the nipple, at the level of the nipple, and above the level of the nipple from left to right. *Bottom row:* Corresponding post-contrast subtracted images demonstrating the abnormal enhancement in the left breast in all the images. Skin thickening and abnormal enhancement of the skin and nipple are also noted. (c) *Dynamic imaging:* Time–intensity curve demonstrates fast uptake of contrast in the initial phase and washout pattern in the delayed phase in keeping with a malignant mass. Postsurgical histology demonstrated grade III invasive ductal carcinoma with ductal carcinoma *in situ* and an extensive intraductal component, with lymphovascular invasion and 2/22 positive axillary lymph nodes.

But perhaps the most important role of breast MRI is to problem-solve equivocal or inconclusive findings of mammography and ultrasound. Asymmetries that look suspicious on mammography with normal ultrasound findings, spontaneous bloody or serous nipple discharge with normal mammography and ultrasound, to make a decision as to which mass to biopsy when multiple masses with varying suspicious characteristics are seen, and to identify a solid mass within ducts with inspissated material making identification of the lesion difficult on ultrasound, are some of the situations where MRI comes to the rescue of the radiologist.

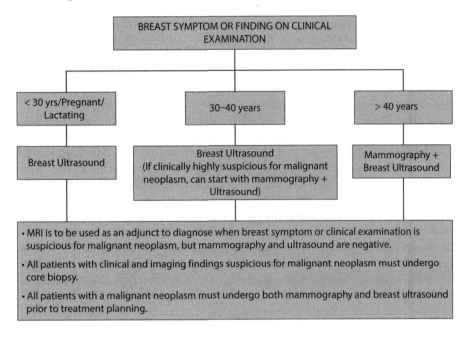

Flowchart on "Algorithm for Breast Imaging."

SYSTEMS OF REPORTING IN BREAST IMAGING

Usage of a standardized reporting system by the radiologist facilitates a better understanding of the radiological findings by the other members of the multidisciplinary team. It is as if a common language is spoken by all! One such system is the Breast Imaging Reporting And Data System (BI-RADS) from the American College of Radiology (34). Other similar systems are also used, such as the Royal College of Radiologists Breast Group breast imaging classification (35). Most importantly, the report must communicate the salient findings to the referring doctor in a clear and unambiguous way.

INTERVENTIONS IN BREAST IMAGING

A radiologist's job is exciting because of the various procedures one can do, both diagnostic and therapeutic, with a kit of a just few needles and wires!

Core biopsy (CB) has been proven to have a lower false-positive rate as well as a lower false-negative rate and is preferred over fine needle aspiration cytology (FNAC) (36). However, fine needle aspiration is very useful for diagnostic aspiration of abscesses for culture and sensitivity assessment or for confirmation of a galactocele. When a mass is predominantly cystic, aspiration of the cystic content prior to obtaining cores of the solid component improves the quality of tissue acquired. A fully automated 14-gauge biopsy gun is the standard device for both ultrasound-guided and mammography-guided stereotactic CB. If a lesion is visualized on ultrasound, it is biopsied under ultrasound guidance, as the procedure is more comfortable for the patient with no radiation risk. It is also quicker, and the needle can be visualized by the radiologist in real time, unlike during the stereotactic biopsy procedure. Hence the most common diagnostic procedure is ultrasound-guided CB of lesions for tissue diagnosis. Only when lesions are not visualized on ultrasound are stereotactic biopsies performed under mammography guidance. A typical example would be small grouped calcifications. However, small masses, asymmetries, and architectural distortions that do not have an ultrasound correlate are also biopsied stereotactically. Vacuum-assisted biopsy (VAB) devices are 7–12 gauge and can acquire all samples in one single percutaneous insertion. It has become the method of choice for very small clusters of calcifications and scanty suspicious calcifications (37). It is performed for rebiopsy of lesions with inadequate sampling or indeterminate reports upon CB (38).

Vacuum-assisted excision (VAE) is an accepted method for therapeutic image-guided excision of small benign masses such as fibroadenomas (39). The concept of VAE of other lesions such as atypical ductal hyperplasia (ADH) that present as a subcentimeter cluster of microcalcifications that are completely excised on VAB is also being explored (40). Excision of small radial scars without atypia on CB or VAB can also be performed by VAE (41). Other therapeutic image-guided procedures include aspiration of breast abscess or a large tender cyst.

It is advisable to leave a marker clip at the site of the lesion that has been excised under image guidance. This is to be able to surgically excise this area if the VAE demonstrates any evidence of malignancy. Marker clips should also be placed into tumors that show a rapid radiological response to neoadjuvant chemotherapy, so that if the mass were to undergo complete radiological response, the marker clip could be localized under image guidance for breast conservation surgery. Clips can be placed under mammography, ultrasound, or MR guidance. Currently, hookwire-guided localization is the most common technique used for preoperative localization of nonpalpable breast lesions. Radioactive seeds, magnetic seeds, radiofrequency identification tags, and nonradioactive radar technology-based devices are other options available (42). After surgery, the excised tissue must be radiographed to confirm the presence of the localizing device and the abnormal tissue in the specimen.

STAGING BREAST CANCER

After establishing the diagnosis of breast cancer with the help of mammography, ultrasound, CB, and in some cases MRI of the breasts, the next important step is to determine the stage of the disease, so that an appropriate treatment plan can be made. Let us look at the radiological investigations deemed appropriate for this step. The stages referred to in this section are as per anatomical staging in the 8th Edition of the American Joint Committee on Cancer (AJCC) Cancer Staging Manual of the American College of Surgeons (ACS) (43).

Routine use of radiological investigations to detect occult distant metastasis is not advised T1 or T2, N1 or N0, in breast cancer due to false-positive studies and the low yield of these investigations (43). A chest X-ray is sufficient. Additional tests should be performed if clinical signs and symptoms raise suspicion of metastases. For example, a Tc99m-methylene diphosphonate (MDP) bone scan can be performed if the patient has local bone pain suggestive of metastasis or if serum alkaline phosphatase is elevated. Abnormal clinical examination findings, elevated serum alkaline phosphatase, or abnormal liver function tests warrant cross-sectional imaging such as contrast-enhanced computed tomography study (CECT) of the abdomen with or without CECT of the pelvis. If there are suspicious chest symptoms or an abnormal chest X-ray, a CECT scan of the chest is advised (43).

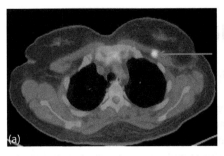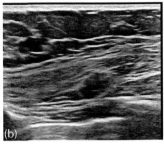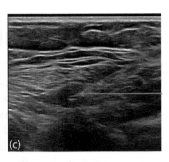

FIGURE 2.3 A 24-year-old woman underwent left breast conservation surgery 1 year ago, had chemotherapy, and completed radiotherapy for invasive ductal carcinoma (IDC). (a) PET-CT demonstrates a single FDG avid left subpectoral mass (*arrow*). No other suspicious lesion is demonstrated. (b) A 1.1 cm × 0.7 cm × 0.8 cm hypoechoic mass (*arrow*) with irregular shape and microlobulated margin, deep to the pectoralis major muscle in the left upper chest is seen on ultrasound. Appearances are suspicious for a malignant lymph node. (c) Ultrasound-guided core biopsy (*arrow shows needle*) demonstrated metastatic adenocarcinoma. Surgical excision confirmed a metastatic lymph node from breast carcinoma.

CECT chest and abdomen and MDP bone scan are advised for patients with stage IIIA and locoregional disease. Alternatively, PET-CT alone could be performed, although this is not routinely advised (43) (Figure 2.3).

It is important to remember that stage migration should be taken into account while planning staging investigations. Triple-negative tumors are generally upstaged in their prognostic stage, and HER2 expression is a downstaging factor. So, a grade 2–3 triple-negative T2N1M0 patient with anatomical stage IIB may get upgraded to a higher clinical prognostic staging of IIIB (43, 44).

MRI of the breast is advised when women present with metastatic breast disease, but no lesion is demonstrated on mammography and ultrasound.

PREGNANCY AND BREAST IMAGING

Ultrasound is the first imaging modality that should be used to assess the breasts of a pregnant woman who presents with a breast lump or other significant symptom. If malignancy is strongly suspected or proven by biopsy, bilateral mammography is advised (45).

Mammography is generally safe during pregnancy (45). However, a few points must be kept in mind regarding the perceived risks of radiation. Pregnancy status of women of childbearing age must be checked for prior to performing mammography, and in case of any doubt, a pregnancy test is advised. The estimated dose to the fetus in the first trimester from an average bilateral two-view mammography is less than 0.03 μGy (0.003 mrad), which can be reduced by at least one-half by wearing a lead apron (46, 47). A lead shield should be offered to all pregnant patients (45). Radiation-related side effects can be classified into deterministic and stochastic effects. Mammography is not expected to cause in utero deterministic side effects such as teratogenic fetal effects, as no deterministic side effects have been reported at radiation less than 50 mGy (5 rad) (47). Stochastic risks have no threshold radiation dose at which cellular damage causing cancer or germ cell mutation occurs. Also, the severity of radiation-induced stochastic effects is independent of the radiation dose (48). Therefore, mammography should be carefully used in pregnant patients, although fear of potential radiation effects on a fetus should not deter us from performing necessary mammographic studies, and a case-based approach to decision making is advised (49).

Routine screening mammography is not performed during pregnancy (45).

Contrast-enhanced breast MRI is not usually performed during pregnancy due to the possibility of gadolinium-related side effects on the fetus (45).

BREAST IMAGING IN MEN

Men presenting with symptoms and signs of a breast lump or nipple discharge are investigated as women are. Gynecomastia is the most common breast disease among men (50). This has a very characteristic appearance on ultrasound, which often suffices to make a diagnosis and reassure the patient. Practice, However, practice varies, and some breast units perform a mammography to confirm gynecomastia (Figure 2.4). Given the high incidence of breast carcinoma in men presenting with suspicious nipple discharge, for men above the age of ≥25 years presenting with this symptom, mammography and breast ultrasound are both advised, as microcalcifications may be missed if only ultrasound is performed (3, 51).

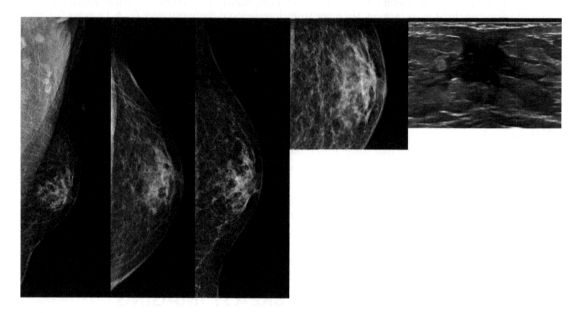

FIGURE 2.4   A 75-year-old man presented with an enlarging left breast. Images from left to right are left MLO, CC, lateral, spot compression mammographic views, and left retroareolar ultrasound view. Mammograms demonstrate dendritic gynecomastia with retroareolar soft tissue density with extensions into deeper adipose tissue. Similarly, the ultrasound image demonstrates characteristic retroareolar hypoechoic tissue with extensions into the deeper adipose tissue.

BREAST IMAGING IN RESOURCE-LIMITED COUNTRIES

Resource-limited refers here to economic resources, as I strongly believe that the so-called resource-limited countries have a more adventurous and resource-unlimited spirited workforce with the inspiration to change the world! Having worked in both resource-rich and resource-limited environments, I have come to realize that at the end of the day, it is a combination of knowledge, hard work, communication, good intention, and attention to detail that saves lives in both environments. In countries with few state-of-the-art tertiary hospitals and many smaller resource-limited hospitals, a hub-and-spoke model could work very well, with basic investigations taking place closer to home and more specialized imaging tests and procedures performed at the hub. In countries where there is a dearth of tertiary hospitals and trained professionals, the solution is to invest resources for the most important basic tools of imaging and to find indigenous intelligent innovations for interventional procedures.

In terms of imaging, the two most basic tools are mammography and breast ultrasound. Although DM has shown better results than analogue (film-screen) mammography, we must not forget that the world at large used analogue mammography and looked after its breast patients quite well for many years before DM was invented! Installation and management of an analogue mammography machine with stereotactic equipment and mammography guided wire localization paddle comes at a fraction of the cost of digital equipment. Many studies have shown that the cancer detection rates for analogue and digital systems are comparable (52, 53). What is more important is a robust quality assurance program to get the best results out of the analogue mammography system. Adjunct screening of dense breasts with ultrasound is effective in mammography-negative dense breasts. Ultrasound can pick up more breast cancers but results in more false positives upon comparison with tomosynthesis as an adjunct to mammography in screening dense breasts (54). It is important to equip ultrasound machines with an appropriate high-resolution probe to perform a good-quality breast ultrasound (25, 34).

Core biopsy is the preferred sampling test. However, FNAC is a reliable tool in the hands of experienced cytopathologists. In resource-limited settings, the pathologists often report a large number of FNAC studies and are very confident and competent in this technique (55, 56).

Hookwire localizations can be performed with indigenously prepared wires that are cost-effective. If the lesion is visualized on ultrasound, localizing in the operation theater with a simple spinal needle after the patient is anesthetized, cleaned, and draped is also an option, as malposition of the needle is less likely. Also, the excised tissue can be scanned in the operation theater to confirm excision of the neoplasm. The other option is to perform ultrasound-guided localization of the hematoma from biopsy; however, this needs to be performed within a narrow time frame before the hematoma becomes invisible on ultrasound (42).

For staging investigations one option is to have a multiple tier system depending on the resources that are available. Some countries have planned such that every breast cancer patient has access to the essential staging investigations as required and attempt is to make available the best staging investigations possible under the circumstances (57).

CONCLUSION

Breast imaging is one of the main pillars of breast health. While the basic concepts of breast imaging are universal, no one radiological model fits all. Depending on the availability of economic resources, level of subspeciality training in breast imaging, and access to pathology resources, each hospital has to put together the best breast imaging unit it can and systematically work toward bettering the services. For those of us who have what is perceived by the world as a state-of-the-art breast unit, it is a constant endeavor to maintain the high standards. For those of us who at present are working toward what we would like to be the world's best breast unit, there is a constant adrenaline rush toward achievement of our dreams. Either way, we are all travelers and let us all enjoy the journey!

REFERENCES

1. Soo MS, Baker JA, Rosen EL. Sonographic detection and sonographically guided biopsy of breast microcalcifications. *AJR Am J Roentgenol.* 2003;180(4):941–48. doi:10.2214/ajr.180.4.1800941.
2. Willett AM, Michell MJ, Lee MJR. Practice diagnostic guidelines for patients presenting with Breast symptoms, November 2010, Document from The Royal College of Radiologists.
3. Expert Panel on Breast Imaging; Lee S-J, Trikha S, Moy L, Baron P, diFlorio RM, et al. ACR Appropriateness Criteria® Evaluation of Nipple Discharge. *J Am Coll Radiol JACR.* 2017 May;14(5S):S138–S53.

4. ACR Appropriateness Criteria® Palpable Breast Masses, Revised 2016. American College of Radiology. Available from: https://org/docacsearch.acr.s/69495/Narrative/ (accessed on 11 September 2020).

5. Tabár L, Dean PB, Chen TH-H, Yen AM-F, Chen SL-S, Fann JC-Y, et al. The incidence of fatal breast cancer measures the increased effectiveness of therapy in women participating in mammography screening. *Cancer.* 2019 15;125(4):515–23.

6. NHS Public Health Functions Agreement 2019–20; Service Specification no. 24, NHS Breast Screening Programme; Public Health England with NHS England and NHS Improvement and NHS Improvement Public Health Commissioning; July 2019.

7. Lee CH, Dershaw DD, Kopans D, Evans P, Monsees B, Monticciolo D, et al. Breast cancer screening with imaging: recommendations from the Society of Breast Imaging and the ACR on the use of mammography, breast MRI, breast ultrasound, and other technologies for the detection of clinically occult breast cancer. *J Am Coll Radiol JACR.* 2010 Jan;7(1):18–27.

8. Buchberger W, Geiger-Gritsch S, Knapp R, Gautsch K, Oberaigner W. Combined screening with mammography and ultrasound in a population-based screening program. *Eur J Radiol.* 2018 [cited 2020 Sep 11];101:24–29. doi:10.1016/j.ejrad.2018.01.022. Available from: https://www.ejradiology.com/article/S0720-048X(18)30030-5/abstract

9. Mainiero MB, Moy L, Baron P, Didwania AD, diFlorio RM, Green ED, et al. ACR Appropriateness Criteria® breast cancer screening. *J Am Coll Radiol.* 2017 Nov;14(11):S383–S90.

10. Chakrabarthi S, Shikha Panwar, Tulika Singh, Shilpa Lad, Jwala Srikala, Niranjan Khandelwal, et al. Best Practice Guidelines for Breast Imaging, Breast Imaging Society, India. Annals of the National Academy of Medical Sciences (India). 2022. DOI: 10.1055/s-0042-1742586.

11. Pisano ED, Gatsonis C, Hendrick E, Yaffe M, Baum JK, Acharyya S, et al. Diagnostic Performance of Digital versus Film Mammography for Breast-Cancer Screening [Internet]. http://dx.doi.org/10.1056/NEJMoa052911. *Massachusetts Medical Society*; 2009 [cited 2020 Sep 13]. Available from: https://www.nejm.org/doi/10.1056/NEJMoa052911

12. Heggie JCP, Barnes P, Cartwright L, Diffey J, Tse J, Herley J, et al. Position paper: recommendations for a digital mammography quality assurance program V4.0. *Australas Phys Eng Sci Med.* 2017 Sep;40(3):491–543.

13. ACR Practice Parameter For the performance of Digital Breast Tomosynthesis (DBT), Adopted 2018 (Resolution 36), American College of Radiology [Internet]. [cited 2020 Sep 14]. Available from: https://www.acr.org/-/media/ACR/Files/Practice-Parameters/DBT.pdf?la=en

14. Tirada N, Li G, Dreizin D, Robinson L, Khorjekar G, Dromi S, et al. Digital breast tomosynthesis: physics, artifacts, and quality control considerations. *Radiogr Rev Publ Radiol Soc N Am Inc.* 2019 Apr;39(2):413–26.

15. Zuley ML, Guo B, Catullo VJ, Chough DM, Kelly AE, Lu AH, et al. Comparison of two-dimensional synthesized mammograms versus original digital mammograms alone and in combination with tomosynthesis images. *Radiology.* 2014 Jun;271(3):664–671.

16. Zuckerman SP, Conant EF, Keller BM, Maidment ADA, Barufaldi B, Weinstein SP, et al. Implementation of synthesized two-dimensional mammography in a population-based digital breast tomosynthesis screening program. *Radiology.* 2016 Dec;281(3):730–6.

17. Aujero MP, Gavenonis SC, Benjamin R, Zhang Z, Holt JS. Clinical performance of synthesized two-dimensional mammography combined with tomosynthesis in a large screening population. *Radiology.* 2017;283(1):70–6.

18. Dromain C, Thibault F, Muller S, Rimareix F, Delaloge S, Tardivon A, et al. Dual-energy contrast-enhanced digital mammography: initial clinical results. *Eur Radiol.* 2011 Mar 1;21(3):565–74.

19. Mori M, Akashi-Tanaka S, Suzuki S, Daniels MI, Watanabe C, Hirose M, et al. Diagnostic accuracy of contrast-enhanced spectral mammography in comparison to conventional full-field digital mammography in a population of women with dense breasts. *Breast Cancer.* 2017 Jan 1;24(1):104–10.

20. Fallenberg EM, Dromain C, Diekmann F, Engelken F, Krohn M, Singh JM, et al. Contrast-enhanced spectral mammography versus MRI: initial results in the detection of breast cancer and assessment of tumour size. *Eur Radiol.* 2014 Jan;24(1):256–64.

21. Iotti V, Ravaioli S, Vacondio R, Coriani C, Caffarri S, Sghedoni R, et al. Contrast-enhanced spectral mammography in neoadjuvant chemotherapy monitoring: a comparison with breast magnetic resonance imaging. *Breast Cancer Res.* 2017 Sep 11;19(1):106.

22. Helal MH, Mansour SM, Ahmed HA, Ghany AFA, Kamel OF, Elkholy NG. The role of contrast-enhanced spectral mammography in the evaluation of the postoperative breast cancer. *Clin Radiol.* 2019 Oct 1;74(10):771–81.

23. Sorin V, Yagil Y, Yosepovich A, Shalmon A, Gotlieb M, Neiman OH, et al. Contrast-enhanced spectral mammography in women with intermediate breast cancer risk and dense breasts. *Am J Roentgenol.* 2018 Nov;211(5):W267–W74.

24. Perry H, Phillips J, Dialani V, Slanetz PJ, Fein-Zachary VJ, Karimova EJ, et al. Contrast-enhanced mammography: a systematic guide to interpretation and reporting. *Am J Roentgenol.* 2018 Nov 1;212(1):222–31.

25. Appavoo S, Aldis A, Causer P, Crystal P, Mesurolle B, Mundt T, et al. CAR Practice Guidelines and Technical Standards for Breast Imaging and Intervention ; 2016 September 17. Canadian Association of Radiologists [Internet]. Available from: https://car.ca/wp-content/uploads/Breast-Imaging-and-Intervention-2016.pdf (accessed on 13th September 2020).

26. D'Orsi CJ, Mendelson EB, Ikeda DM, et al. Breast Imaging Reporting and Data System: ACR BIRADS Breast Imaging Atlas. Reston (VA): American College of Radiology; 2003 [Internet]. [cited 2020 Sep 13]. Available from: https://www.acr.org/Clinical-Resources/Reporting-and-Data-Systems/Bi-Rads

27. Youk JH, Gweon HM, Son EJ. Shear-wave elastography in breast ultrasonography: the state of the art. *Ultrasonography*. 2017 Oct 1;36(4):300–9.: 300–9.

28. Wojcinski S, Farrokh A, Hille U, Wiskirchen J, Gyapong S, Soliman AA, et al. The Automated Breast Volume Scanner (ABVS): initial experiences in lesion detection compared with conventional handheld B-mode ultrasound: a pilot study of 50 cases. *Int J Womens Health*. 2011 Oct 11;3:337–46.

29. Kelly KM, Richwald GA. Automated whole-breast ultrasound: advancing the performance of breast cancer screening. *Semin Ultrasound CT MR*. 2011;32(4):273–80. doi:10.1053/j.sult.2011.02.004.

30. DeMartini WB, Rahbar H. Breast magnetic resonance imaging technique at 1.5 T and 3 T: requirements for quality imaging and American College of Radiology Accreditation. *Magn Reson Imaging Clin N Am*. 2013 Aug 1;21(3):475–82.

31. Macura KJ, Ouwerkerk R, Jacobs MA, Bluemke DA. Patterns of enhancement on breast MR images: interpretation and imaging pitfalls. *RadioGraphics*. 2006 Nov 1;26(6):1719–34.

32. Abe H, Schmidt RA, Shah RN, Shimauchi A, Kulkarni K, Sennett CA, et al. MR-directed ("Second-Look") ultrasound examination for breast lesions detected initially on MRI: MR and sonographic findings. AJR Am J Roentgenol. 2010 Feb;194(2):370–7.

33. Argus A, Mahoney MC. Indications for breast MRI: case-based review. *Am J Roentgenol*. 2011 Mar 1;196(3_supplement):WS1–WS14.

34. D'Orsi CJ, Mendelson EB, Ikeda DM, et al. Breast Imaging Reporting and Data System: ACR BIRADS Breast Imaging Atlas. Reston (VA): American College of Radiology; 2013.

35. Maxwell AJ, Ridley NT, Rubin G, Wallis MG, Gilbert FJ, Michell MJ. The Royal College of Radiologists Breast Group breast imaging classification. *Clin Radiol*. 2009 Jun 1;64(6):624–7.

36. Vimpeli S-M, Saarenmaa I, Huhtala H, Soimakallio S. Large-core needle biopsy versus fine-needle aspiration biopsy in solid breast lesions: comparison of costs and diagnostic value. *Acta Radiol Stockh Swed*. 2008 Oct;49(8):863–9.

37. Wilkinson L, Thomas V, Sharma N. Microcalcification on mammography: approaches to interpretation and biopsy. *Br J Radiol* [Internet]. [cited 2020 Nov 8];90(1069). Available from: https://www.ncbi.nlm.nih.gov/pmc/articles/PMC5605030/

38. Borrelli C, Cohen S, Duncan A, Given-Wilson R, Jenkins J, et al. Clinical Guidance for Breast Cancer Screening Assessment, NHS Breast Screening Programme. NHSBSP publication number 49, fourth edition; November 2016.

39. Image-Guided Vacuum-Assisted Excision Biopsy of Benign Breast Lesions. Interventional Procedures Guidance, National Institute for Health and Care Excellence. Published: 22 February 2006. Available from: www.nice.org.uk/guidance/ipg156

40. Schiaffino S, Massone E, Gristina L, Fregatti P, Rescinito G, Villa A, et al. Vacuum assisted breast biopsy (VAB) excision of subcentimeter microcalcifications as an alternative to open biopsy for atypical ductal hyperplasia. *Br J Radiol* [Internet]. 2018 May [cited 2020 Nov 8];91(1085). Available from: https://www.ncbi.nlm.nih.gov/pmc/articles/PMC6190792/

41. Pinder SE, Shaaban A, Deb R, Desai A, Gandhi A, Lee AHS, et al. NHS breast screening multidisciplinary working group guidelines for the diagnosis and management of breast lesions of uncertain malignant potential on core biopsy (B3 lesions). *Clin Radiol*. 2018 Aug;73(8):682–92.

42. Cheang E, Ha R, Thornton CM, Mango VL. Innovations in image-guided preoperative breast lesion localization. *Br J Radiol* [Internet]. 2018 May [cited 2020 Nov 8];91(1085). Available from: https://www.ncbi.nlm.nih.gov/pmc/articles/PMC6190760/

43. American Joint Committee on Cancer (AJCC) Cancer Staging Manual, 8th Edition, The American College of Surgeons (ACS). [Internet]. [cited 2020 Nov 8]. Available from: https://cancerstaging.org/references-tools/deskreferences/Documents/AJCC%20Cancer%20Staging%20Form%20Supplement.pdf

44. Kalli S, Semine A, Cohen S, Naber SP, Makim SS, Bahl M. American Joint Committee on Cancer's Staging System for Breast Cancer, 8th Edition: what the radiologist needs to know. *RadioGraphics*. 2018 Sep 28;38(7):1921–33.

45. Breast imaging of the pregnant and lactating patient: imaging modalities and pregnancy-associated breast cancer. *Am J Roentgenol.* [cited 2020 Jun 30]. 200(2) (AJR) [Internet]. Available from: https://www.ajronline.org/doi/full/10.2214/ajr.12.9814

46. Sechopoulos I, Suryanarayanan S, Vedantham S, D'Orsi CJ, Karellas A. Radiation dose to organs and tissues from mammography: Monte Carlo and Phantom Study. *Radiology.* 2008 Feb;246(2):434–43.

47. ACR–SPR Practice Parameter for Imaging Pregnant or Potentially Pregnant Adolescents and Women with Ionizing Radiation R 2018 (Resolution 39). Pregnant-Pts.pdf [Internet]. [cited 2020 Jun 29]. Available from: https://www.acr.org/-/media/ACR/Files/Practice-Parameters/Pregnant-Pts.pdf

48. Wieseler KM, Bhargava P, Kanal KM, Vaidya S, Stewart BK, Dighe MK. Imaging in pregnant patients: examination appropriateness. *Radiogr Rev Publ Radiol Soc N Am Inc.* 2010 Sep;30(5):1215–29; discussion 1230–1233.

49. Wagner LK, Applegate KE. Re: More cautions on imaging of pregnant patients. *Radiogr Rev Publ Radiol Soc N Am Inc.* 2011 Jun;31(3):891; author reply 891–892.

50. Iuanow E, Kettler M, Slanetz PJ. Spectrum of disease in the male breast. *Am J Roentgenol.* 2011 Mar 1; 196(3):W247–59.

51. Muñoz Carrasco R, Álvarez Benito M, Rivin del Campo E. Value of mammography and breast ultrasound in male patients with nipple discharge. *Eur J Radiol.* 2013 Mar;82(3):478–84.

52. Kerlikowske K, Hubbard RA, Miglioretti DL, Geller BM, Yankaskas BC, Lehman CD, et al. Comparative effectiveness of digital versus film-screen mammography in community practice in the United States. *Ann Intern Med.* 2011 Oct 18;155(8):493–502.

53. Song SY, Park B, Hong S, Kim MJ, Lee EH, Jun JK. Comparison of digital and screen-film mammography for breast-cancer screening: a systematic review and meta-analysis. *J Breast Cancer.* 2019 May 13;22(2):311–25.

54. Tagliafico AS, Mariscotti G, Valdora F, Durando M, Nori J, La Forgia D, et al. A prospective comparative trial of adjunct screening with tomosynthesis or ultrasound in women with mammography-negative dense breasts (ASTOUND-2). *Eur J Cancer Oxf Engl 1990.* 2018;104:39–46.

55. McHugh KE, Bird P, Sturgis CD. Concordance of breast fine needle aspiration cytology interpretation with subsequent surgical pathology: an 18-year review from a single Sub-Saharan African institution. *Cytopathol Off J Br Soc Clin Cytol.* 2019;30(5):519–25.

56. Kazi M, Suhani, Parshad R, Seenu V, Mathur S, Haresh KP. Fine-needle aspiration cytology (FNAC) in breast cancer: a reappraisal based on retrospective review of 698 cases. *World J Surg.* 2017;41(6):1528–33.

57. National Cancer Grid Breast Cancer Management Guidelines, National Cancer Grid, India [Internet]. [cited 2023 October 22]. Available from: https://tmc.gov.in/ncg/docs/pdf/NCG_Guidelines_%202019/NCG%20 Guidelines%20for%20Breast%20Cancer-2019.pdf

CORE AREA III: PHYSIOLOGY AND BENIGN CONDITIONS

Developmental Anomalies of the Breast

3

Agnimita Giri

INTRODUCTION

The mammary glands are modified apocrine glands. The development occurs from two sources. The surface ectoderm forms the epithelial lining of the ducts and alveoli, while the mesoderm forms the fibrofatty stroma.

During 4th to 6th week of intrauterine life, two ectodermal mammary ridges appear on each side of the body wall from the future axilla to inguinal region. These ectodermal ridges usually regress, except the one located in the 4th or 5th intercostal space, which develops into mammary glands. The axillary tail of the gland may be due to the persistence of the cephalic end of the ridge. The bud at the 4th or 5th intercostal space presents a depression known as the mammary pit. Fifteen to twenty epithelial cords from the bottom of the pit grow into underlying mesoderm and subdivide further to form the ducts and terminate as ampullated ends. This occurs by 15–20 weeks of fetal life when the areola becomes apparent. The cords are canalized by the end of intrauterine life. As the underlying mesoderm develops, the mammary pit evaginates to form the nipple shortly before birth.

POSTNATAL DEVELOPMENT OF BREAST

Breast maturation and involution occur in the first 2 years of life. The normal gland then remains quiescent from 2 years of age until puberty. The breast is usually palpable in the newborn, irrespective of gender, due to varying amounts of tissue. The nipple becomes everted around this time. The areolar

DOI: 10.1201/9780367821982-3

pigmentation increases, and erectile tissue develops in the nipple–areolar complex. In a few cases the nipples remain inverted until puberty. The morphological changes in the postnatal period do not follow a linear progression, and three different morphological types (I–III) can occur. The functional changes are linear. There is a stage of apocrine metaplasia prior to involution. There are small ducts in a fibroblastic stroma in the infant breast by the age of 2 years.

PUBERTAL DEVELOPMENT OF THE FEMALE BREAST

The breast development begins in females as the first sign of puberty mainly under the influence of estrogen. Tanner's stages of development of the breast can be stated as follows:

- *Stage 1*: Elevation of papilla. This preadolescent stage has no additional development of stroma or parenchyma beyond what has occurred in infancy. The estrogen surge depends on pituitary growth hormone and ability of growth hormone to stimulate production of insulin-like growth factor 1 in the breast during puberty. This stimulates breast development. This occurs between 8.5 and 13.5 years of age. Nondevelopment of breasts by 14 years of age in females will require further investigation.
- *Stage 2*: Formation of breast bud with nipple elevation, a small mound of breast tissue, and areolar diameter enlargement occurs. This occurs at the average age of 11 years. The normal age of thelarche is from 8.5 to 13 years.
- *Stage 3*: Specifies further enlargement the breast and areola with no separation of contours, which occurs at an average age of 12.5 years.
    Between Tanner stages 2 and 3, there may be a discrepancy in size between the breasts of a female at puberty.
- *Stage 4*: There is nipple and areolar enlargement, leading to the formation of a secondary mound on the breast, with the average age being 13–14 years.
    Between Tanner stages 3 and 4, menarche usually occurs.
- *Stage 5*: Recession of the areola on to the breast, resulting in loss of the separation of the contours. This stage occurs around 15 years of age.

The average time spent between Tanner stages 2 and 5 is 4–4.5 years. The average increase in the size of diameter of the nipple between Tanner stages 1 and 5 is 5–6 mm.

Cellular changes: Increase in stromal and parenchymal growth occurs first. It is followed by ductal elongation and dichotomous branching under the influence of estrogen. During puberty, the epithelium forms a branching bilayer ductal structure with an outer basal layer of myoepithelial cells and an inner layer of luminal cells. There are two types of luminal cells: Ductal luminal cells lining the ducts and alveolar luminal cells (for lactation). At the terminal end of the bud, ductal elongation and complex branching take place. There are mammary stem cells in the cap cell layer of the terminal bud.

The primary ducts divide into segmental and subsegmental ducts and form terminal ducts, which further divide to form terminal ductules or acini. A collection of acini arising from one terminal duct with surrounding intralobular stroma is called a terminal duct lobular unit (TDLU). This is the functional unit of the breast. The elongation of the duct continues and the remaining space in the breast is occupied by adipose tissue with blood vessels, immune cells, and fibroblasts.

Lobular development is of four types. Type 1 is a short terminal duct that ends in a cluster of secretory cells called alveoli. Types 2–4 represent the branching of terminal ducts into several ductules and an increasing number of alveoli. The adult nulliparous breast completely matures (ductal and stromal) by 18–20 years of age and consists of type 1 lobules. The gland remains in a mature but inactive stage until pregnancy.

PUBERTAL DEVELOPMENT OF THE MALE BREAST

In males, due to raised testosterone concentration at puberty, there is no development of breasts, but up to 40% of males may have transient gynecomastia, probably due to estrogenic dominance. A pubertal increase in nipple diameter occurs in males. Males and females can have the same nipple diameter until pubic hair stage 3.

REGULATION OF BREAST DEVELOPMENT

Prenatal infant and pubertal breast development is due to interactions between epithelial components and mesenchymal stromal cells. The local migration and changes in epithelial cell adhesion take place under the influence of the inductive properties of the mesenchyme. At all stages of development there are hormonal influences on the paracrine interaction between the mesenchyme and parenchyma. Placental hormones entering fetal circulation influence the formation of lactiferous ducts.

The other hormones that might help prenatal and pubertal breast development are growth hormone, insulin-like growth factors, estrogen, prolactin, adrenal corticoids, and triiodothyronine.

Ductal morphology and branching seem to be influenced by some regulators like ErbB2. Another regulator, bcl-2, acts as an inhibitor of apoptosis of the fetal and infant breast.

Hormone receptors are not expressed in the mammary stem cells and progenitors; there is no proliferation of hormone receptor–positive stem cells. Thus, hormone-mediated morphological changes occur through a complex regulatory network of paracrine signals and transcription factors to control the mammary stem cell activity.

The human breast ultimately reaches adulthood after undergoing extensive remodeling under the influence of hormonal signals in different stages of development.

Dysregulation may lead to congenital and developmental anomalies of the breast.

Congenital Anomalies

1. **Amastia and athelia**
   - Amastia is bilateral agenesis of the mammary gland. It may be unilateral.
   - Athelia is the absence of the nipple and areola. It may be bilateral or unilateral.
   - Amastia and athelia may be associated with Poland syndrome (breast anomalies may include absent chest wall muscles with the absence of 2nd to 5th ribs, webbed fingers, vertebral anomalies, radial nerve palsy, and pectus excavatum).

Treatment: Amastia can be treated by augmentation mammoplasty using implants or an expander implant. In expander implants, the volume of the implant is adjusted with time to match the volume of the contralateral breast.

2. **Polymastia and polythelia**
   - The incidence in the general population is approximately 1%. This condition may be inheritable.
   - Polythelia is more common in males than in females.
   - Polymastia refers to extra or accessory breast tissue, and polythelia refers to extra or supernumerary nipples, most commonly occurring along the milk line underneath the normally located breast or nipples.
   - They rarely can occur in ectopic sites like back or the buttocks.

Treatment: Accessory or ectopic breast tissue may cause discomfort during menstrual cycles and the postpartum period. Surgery is indicated for cosmetic reasons only.

DISORDERS IN PREPUBERTAL CHILDREN

Witch's Milk

In 60% of normal newborns, there may be unilateral or bilateral enlargement of the breast under the influence of maternal hormones. These changes may be sometimes associated with secretion of an opaque liquid, which is often termed witch's milk. It resolves spontaneously and no treatment is needed.

Benign Premature Thelarche

Isolated breast development may occur in females between the ages of 6 months and 9 years. The diagnosis of precocious puberty is considered if there are signs of puberty like hair growth and accelerated bone age. This should be carefully examined, as it may indicate ovarian or adrenal tumors.

Treatment of isolated thelarche is reassurance and re-evaluation every 6–12 months. If breast development does not regress or shows progression within 1–2 years, endocrine workup is required. If there are other signs of puberty, then precocious puberty must be excluded. Precocious puberty may be peripheral (gonadotropin-releasing hormone [GnRH]-independent) or incomplete and central (GnRH-dependent).

Secretion of sex steroid independent of GnRH release is responsible for peripheral precocious puberty. Serum follicle-stimulating hormone (FSH) and luteinizing hormone (LH) levels are normal or low. Administration of steroids exogenously, secretion of endogenous steroids from an adrenal or ovarian tumor, and McCune–Albright syndrome are the main causes.

Early-onset puberty is often mediated centrally by premature activation of the hypothalamic-pituitary-gonadal axis. It occurs mostly in females. The common cause of central precocious puberty is idiopathic. Other causes may be central nervous system (CNS) lesions, trauma, and hypothalamic hamartomas. The GnRH stimulation test is diagnostic.

Treatment: Continuous administration of exogenous GnRH to suppress FSH and LH release, along with resection of the lesion responsible for precocious puberty.

Inflammations of the Breast

Breast abscesses can occur in prepubertal children and adolescents due to *Streptococcus* and *Staphylococcus* as the infective agents. Treatment is needle aspiration rather than incisional drainage in order to minimize the risk of breast bud damage, followed by oral antibiotics. Nowadays, due to nipple piercing, infection may occur around 7 months afterward in 10%–20% of cases. Treatment requires removal of the foreign body and drainage of pus. Healing is delayed for 6–12 months due to formation of a tract. In newborns, mastitis neonatorum can occur in the second and third week of life. Cellulitis occurs with or without an abscess. Treatment is antibiotics, but if the abscess doesn't resolve, drainage is required.

DISORDERS DURING PUBERTY

Breast asymmetry: One breast develops rapidly before the other breast. On clinical examination there is homogenous single breast enlargement with or without tenderness and without a palpable mass. Ultrasonography reveals breast tissue without a mass. In most cases the asymmetry resolves with time. If the asymmetry persists even after full development of the breast, then reduction or augmentation mammoplasty is needed.

Enlarged breasts or macromastia: This is commonly associated with mastalgia, back pain, painful shoulder grooving, poor posture, and loss of body image. It occurs in adolescence and is mostly associated with obesity. Treatment is weight reduction, physical therapy, improved posture, support brassiere and nonsteroidal antiinflammatory drugs (NSAIDs). After breast development is complete, reduction mammoplasty may be done.

Juvenile breast hypertrophy: It is an extreme form of bilateral diffuse symmetrical breast enlargement occurring during menarche. It is associated with neck, shoulder, and back pain. During thelarche there is an abnormal response of breast tissue under hormonal influence, but the levels of estradiol and progesterone are normal. There is an increase in connective tissue with moderate ductal proliferation in the breast. Treatment may be hormonal, but definitive treatment is reduction mammoplasty or subcutaneous mastectomy with prosthesis.

Breast atrophy: This can occur in puberty due to poor eating habits. In this case, there is loss of fat and tissues supporting the breasts. It can be associated with polycystic ovarian syndrome (PCOS) due to hyperandrogenism. Anorexia nervosa or chronic disease can also be a cause. Treatment depends on the situation but includes estrogen, antiandrogen, proper nutrition, and weight gain.

Tuberous breast: It is a reduced basal diameter of the breast both in horizontal and vertical levels due to breast hypoplasia, along with herniation of the nipple–areolar complex through a constricting ring. This results in protuberation of the areola causing cosmetic deformity. The treatment is reassurance, but surgical reconstruction is required in severe cases.

Gynecomastia: It occurs in 50%–60% of males in early adolescence and is usually seen 1 year after the onset of puberty. Gynecomastia rarely occurs secondary to endocrine syndromes or tumors and can present before puberty. Clinically it presents as diffusely enlarged and painful breasts or discreet mobile subareolar masses. Eccentric breast masses require evaluation. Testicular examination is mandatory in cases of gynecomastia. Simple gynecomastia is most common, but less common secondary causes include Klinefelter's syndrome, testicular feminization, hormone-secreting tumors, hyperthyroidism, hypothyroidism, cirrhosis, drug use like marijuana, cimetidine use, and familial predisposition. Pseudogynecomastia is associated with obesity, and weight loss with reassurance can resolve the condition. Mild to moderate cases of simple gynecomastia should be reassured that the condition is self-limiting. But in severe cases where the breast enlargement is more than 4 cm, chances of spontaneous resolution are rare, and breast pain or discomfort and psychological trauma are possible, surgical correction is recommended. Surgical correction is done by subcutaneous mastectomy through a subareolar incision with or without liposuction.

NEOPLASTIC DISORDERS OF THE BREAST

Fibroadenomas account for 68% of breast masses in adolescents. They can be simple fibroadenomas, giant or juvenile fibroadenomas, and phyllodes tumor.

- *Simple fibroadenomas*: are the most common lesion in adolescent girls. This is often a painless and asymptomatic breast lump. Sometimes pain occurs before the menstrual cycle. Clinically the breast configuration is not distorted; the lump occurs mostly single but can be multiple; and it is rubbery in consistency, well circumscribed, and mobile and not fixed to surrounding tissues. Juvenile or giant fibroadenomas are characterized by painless progressive lumps.

Histologically, they contain proliferating stroma around elongated ducts. Ultrasonography confirms the diagnosis and shows a solid, well-circumscribed avascular mass. Triple assessment is needed for diagnostic confirmation. ***Treatment*** in small lesions is reassurance. In a few large lesions surgical excision may be done.

- *Phyllodes tumor*: This comprises 0.4% of breast masses in adolescence. They can be benign or malignant. The lump is mobile with the overlying skin thin, shiny, and with increased vascularity. There is no nipple retraction or nipple discharge and no dimpling of overlying skin, but there can be a painless, rapidly growing breast lump. Histologically, they are not fully encapsulated and extending into surrounding breast tissue. Benign lesions have a hyperplastic and cellular stromal component. Malignant lesions have cellular atypia anaplasia with high mitotic activity in the cells of the stromal component.

Treatment in adolescence is excision with a rim of normal tissue. Breast conservation is recommended in this age group. Systemic therapy is usually not recommended. The local recurrence rate can be as high as 20%–30%.

Malignant lesion is rare in this age group.

FURTHER READING

1. Asma Javed, Aidia Lteif: Development of Human Breast: Semin Plast Surg. 2013 February; 27(1): 5–12
2. Marjorie J.Arca et al: Breast Disorders in the Adolescent Patients; Adolesc Med Clin. 2004 Oct,15(3):473–85
3. Kliegman, St Geme, Blum,Shah, Tasker, Wilson: Nelson Text Book of Paediatrics : 21st Edition 2019

Pathophysiology and Hormonal Factors Involved during Pregnancy and Lactation and Their Effects on Lactogenesis

4

Agnimita Giri

BACKGROUND

All newborns from 0 to 6 months of age should receive exclusive breastfeeding for their proper growth and development. However, only 44% of mothers can achieve exclusive breastfeeding for the first 6 months (1). If optimal, breastfeeding can be continued until 0–23 months of age of the baby; then it is estimated that 820,000 under-5 deaths can be prevented. Breastfeeding is associated with a higher level of IQ, better school attendance, higher studies, and higher income in adult life (2). The factors responsible for delayed lactation and nonlactation are anatomical abnormalities of the nipple, anatomical abnormalities in newborn, separation between mother and newborn, faulty feeding technique, and early introduction of formula feeding. However, even after correction of these factors, a large percentage of newborns are unable to receive breast milk. Hormonal factors can be attributed to these cases (3). This is because hormonal factors play a crucial role in stage 2 lactogenesis (3).

Delayed lactation refers to the condition when onset of lactation is delayed beyond 3 days of age of the baby (4). Nonlactation is the condition where lactation could not be established. Though delayed lactation may occur, the chances of nonlactation are much lower, as by 7 days postpartum lactation can be established in most cases (4).

DOI: 10.1201/9780367821982-4

MICROSCOPIC ANATOMY OF THE BREAST

The breast microscopic structure is formed by 15–20 large ducts, which just before opening into the areola, are dilated, forming lactiferous sinuses. These ducts branch and rebranch within the breast tissue and ultimately are connected to rounded structures called acini. The terminal duct along with the acini is the functional unit of the breast called terminal duct lobular unit (TDLU). The lobules are responsible for milk production.

The basement membrane surrounding the entire ductal system of the breast, including the lobules, separates the epithelial cells from the breast tissue. This basement membrane also extends to the basement membrane of the skin, making it continuous. There are two types of epithelial cells lining the ducts: Luminal cells and myoepithelial cells. Luminal cells form the innermost epithelial cell layer of the ducts and TDLU. These luminal cells undergo changes during lactation to secrete milk in smaller ducts and TDLU, but not in larger ducts. The myoepithelial cells form the outermost lining between the basement membrane and luminal cells. These cells do not cover the basement membrane completely and possess a contractile meshwork, which is active during the ejection of milk in lactation. The breast stroma consists of two types: Interlobular, which forms the major volume of breasts and contains fibroblasts, myofibroblasts, blood vessels, and lymphatic system. The other type of stroma is intralobular, which supports the lobules and TDLU (5).

Changes in the breast occur during pregnancy and lactation under the influence of hormones. These anatomical and physiological changes in the breast ultimately bring the development of the breast to complete maturity. During the prepregnant stage, the ratio of adipose tissue to glandular and ductal tissue is higher than during pregnancy and lactation. During ovulation, due to the raised level of estrogen, there is an increase in alveolar epithelium and secretion of different constituents of milk. Following conception, the corpus luteum secretes estrogen and progesterone during the second week of pregnancy, an action which is later maintained by the placenta. Under the influence of estrogen there is an increase in the growth of ductal tissue and a decrease in adipose tissue. The increased level of progesterone induces lobular growth. The estrogen level rises from 2 ng/mL to 22 ng/mL, and progesterone rises from 27 ng/mL to 138 ng/mL during early to term pregnancy (6).

The high level of estrogen stimulates the anterior pituitary gland, which induces the production of prolactin hormone by the lactotroph cells of the gland. Prolactin stimulates the alveolar cell to produce different components of milk. By the 20th week of gestation there is sufficient prolactin secretion to produce milk. But under the influence of elevated levels of estrogen and progesterone, milk secretion is suppressed. The acini of the breast are filled with colostrum starting with the second trimester of pregnancy. Colostrum contains large quantities of antibodies produced from lymphocytes compared to lower quantity of lipids which is produced from epithelial cells. Antibacterial factors are secreted by lymphocytes, plasma cells, and eosinophils into the alveoli under the hormonal influence. Gradually, aggregation of the immune cells and plasma cells ceases and lipid-rich breast milk is secreted. Further ductal proliferation filled with colostrum occurs during the 3rd trimester of pregnancy under the influence of hormones. After delivery there is withdrawal of the progesterone, which stimulates prolactin and oxytocin. Prolactin stimulates milk secretion, and oxytocin helps in milk ejection by the contraction of myoepithelial cells.

There is an increase in the size of the breasts, increase in pigmentation of the areola, and hypertrophy of the Montgomery's tubercle, which indicate the pregnancy changes of the breast preparing for lactation. Failure of these changes is associated with scanty milk flow and difficulty in breastfeeding (6).

CURRENT KNOWLEDGE OF LACTOGENESIS

During early pregnancy, lobular growth of breast occurs under the influence of Human Chorionic Gonadotrophin liberated from the syncytiotrophoblast. HCG maintains the corpus luteum which initially secretes progesterone and estrogen. Thereafter, lobular growth and ductal proliferation occurs under the influence of placental progesterone and estrogen respectively.

Stage 1 lactogenesis: This starts from the mid-trimester of pregnancy under the influence of estrogen and progesterone. Colostrum is secreted in the acini, but milk secretion does not occur due to presence of progesterone. The alveolar cells are converted into lactocytes, which are capable of secreting immunoglobulin-rich colostrum.

Stage 2 lactogenesis: This occurs after withdrawal of the placenta and fall in the level of progesterone following delivery of the newborn. This is followed by a rise in prolactin level, which along with the influence of other hormones like insulin and cortisol, stimulates the synthesis of milk. Milk is secreted by the mammary epithelial cells. It contains carbohydrate (mainly lactose), protein, lipids, vitamins, minerals, and water. In the presence of prolactin, insulin, and glucocorticoids, the mammary cells synthesize proteins, certain amino acids, and fat (7).

Stage 3 lactogenesis: This is characterized by the milk let-down reflex. As there is stimulation of the nipple–areolar complex when the baby sucks the nipple, it liberates oxytocin from the posterior pituitary gland of the mother. Oxytocin helps to contract the myoepithelial cells, and milk ejection occurs (8).

ROLE OF INSULIN IN THE MAMMARY GLANDS

Early research on the role of insulin influencing lactogenesis by stimulation of the mammary glands was concluded to be contradictory.

Neville and Picciano pointed out that during lactation, the plasma insulin level is low, and studies in animals and humans did not show any effect of increase in the plasma glucose–insulin level on milk production (9).

Other researchers also rejected the idea of a direct role of insulin in lactogenesis. It was argued that lactose formation within the acini occurs via glucose transport across the basolateral membrane of the lactocyte, and this occurs via non-insulin-dependent transport of molecules (10).

Current evidence has established the role of insulin in lactogenesis. Insulin influences metabolic processes, including lipid and protein synthesis, in addition to cell growth and differentiation. Insulin helps in *de novo* synthesis of lipids, proteins, and carbohydrates. It stimulates the expression of genes directly involved in milk protein synthesis by increased expression of milk protein transcription and translation factors (11). Menzies et al. concluded that insulin, hydrocortisone, and prolactin are the key hormones responsible for milk protein gene expression. However, they could not delineate the exact pathway of insulin in the whole process. They did a mammary explant culture and combined it with lactogenic hormones, followed by the study of global changes of gene expression using Affimatrix Microarray. They found that 164 genes are responsive to insulin and 18 of them are important in protein synthesis at the level of transcription and post-transcription amino acid uptake and metabolism. Folate metabolism is also an important and pivotal factor for protein synthesis. Further analysis of cell lines reveals that transcription factors STAT5a and ELF5, key components of protein synthesis, require signaling. STAT5a and ELF5 could be induced even in the absence of prolactin and in the presence of insulin. Prolactin plays an important role

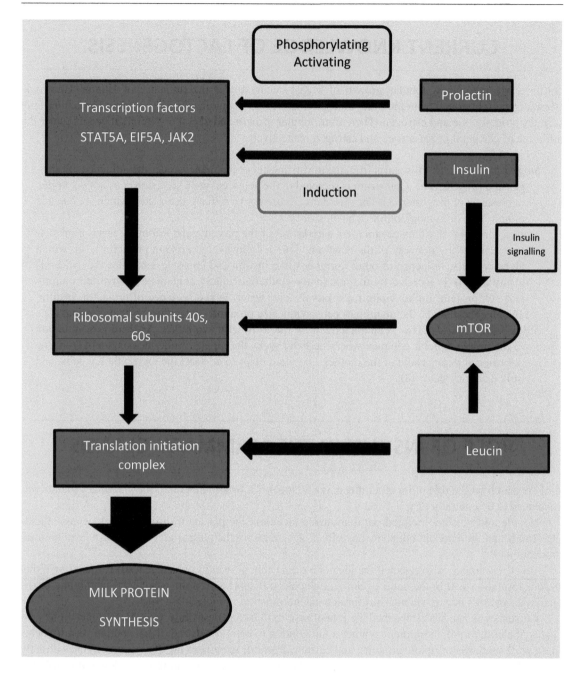

FIGURE 4.1   Pathway for milk protein synthesis: Role of insulin and prolactin (22).

in phosphorylating and activating STAT5a, but the expression is only induced by insulin. This established the crucial role of insulin in the transcription of milk protein genes (11, 12) (Figure 4.1).

Pathbreaking research between 2009 and 2011 (13–16) established mammary gland sensitivity to insulin throughout the reproductive cycle. This is due to differential gene expression of insulin receptors (INSRs), which are present in two different isoforms: INSR-A and INSR-B (13, 14). During early pregnancy, the role of INSR-A is more prominent. INSR-A combines with insulin or with insulin-like growth factor II (IGFII) and activates the GTP protein (RAS) MAPK signaling pathway (15, 16). This directly

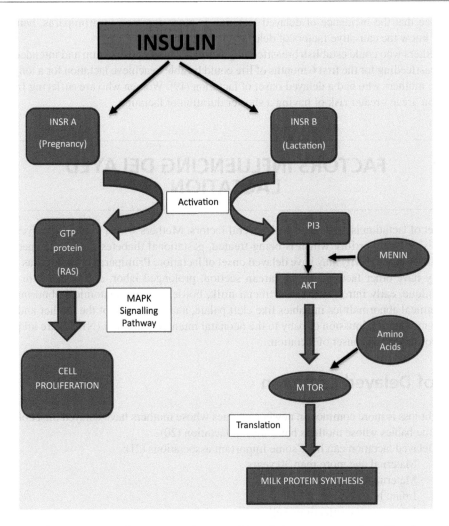

FIGURE 4.2   Insulin receptors and PI3-AKT pathway and its role in mammary cell proliferation and milk protein synthesis (21, 23, 13, 14).

leads to cell proliferation. INSR-B is overexpressed during lactation. Berlato and Doppler (13) demonstrated that there is 2.5-fold increase in INSR-B expression during this phase. INSR-B combines with insulin and activates the phosphatidylinositol-3-OHkinase-protein kinase Bα (PI3-AKT) signaling pathway, which leads to nutritional metabolism (15) (Figure 4.2).

Insulin influences lactose synthesis and milk fat synthesis by the same pathways (17).

Thus, the current evidence suggests that the mammary glands show a transformation from cell proliferation to lactogenesis directly under the influence of INSR. Therefore, insulin has presently been designated as a key factor in the whole process.

DELAYED LACTOGENESIS: GLOBAL DATA

Delayed lactation can be defined as when lactation is established 72 hours after the delivery of the newborn. The incidence of delayed lactation in primiparas and in multiparas are 33% and 8%, respectively (18).

As we see that the incidence of delayed lactation is more common in primiparas, hence it is very important to know the causative factors of delayed lactation in primiparas.

Also mothers who could establish breastfeeding within 72 hours postpartum and intended to continue exclusive breastfeeding for the first 6 months of life could be able to achieve lactation for a longer period of time than the mothers who had a delayed onset of lactation (19). Women who are suffering from delayed-onset lactation are at greater risk of having a shorter duration of lactation.

FACTORS INFLUENCING DELAYED LACTATION

Delayed onset of lactation is associated with several factors. Mothers with a history of polycystic ovarian syndrome, history of infertility which is being treated, gestational diabetes mellitus, hypertension, and raised body mass index (BMI) may have delayed onset of lactation. Primiparas or multiparas with delayed lactation may have other factors like caesarean section, prolonged labor, and peripartum pain. Faulty feeding technique, early introduction of artificial milk, bottle feeding, anatomical abnormalities of the nipple, anatomical abnormalities in babies like cleft palate, and separation of the mother and baby due to illness of the mother or admission of baby to the neonatal intensive care unit (NICU) are all predisposing factors promoting delayed onset of lactation.

Impact of Delayed Lactation

- Weight loss is more common in newborn babies whose mothers have delayed onset of lactation than the babies whose mothers have normal lactation (20).
  - Delayed lactation can have some important associations (21):
    - Maternal age more than 30 years
    - Maternal obesity
    - Infant birth weight > 3.6 kg
    - Infant not breastfeeding well
    - Lack of nipple discomfort
    - Presence of edema in the postpartum period

CONCLUSION

The science of lactogenesis has evolved rapidly in the last 50 years. Traditionally, the model was based on a simplistic triangular interaction between prolactin, milk stimulation, and oxytocin. The full effort to achieve exclusive breastfeeding in infants 0–6 months of age did not achieve its target. Looking at the evidence, it was obvious that there are factors beyond maternal motivation that are elusive. The end of the last century saw the first hint of insulin and other hormones as subtle but key factors in achieving lactogenesis. Though the initial research could not demonstrate a direct linkage between insulin and lactogenesis, the evolution of molecular biology and genetics changed the understanding of delayed/nonlactation (22). As the genetic sequence of milk proteins and cell signaling pathways were deciphered, it became evident that insulin and INSR play a pivotal role in breast development during pregnancy, synthesis of milk, and its secretion.

As obesity and the resultant insulin resistance is the new epidemic which has led to multiple diseases, the effect is also obvious during the life of a mother in pregnancy and lactation.

FUTURE DIRECTIONS

Obesity is a lifestyle disorder. Obesity predisposes to carcinogenesis, cardiovascular illness, diabetes mellitus, and multiple other diseases. That it is a key factor in restricting lactogenesis has only recently been exposed. The impact in these cases is likely to affect the next generation and set in an irreversible vicious cycle. Nonlactation or delayed lactation will lead to early introduction of artificial feeds. The combination of lack of breastfeeding and consumption of artificial feeds is likely to have multiple short-term and long-term effects in the newborn. The need of the hour is to have clinical and translational research to address the issue. Public health strategies based on lifestyle modification and reduction of maternal obesity can lead to reduced insulin resistance. This can therefore lead to achievement of exclusive breastfeeding in infants between 0 and 6 months.

REFERENCES

1. https://www.who.int/news-room/fact-sheets/detail/infant-and-young-child-feeding 9, June
2. Victora CG et al. Breastfeeding in the 21st century: epidemiology, mechanisms, and lifelong effect. Lancet 387(10017):475–90. http://www.thelancet.com/journals/lancet/article/PIIS0140-6736(15)01024-7/abstract
3. Yong Joo Kim. Pivotal roles of prolactin and other hormones in lactogenesis and the nutritional composition of human milk. Clinical and Experimental Pediatrics 2020 Aug;63(8):312–3. Published online 2020 Aug 15. doi: 10.3345/cep.2020.00311
4. Elizabeth B, Cynthia RH, Ann MD, et.al. Does delayed onset lactogenesis II predict the cessation of any or exclusive breastfeeding? Journal of Pediatrics 2012 Oct;161(4):608–14. Published online 2012 May 9. Author manuscript; available in PMC 2013 Oct 1., Published in final edited form as: J Pediatr.
5. Alex A, Bhandary E, McGuire KP. Anatomy and Physiology of the Breast during Pregnancy and Lactation. In: Alipour, S., Omranipour, R. (eds) Diseases of the Breast during Pregnancy and Lactation. Advances in Experimental Medicine and Biology 2020;1252:3–7. PMID: 32816256 Review.
6. Schock H, Zeleniuch-Jacquotte A, Lundin E, Grankvist K, Lakso HÅ, Idahl A et al. Hormone concentrations throughout uncomplicated pregnancies: a longitudinal study. BMC Pregnancy Childbirth 2016;16(1):146
7. Reza Rezaei, Zhenlong Wu, Yongqing Hou, Fuller W. Bazer & Guoyao Wu. Amino acids and mammary gland development: nutritional implications for milk production and neonatal growth. Journal of Animal Science and Biotechnology 2016;7(20).
8. Physiology, Lactation. StatPearls. NCBI Bookshelf. https://www.ncbi.nlm.nih.gov › books › NBK499981
9. Neville MC, Picciano MF. Regulation of milk lipid secretion and composition. Annual Review of Nutrition 1997;17:159–83. [PubMed]
10. Shennan DB, Peaker M. Transport of milk constituents by the mammary gland. Physiological Reviews 2000;80:925–51. [PubMed]
11. Menzies KK, Lee HJ, Lefevre C, Ormandy CJ, Macmillan KL, Nicholas KR. Insulin, a key regulator of hormone responsive milk protein synthesis during lactogenesis in murine mammary explants. Functional & Integrative Genomics 2010;10:87–95. [PubMed].
12. Menzies KK, Lefevre C, Macmillan KL, Nicholas KR. Insulin regulates milk protein synthesis at multiple levels in the bovine mammary gland. Functional & Integrative Genomics 2009;9:197–217. [PubMed] [Google Scholar]
13. Berlato C, Doppler W. Selective response to insulin versus insulin-like growth factor-I and -II and up-regulation of insulin receptor splice variant B in the differentiated mouse mammary epithelium. Endocrinology 2009;150(6):2924–33. [PubMed] [Google Scholar]
14. Rowzee AM, Ludwig DL, Wood TL. Insulin-like growth factor type 1 receptor and insulin receptor isoform expression and signaling in mammary epithelial cells. Endocrinology 2009;150(8):3611–9. [PMC free article] [PubMed] [Google Scholar]

15. Belfiore A, Frasca F, Pandini G, Sciacca L, Vigneri R. Insulin receptor isoforms and insulin receptor/insulin-like growth factor receptor hybrids in physiology and disease. Endocrine Reviews 2009;30(6):586–623. [PubMed] [Google Scholar]

16. Kalla Singh S, Brito C, Tan QW, De LM, De LD. Differential expression and signaling activation of insulin receptor isoforms A and B: a link between breast cancer and diabetes. Growth Factors 2011;29:278–89. [PMC free article] [PubMed] [Google Scholar]

17. Osorio J, Lohakare J, Bionaz M. Biosynthesis of milk fat, protein, and lactose: roles of transcriptional and posttranscriptional regulation. Medicine Physiological Genomics. Published 26 January 2016 Biology. doi: 10.1152/physiolgenomics.00016.2015 Corpus ID: 1426116

18. Dewey KG, Nommsen-Rivers LA, Heinig MJ, Cohen RJ. Risk factors for suboptimal infant breastfeeding behavior, delayed onset of lactation, and excess neonatal weight loss. Pediatrics 2003;112:607–19.

19. Chapman DJ, Perez-Escamilla R. Does delayed perception of the onset of lactation shorten breastfeeding duration? Journal of Human Lactation 1999;15:107–11, quiz 137–9

20. Chantry CJ, Dewey KG, Nommsen-Rivers LA, Peerson JM, Cohen RJ. Excess weight loss in breastfed newborns relates to intrapartum fluid delivery to the mother. Pediatric Academic Society 2009;3680:3 (meeting abstr).

21. Laurie A Nommsen-Rivers, Caroline J Chantry, Janet M Peerson, Roberta J Cohen, Kathryn G Dewey. Delayed onset of lactogenesis among first-time mothers is related to maternal obesity and factors associated with ineffective breastfeeding. American Journal of Clinical Nutrition 2010 September;92(3):574–84. doi: 10.3945/ajcn.2010.29192. Published: 23 June 2010.

22. Honghui L, Xue L, Zhonghua W. MEN1/Menin regulates milk protein synthesis through mTOR signaling in mammary epithelial cells. Scientific Reports 2017 December;7(1). doi: 10.1038/s41598-017-06054-w LicenseCC BY 4.0, Florida International University, Xueyan L.

23. Milk Protein Synthesis in the Lactating Mammary Gland: Insights from Transcriptomics Analyses September 2012 DOI:10.5772/46054, In book: Milk Protein (pp.285-324) Chapter: 11 Publisher: In TechEditors: Walter Hurley, Authors: Massimo Bionaz, Oregon State University; Walter L Hurley, University of Illinois, Urbana-Champaign

Benign Breast Diseases

5

Diptendra Kumar Sarkar

ABERRATION OF NORMAL DEVELOPMENT AND INVOLUTION OF THE BREAST

The nonmalignant diseases of the breast were grouped under the nomenclature benign breast disease. However, clinicians and patients refuse to accept the word "disease," as most cases are due to physiological variations. The nomenclature aberration of normal development and involution (ANDI) was formulated by the Cardiff Breast Clinic. It encompasses all the terminologies like benign breast disease, fibrocystic disease, fibroadenosis, chronic mastitis, and mastopathies.

- *Etiology*: The female breast during the lifetime undergoes various changes under the influence of hormones. It can be divided into premenarche, reproductive period, and postmenopausal phases. During the reproductive period, there is also superimposed hormone-induced physiological variations during the menstrual cycles.
- *Pathology*
  - Normally, in spite of the hormonal changes, the subtle changes in breast histology are insignificant. The wider physiological variations may lead to:
    - Proliferation of breast parenchymal tissue leading to discrete lump formation clinically.
    - *Effacement of the fat and elastic tissue with development of fibrosis*: It is often accompanied by the presence of chronic inflammatory cells (nodularity of the breast).
    - Sequestration of the secretion within the breast parenchyma leading to cyst formation.
    - The lining epithelium of the ducts and the acini may proliferate leading to hyperplasia. Excessive proliferation can give rise to atypia.
    - Extensive proliferation of the lining epithelium of the ducts can lead to papillomatous projection within the ducts, known as papillomatosis.

Risk of malignancy associated with benign breast diseases:

- *No risk*
  - Adenosis, sclerosis or florid
  - Apocrine metaplasia
  - Cysts macro and/or micro
  - Duct ectasia
  - Fibroadenoma
  - Fibrosis

DOI: 10.1201/9780367821982-5

- Hyperplasia
- Mastitis (inflammation)
- Periductal mastitis
- Squamous metaplasia
- *Slightly increased risk (1.5–2 times)*
  - Hyperplasia, moderate or florid, solid or papillary
  - Papilloma with a fibrovascular core
- *Moderately increased risk (5 times)*
  - Atypical hyperplasia (ductal or lobular)
- *Insufficient data to assign a risk*
  - Solitary papilloma of lactiferous sinus
  - Radial scar lesion

Clinical presentations:

1. Mastalgia
2. Nodularity or lumpy breast
3. Discrete lump
4. Nipple discharge

MASTALGIA

Breast pain is possibly the most common reason for presentation of a female in breast clinics. Broadly it can be divided into:

1. *Cyclical mastalgia*: Mostly caused due to physiological variations in hormonal levels.
2. *Noncyclical mastalgia*: It can again be divided into two groups:
   a. *Breast causes*: Duct ectasia, periductal mastitis, inflammation of the breast, traumatic fat necrosis, Mondor's disease, breast cancer (rarely).
   b. *Non-breast causes*: Myalgia, costochondritis (Tietze's syndrome), cardiac and lung causes.

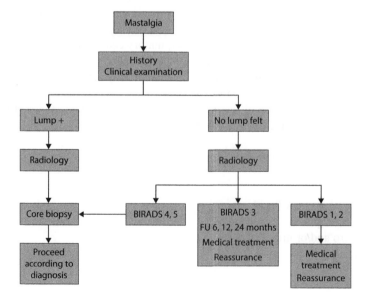

Treatment of Mastalgia

Cyclical mastalgia

1. Repeated reassurance
2. Maintenance of breast pain chart
3. *Medicines with moderate evidence*: Tamoxifen at a dose of 10 mg on alternate days for a period of 3–6 months
4. *Medicines with weak/No evidence*: Danazol (100 mg twice daily for 2 months), evening primrose oil (3–6 months)
5. Optimum breast support
6. Reduction of coffee, tea

Noncyclical mastalgia

1. *Breast causes*: Reassurance and analgesics
2. *Non-breast cause*: To be evaluated and treated accordingly

LUMPY BREAST/FIBROADENOSIS

It is characterized clinically by a lumpy (nodularity) breast with or without mastalgia and nipple discharge. High-resolution ultrasonography (HRUSG) of the breast shows variable features ranging from a normal breast to focal nodularity of the breast with or without cystic changes. Core biopsy is recommended if a discrete lump (BI-RADS 4 onwards) is detected. Reassurance is the mainstay of the diagnosis. Surgery is usually not done. In patients with high-risk pathological lesions (proliferative and atypical), excision is recommended.

Discrete Lumps

The most common causes of benign discrete lumps of the breast include fibroadenoma and cystic lesions of the breast.

Fibroadenomas

These are currently thought of as minor aberration of the normal process of lobular development, which usually occurs between 15 and 35 years of age. Fibroadenomas shrink after menopause.

Pathology

It is characterized by proliferation of stroma and glands. The stroma shows spindle-shaped cells with oval or elongated nuclei. The glandular proliferation has two layers. The outer layer comprises myoepithelial cells (nondisrupted) and inner cuboidal to columnar cells. The growth pattern can be of two types:

a. *Intracanalicular*: The stroma overgrows and compresses the glands giving rise to cleft-like spaces.
b. *Peri-canalicular*: The stroma surrounds the gland without compressing it. The glandular architecture remains nondistorted.

Histological Variants of Fibroadenoma

TYPE	CHARACTER
Myxoid fibroadenoma	• Blue-tinged myxoid changes in the stroma • May be associated with Carney complex (autosomal dominant disorder characterized by endocrine tumors, myxomas, skin hyperpigmentation, and blue nevi)
Cellular fibroadenoma	• Increased stromal cellularity
Juvenile fibroadenoma	• Increased stromal cellularity • There is increased epithelial hyperplasia
Complex fibroadenoma	• Sclerosing adenosis, epithelial calcification, and papillary apocrine changes

Natural History of Fibroadenomas

Fibroadenomas can be single or multiple. Based on their growth kinetics they can be classified as follows:

1. *Nonprogressive fibroadenomas*: Most lesions achieve a static phase in 2 years. Some of them involute during pregnancy and lactation. A small proportion of them persist and may become calcified.
2. *Progressive fibroadenomas*: A fraction of fibroadenomas may show growth spurts and may achieve large proportions (known as giant fibroadenomas >5 cm in size). These lesions may be confused with phyllodes tumors.

Clinical Presentation

A painless lump in the breast usually between the second and third decades of life. The progression of the lesion has to be noted to assess the growth kinetics of the fibroadenoma.

Diagnosis: Triple assessment forms the cornerstone of diagnosis
1. *Clinical breast examination*: A firm mobile lump is detected. The free mobility of fibroadenomas has earned the name of a "breast mouse."
2. *HRUSG breast*: The lesions are wider than taller (they are parallel to the overlying skin). The surface is smooth but may show lobulations. Presence of a perilesional halo confirms the diagnosis of a benign lesion. Often it may be difficult to distinguish a fibroadenoma and a phyllodes tumor. Phyllodes tumors typically show gross lobularity and are frequently associated with intralesional clefts.
3. *Core biopsy*: Confirms the diagnosis. It can also distinguish between fibroadenoma and phyllodes lesions.

Treatment
1. *Follow-up*: Multiple fibroadenomas, small (<3 cm) lesions, nonprogressive lesions, and involuting/calcified fibroadenomas should not be offered surgical interventions. However, triple assessment confirmation is essential before endorsing a nonoperative strategy.
2. *Surgery*: Enucleation is the procedure of choice in indicated lesions. However, it is essential to confirm the diagnosis of fibroadenoma before planning surgery.

INFECTIONS OF THE BREAST

Bacterial mastitis is the most common variant of breast infection.

Etiology

1. *Lactational mastitis*: Caused by milk congestion and engorgement of the breast. It may be due to maternal factors like nipple abnormalities (anatomical defects, cracked or sore nipple) leading to milk stagnation coupled with ascending infection from the oral cavity of the child. *Staphylococcus aureus* is the most common organism.
2. *Nonlactational mastitis:* Usually occurs after the fourth decade of life. This can be central (periareolar) or peripheral. It is caused due to duct ectasia followed by periductal mastitis. This leads to abscess formation, which commonly ruptures to form a sinus tract with communication with lactiferous ducts. Rheumatoid arthritis, diabetic mastopathy, and chronic smokers are associated with increased risk of nonpuerperal breast abscess.

Presentation

1. *Stage of cellulitis*: Presents with pain with fever. On examination, features of inflammation are present.
2. *Stage of abscess formation*: There is accumulation of pus within the breast parenchyma. The features of localization start becoming obvious.
3. *Stage of chronic abscess:* Untreated or inappropriately treated breast abscess ends up forming an indurated mass with multiple pockets of pus.

Evaluation

1. *Clinical breast examination*: It is often difficult for the clinician to differentiate between cellulitis and abscess.
2. *HRUSG*: Mastitis can be diagnosed as an ill-defined area of altered echogenicity and hypoechoic areas in the breast parenchyma. There is thickening of overlying skin. Diagnosis is made by the presence of a hypoechoic collection. In some cases, it is unilocular, while in others multilocularity is found. The periphery of the abscess has a thick echogenicity along with vascularity. The location, number, and size (volume) of the collection are noted. In long-standing undetected cases there is gross induration (solidification) of the abscess contents with multiple small pockets of collection. There may be lactiferous duct fistula.
3. *Core biopsy/Aspiration*: If ultrasound guidance (USG) demonstrated a pyogenic collection, pus is aspirated and send for culture sensitivity. In tuberculosis (TB)-endemic countries staining for acid-fast bacilli with or without core biopsy nucleic acid amplification testing (CB NAAT) for TB may be done. A chronic breast abscess can lead to diagnostic confusion with malignancy. In such cases USG core biopsy may be done to exclude malignancy.

Treatment

1. *Stage of cellulitis*: Treatment with empirical antibiotics, breast support, and analgesics. HRUSG should be done at regular intervals to exclude breast abscess.
2. *Stage of abscess formation*: HRUSG aspiration is the treatment of choice. In case of a large or multiloculated abscess, multiple aspirations may be needed. Open drainage is indicated if USG aspiration fails.

3. *Stage of chronic abscess*: If there is loculated pus, aspiration under antibiotic coverage is the first choice. If the collection is thick, open drainage may be done. Surgery is preferred in patients with lactating duct fistula or nonresolving lesions.

Tuberculosis of the Breast

TB of the breast is not an uncommon entity in TB-endemic countries. The presentation ranges from a solitary lump to breast ulcers with or without axillary lymph nodes. Diagnosis is done using HRUSG (nonspecific findings), aspiration of pus and culture (positive staining for acid-fast bacilli, positive CB NAAT, and mycobacterial culture). Treatment comprises antitubercular therapy. In most cases there is no residual disease. Surgery is offered if there is persistent disease after ATD.

Duct Ectasia and Periductal Mastitis

Duct ectasia is defined as dilatation of the lactiferous duct. The exact cause is not known. Age-related changes, smoking, and arteriopathies have been suggested as contributing factors.

- **Pathogenesis**
  - *Stage of ductal dilatation*: There is focal eccentric or saccular dilatation of the lactiferous duct.
  - *Stage of intraductal stasis*: The secretion stagnates within the dilated segment of the lactiferous duct. This sets in intraductal inflammation.
  - *Stage of periductal mastitis*: The intraductal cytokines and oxygen free radicals escape through the gap in the lining ductal epithelium and initiate periductal inflammation.
  - *Stage of complication*: The periductal mastitis can give rise to abscess formation and rupture to produce the sinus or fistula.
- **Clinical presentation**
  - In the initial phase, nipple discharge (of any type) accompanied with noncyclical mastalgia is the prominent feature.
  - In later stages, a painful inflammatory mass with or without mammary duct fistula is present. Quite often, nipple retraction and peau d'orange–like features may appear mimicking a locally advanced breast cancer.
- **Diagnosis**
  - Triple assessment remains the cornerstone.
  - HRUSG may demonstrate the presence of an inflammatory pocket-like collection along with ductal dilatation and delineation of ductal fistula.
  - Core biopsy is required in the presence of a lump to differentiate from carcinoma.
- **Treatment**
  - In early stages, reassurance is only needed.
  - Empirical antibiotics with an amoxycillin and clavulanic acid combination may be used.
  - USG aspiration of the abscess is done when there is a well-localized pus collection.
  - Mammary duct fistula is treated by en bloc excision of the fistula with partial or complete duct excision.

Granulomatous Mastitis

Granulomatous mastitis is an evolving entity in benign breast disease.

- **Etiologies**
  - *Idiopathic granulomatous mastitis (IGM)*: It may or may not be associated with:
    - Diabetic mastopathy
    - Wegener's granulomatosis
    - Sarcoidosis
    - Collagen vascular disease
  - Secondary granulomatous mastitis
    - Corynebacterial infection
    - Tuberculosis
- **Pathogenesis**
  - The inflammatory process initiates within the dilated and deformed duct.
  - The initiation factor is often unknown. IGM, thought to be an autoimmune reaction, is associated with polymorphism of the prolactin gene. The subsequent progression of the disease mimics periductal mastitis.
  - Diabetes and all the collagen vascular diseases may initiate similar autoimmune reactions.
- **Clinical presentation**
  - Most patients present with noncyclical mastalgia associated with an indurated breast lump.
  - In late stages, there is nipple retraction, peau d'orange, and single or multiferous duct fistula.
  - Many patients present with recurrent abscess formation, nonhealing ulcers, and reactive arthritis.
  - In late stages, the entire breast can be involved and is deformed.
  - Many a time it mimics malignancy.
  - The majority of patients have a history of diabetes and breastfeeding within 2 years.
- **Diagnosis**
  - Triple assessment
    - USG demonstrates nonspecific lesions, micro-abscesses, or focal pus collection. Ductal dilation and lactiferous fistula and dermal thickening are seen in late cases.
    - Core biopsy can demonstrate, in early cases, noncaseating granulomatous lesions. In late cases, the primary pathological findings are often obscured due to secondary inflammation.
  - Pus, if present, may be aspirated and is sent for culture sensitivity and including demonstration of acid-fast bacilli. CB NAAT for *Mycobacterium tuberculosis* may be done to exclude TB.
  - In case of chronic abscess or nonhealing ulcers, open incisional biopsy or biopsy from the wall of the abscess cavity may establish the diagnosis.
  - Each patient should be evaluated for diabetes mellites and an entire rheumatological profile be done to rule out collagen vascular disease.
- **Treatment**
  - Isolated lump without infection is treated with corticosteroids.
    - Oral prednisolone at a dose of 20 mg/day can be started, and gradually the dose can be increased up to 40 mg/day. It can be continued up to 8–12 weeks depending on the response and then tapered off.
    - In case of failure methotrexate is used.
  - *Lump with secondary infection*: Empirical antibiotics along with USG or open drainage is done at primary setup. When infection subsides, steroids can be started.
  - *Presence of sinus/Fistula*: Control of infection with empirical antibiotics followed by steroid therapy is the preferred method. In patients with lactiferous duct fistula, excision of the sinus with en bloc partial or total duct excision may be curative.

NIPPLE DISCHARGE

Nipple discharge is a common problem faced by women across all ages.

Types of discharge

1. *According to number of ducts*: Single or multiple.
2. *According to nature of discharge*: Serous, blood stained, grumous, purulent, and milky.

Causes of nipple discharge

1. *Lactation*: It is the most common physiological cause of nipple discharge.
2. *Galactorrhea*: It is defined as milky discharge unrelated to breastfeeding. This is usually bilateral and from multiple ducts.
   a. Physiological and may persist even after cessation of lactation.
   b. *Drug induced*: Antidopaminergic agents (tricyclic antidepressants, reserpine, methyl-dopa, cimetidine, benzodiazepines), dopamine receptor blockers (phenothiazines, metoclopramide, haloperidol), and estrogenic (digitalis).
   c. Hypothyroidism.
   d. Prolactinoma.
3. *Pathological nipple discharge*: Nipple discharge that is bloody and from a single duct requires evaluation. Normal physiological discharges are usually nonbloody (serous, grumous, or yellowish). Though rare, serous discharges may have coincidental malignancies.
   a. Malignancy is found in 10% of cases.
   b. Benign conditions like duct papillomas, duct ectasias, and fibrocystic diseases can also produce nipple discharge.
   c. Trauma to nipple and infections in lactating mothers can also produce bloody discharge from the nipple.

Evaluation of nipple discharge

1. Triple assessment is the cornerstone of evaluation. The patient is asked to radially massage the breast to demonstrate the type of nipple discharge. Pressing the nipple is a wrong technique for eliciting nipple discharge. It can produce micro trauma leading to false bloody discharge. HRUSG may demonstrate ductal or extraductal pathologies. If a lump or suspicious lesion is felt, core biopsy is recommended.
2. Occult blood (guaiac) test is a sensitive and specific test to differentiate between bloody and nonbloody discharge.
3. Ductal fluid cytology is extremely insensitive and is not recommended.
4. Ductogram and ductoscopy are performed in limited circumstances.

Management

1. Physiological discharges are treated with reassurance. Correction of hypothyroidism or hyperprolactinemia is helpful. In persistent hyperprolactinemia, MR of the pituitary is done to exclude prolactinoma. Prolactinomas are treated by bromocriptine or surgery.
2. In the case of bloody discharge without demonstrable underlying pathology, ductal surgery is recommended. In young patients microdochectomy is recommended. It is diagnostic as well as therapeutic in many circumstances. In elderly patients (who do not plan for pregnancy and lactation) major (total) duct excision is the treatment of choice.

3. Post-surgery if malignancy is detected in HPE, appropriate treatment is suggest depending on the situation.

GYNECOMASTIA

Definition: It is defined as enlargement of the male breast caused by an imbalance between estrogen and androgen levels.

Types

1. *Physiological*: Extremes of age, puberty.
2. *Medications*: Antiandrogens, Aldactone, anabolic steroids, antiretroviral, antidepressants, anti-cancer drugs, alcohol, digitalis.
3. *Diseases*: Hypogonadism, testicular tumors, adrenal tumors, pituitary tumors.
4. *Organ-specific diseases*: Hyperthyroidism, chronic kidney disease (CKD), chronic liver disease (CLD).

Clinical

1. *True gynecomastia*: Characterized by proliferation of breast tissue under the NAC.
2. *Pseudogynecomastia*: Characterized by deposition of fat in the breast. It is commonly associated with obesity.

Triple assessment: In most patients, the diagnosis of gynecomastia is obvious in HRUSG and further evaluation is not essential. However, core biopsy is needed in case of any doubt.

Grades of Gynecomastia

GRADE	NODULE	STRETCHING	PTOSIS
1	+	−	−
2	++	+	−
3	+++	++	+

Differentiation with Malignancy

Malignant nodules are mostly eccentric in terms of location, whereas nodular gynecomastia is usually symmetrical and NAC-centric. Features of malignancy like skin tethering, irregularity, and immobility are absent in gynecomastia.

Management

Most cases of gynecomastia do not require surgical interventions. Tamoxifen is used in some cases. The response rate is unpredictable. Grade 1 gynecomastia is treated by reassurance, while the rest may be treated for cosmetic reasons. Subcutaneous NAC-preserving mastectomy/mastopexy is the treatment of care. Patients with nonptotic pseudogynecomastias may be treated with liposuction.

CORE AREA IV: ETIOLOGY, MOLECULAR BASIS, AND SCREENING

Etiopathogenesis, Risk Factors, and Genomics in Breast Cancer

6

Diptendra Kumar Sarkar

EPIDEMIOLOGY

Breast cancer (BC) is the most common cancer in females worldwide. The GLOBOCAN 2018 data suggest an annual incidence of 2,088,849 cases. The crude rate (CR) and the age standardized rate (ASR) is 55.2 and 46.3 per 100,000 population, respectively. The CR and ASR mortality rate is 16.6 and 13 per 100,000 population, respectively. In India, the ASR is 25.8 per 100,000 population with a mortality of 12.1 per 100,000 population (1). The global mortality rate in breast cancer is approximately 29%, but in India it is 46.8%. BC tops the list with a contribution of 14% of all cancers in India.

RISK FACTORS

Various factors can be attributed to the increased risk of BC.

Nonmodifiable factors associated with increased risk (strong evidence)

    1. *Sex*: The ratio of female:male BC is 99:1.

DOI: 10.1201/9780367821982-6

2. *Age*: Increasing age is associated with higher risk of BC. One in eight women carries a lifetime risk for the development of breast cancer (80 years). There are hospital-based data to suggest that BC in India occurs 15 years younger than in Western counterparts. Whether it is due to a relatively younger Indian population or a true phenomenon remains to be proven.

3. *Inherited BC*: There is strong evidence to suggest that 5%–10% of cancers are caused by identifiable and named inherited genetic mutations. Such cancers are known as **hereditary BCs**. There can also be a familial cluster of cases which is higher in incidence than the healthy population, but no named mutation can be identified. Such BC is known as **familial cancer**. The third variety comprises the majority and is named **sporadic BC**.

4. *Breast density*: Women with increased breast density carry a higher risk of BC. Breast density is dependent on familial predisposition, reproductive pattern, and alcohol intake. The relative risk of BC varies from 1.79 (for mild increase in density) to 4.64 (for severely dense breasts) (2).

5. *High-risk breast lesions*: The presence of ductal carcinoma *in situ* (DCIS) predisposes to the occurrence of invasive BCs. Lobular carcinoma *in situ* (LCIS) is looked upon as a marker for BC. A previous history of breast biopsy showing evidence of proliferative lesions or lesions with atypia increases the risk of BC.

Modifiable factors associated with increased risk (strong evidence)

1. *Late pregnancy*: Woman with a first childbirth before the age of 20 years has a lower risk for BC. Nulliparity and age of first pregnancy after 35 years of age are associated with a 50% increase in the incidence of BC.

2. *Menstruation*: Early menarche (< 11 years) and late menopause (> 51 years) increase the risk of BC.

3. *Nonlactation*: Past evidence shows nonlactation is associated with increased incidence of BC (the relative risk [RR] of breast cancer is decreased 4.3% for every 12 months of breastfeeding, in addition to 7% for each birth) (3). However, there is contradictory evidence suggesting that not all subsets of individuals would be in accordance with this finding.

4. *Exercise*: Weekly exercise for more than 4 hours is associated with a 30%–40% reduction of BC risk.

5. *Oral contraceptives*: Oral contraceptive pills (OCPs) with high estrogen content (used 2–3 decades back) were associated with a higher risk of BC. Presently the OCPs are progesterone-predominant ones and carry minimum/no risk of BC.

6. *Hormone replacement therapy (HRT) using estrogen*: The evidence is conflicting. While a major randomized controlled trial (RCT) shows a 23% reduction in BC 6.8 years after estrogen use for 5.8 years, another observational trial shows a 30% increased incidence of BC. Therefore, HRT should preferably be used wisely and under supervision and surveillance.

7. *Ionizing radiation*: The risk of BC increases 10 years after exposure of the breast to ionizing radiation and persists throughout the lifetime. The risk is increased if exposure occurs during puberty and the developmental period of the breast.

8. *Obesity*: Postmenopausal obesity is associated with a RR of 2.85 in terms of risk in development of BC (82 kg vs. 58 kg).

9. *Alcohol*: Increases risk of BC in dose-dependent manner. It is uncertain whether the risk reduces with cessation of alcohol. (Increase in RR by 7% for each drink per day.)

Factors (interventions) that reduce the risk of breast cancer (strong evidence)

1. *Selective estrogen receptor modifiers (SERMs)*: Both tamoxifen and raloxifene reduce the incidence of BC in the postmenopausal age group. In addition to this, tamoxifen reduces the risk of BC in high-risk individuals in the premenopausal age group (30%–50% risk reduction in estrogen receptor [ER]–positive women). The protective effect persists even after cessation of

SERMs, with a longer effect with tamoxifen compared to raloxifene. Tamoxifen increases the risk of thrombotic events, endometrial cancer, and cataract. Raloxifene increases the risk of thrombotic events and cataract but not endometrial carcinoma.

2. *Aromatase inhibitor*: Exemestane use is associated with a reduction of breast cancer.

HEREDITARY BREAST CANCER AND RISK ASSESSMENT

Familial characteristics and risks that identify an individual to have an increased risk of occurrence for hereditary breast cancer (HBC) are as follows:

- Family characteristics
- Software analysis
- Genetic analysis

Familial characteristics

A. Patients diagnosed with cancer (4)

- Personal diagnosis of DCIS or invasive breast cancer plus one or more of the following:
  - Diagnosed at 50 years or younger.
  - Triple-negative breast cancer diagnosed at 60 years and younger.
  - At any age
    - Known mutation in cancer susceptibility gene within the family.
    - An additional breast cancer primary.
    - One or more first- to third-degree relatives with breast cancer 50 years and younger.
    - One or more first- to third-degree relatives with ovarian cancer at any age.
    - Two or more close blood relatives with BC, pancreatic cancer, or prostate cancer (Gleason score 7 or metastatic) at any age.
    - While these criteria adhere to the Western population data, such findings are not compatible with Indian data. This is largely because of the large volume of cases in the fourth decade of life. Most Indian studies report a higher incidence of Triple Negative Breast Cancer (TNBC) compared to Western data.
  - An individual of Ashkenazi Jewish ancestry.
  - Male BC.
- Personal history of other cancers

B. Patients not diagnosed with cancer (4)

- A close relative with a known genetic mutation.
- A first- or second-degree relative with cancer at less than 45 years of age.
- A family history of three or more of the following:
  - Breast, pancreas, prostate, melanoma, sarcoma, adrenocortical carcinoma, brain tumors, leukemia, diffuse gastric cancer, colon cancer, endometrial cancer, thyroid cancer, kidney cancer, dermatological manifestations, and/or macrocephaly and hamartomatous gastrointestinal (GI) polyps.

Software used for risk evaluation of individuals with high familial risk for BC (5)

- *Empiric models*: These models use a large number of variables, typically a combination of personal and/or family history factors. These include GAIL, PENN1 and 2, Myriad 1 and 2, and others.
- *Genetic models*: These models focus on exact familial predispositions and factors. These include CLAUS, BRCAPRO, BRODICEA, and IBIS (Cuzick model).

These software types use global data and calculate the risk of an individual compared to their ethnic base population. None of the software programs mentioned here have been validated in the Indian subcontinent.

Genetic analysis

Indications for genetic testing

1. Strong familial predisposition
2. Statistically higher risk for occurrence of BC in an individual (as compared to normal healthy population of her age and race)

Genetic counseling: This is the cornerstone in the genetic risk assessment process. It is mandatory to explain the indications, risk involved, the predictability of the genetic assessment, the penetrance of the gene, and the interventions that can be offered if the individual is detected to have one of the identified genetic mutations.

Genomics of breast cancer

Initiation of cancer: It usually originates from cells at the terminal duct lobular unit and is caused due to hereditary (germline) or sporadic (somatic) cancers (Figure 6.1).

- *Hereditary cancers*: It may be due to a germline mutation (explained earlier) in 5%–10% of cases. Characteristically there is a mutation in the *BRCA* genes. The *BRCA* genes are mismatch repair genes and correct any new mutations. When the mismatch repair genes are mutated, the mutations remains uncorrected leading to BC.
- *Sporadic cancers*: Caused due to somatic mutations in 90%–95% of cases. Many of these mutations are caused due to methylation-induced epigenetic changes in mismatch repair or tumor suppressor genes. Our study at IPGMER shows that decreased *BRCA2* gene expression accelerates sporadic BC progression (7, 8). This results in silencing of the mismatched repair gene without any mutation. Any further mutations remain uncorrected.
  - The majority of BC cases are sporadic in nature and can be attributed to numerous somatic gene mutations. When complete genetic sequencing of a sporadic BC is done, one can find somewhere between 50 and 80 different mutations. Such mutations can be further subdivided into:
  - *Passenger mutations*: These are temporary mutations and are unlikely to play any significant role in carcinogenesis.
  - *Driver mutations*: These are significant mutations and play an impactful role. Traditionally, a large number of mutations are observed (TP53, CDH1, PI3K, Cyclin D, PTEN, AKT) in large volumes and are known as gene mountains. A small volume of mutations are also observed (approximately 5%) and are known as gene hills. All these mutations make a sporadic cancer heterogeneous genetically. This also explains the different biological behavior of the cancers and the differential responsiveness to treatment.

TABLE 6.1   Genes involved in causation of hereditary breast cancer

GENES	LOCATION	PENETRANCE	INCIDENCE	CANCERS CAUSED
BRCA1	17q21	High 60%–85% (Lifetime for BC) 15%–40% Ovarian cancer	1/1,400	HOBC (Breast, prostate, colon, liver, bone)
BRCA2	13q12.3	High 60%–85% (Lifetime for BC) 15%–40% Ovarian cancer	1/400	HOBC (Male BC, pancreas, gallbladder, pharynx, stomach, melanoma, prostate, D1 Fanconi anemia
TP53	17q13.1	High 50%–90% (by 50 years)	<1/1,000	Li–Fraumeni syndrome BC, STS, CNS tumors, adrenocortical, leukemia, prostate
PTEN	10q23.3	High 25%–50%	<1/10,000	Cowden syndrome BC, thyroid, oral mucosa, endometrial, brain
CDH1	16q22.1	High	<1/10,000	Familial diffuse gastric cancer (Lobular BC)
STK11/ LKB1	19P13.3	High 30%–50% (by 70 years)	<1/10,000	PJ syndrome
CHEK2	22q12.1	Moderate or 2.6	1/100–200	Li–Fraumeni BC, prostate, colon, brain, STS
BRIP1	17q22	Moderate	<1/10,000	BC, Fanconi anemia
ATM	11q22.3	Moderate	1/33–333	Ataxia telangiectasia: HOBC, leukemia, lymphoma, stomach, pancreas, bladder, immunodeficiency
PALB2	16p12	Moderate	<1/1,000	BC, pancreas, prostate
Others	Multiple genetic locations	Low	Variable	BC
Microsatellite instability	MMR genes MLH1 MSH2 MSH5 PMS2		2- to 18-fold increase in population	Lynch syndrome

Source: From Reference (4).

Thus with time there is accumulation of various lethal and nonlethal mutated genes. These mutations are nurtured by endogenous and exogeneous estrogen via crosstalk through transforming growth factor (TGF).

- **Progression of cancer**

     The mutations are responsible for the initiation of the cancer. Subsequently, these mutations work through some cell signaling pathways and are responsible for the progression of the cancer (interferon signaling, cell cycle check points, mismatch repair gene pathways, p53 pathways, AKT pathways, TGF B signaling, Notch pathways, EGFR pathways, fibroblast growth factor, ERBB2, and RAS and PI3K pathways).

TABLE 6.2   Preventive strategies for hereditary breast cancers

METHODOLOGY	RISK REDUCTIONS	LEVEL OF EVIDENCE
Breast self-examination	• No reduction in population mortality (no study for high-risk population)	Weak
Clinical breast examination	• 30% reduction in population mortality (no study for high-risk population)	Strong
Tamoxifen Breast cancer prevention trial	• 49% reduction in breast cancer in high-risk group (effects persists 11 years after cessation) • Reduced fracture • Increased thrombosis and PE • Increased endometrial carcinoma (persists 5 years after cessation) • No overall improvement in mortality after 7 years	Strong
Bilateral risk-reducing mastectomy with or without primary reconstruction	• 90% reduction in breast cancer in high-risk group	Strong
Intensified annual screening starting 5 years earlier than the youngest detected breast cancer in the family	• Annual radiological evaluation using mammography or MRI	Strong

Source: From Reference (6).

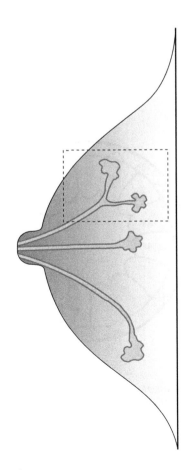

FIGURE 6.1   Terminal duct lobular unit.

- **Role of amplicon in BC progression**

    In most BCs, there are zones in the genetic sequence that amplify the proliferation process (very much like polymerase chain reaction [PCR] artificially). The HER2-neu in chromosome 17 is one such amplicon that aggravates the proliferation of the cancer. Apart from HER2-neu, other amplicons (e.g., CCDN1, MYC, EGFR, ZNF217, and others) also play an important role in proliferation and antiapoptosis.

- **Molecular portraits in BC and their significance**

    The mutated DNA encodes for a protein through mRNA. In a tumor mass there is a large group of heterogeneous DNA and the resultant proteins. These bear the genetic signature of a particular cancer. The genetic signature determines the biological behavior of the cancer and can predict the possibility of response to various forms of treatment.

- **Molecular subtypes:** Based on the work done by Perou and Sorlie, BC can be subdivided into the following types (Figure 6.2):
    - *Luminal cancers*: These cancers originate from the inner lining luminal cells and express the luminal patterns of genes. These include cytokeratin 8 and 18, ER ESR1, GATA, GATA3, FOXA1, XPB1, and MYB. They are further divided into:
        - *Luminal A*: High expression of ER-related genes, low expression of proliferation-related genes, and HER2-neu clusters.
        - *Luminal B*: Relatively lower expression of ER-related genes, higher expression of proliferation-related genes, and HER2-neu clusters.
    - *HER2-neu–enriched cancers*: Classically BC that has a high expression of HER2-neu and proliferation-related gene expression is known as HER2-neu–enriched cancer. These cancers have low or no expression of ER and/or PR. Though this can make it difficult to differentiate between the luminal B and HER2-neu variety, a true HER2 variant will not express ER and PR. It is prognostically a bad biological variant but shows extremely good response to trastuzumab.

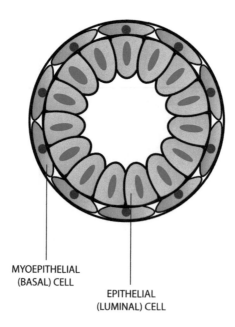

MYOEPITHELIAL
(BASAL) CELL

EPITHELIAL
(LUMINAL) CELL

FIGURE 6.2   Neoanatomy of the breast.

- *Normal variant*: Close to luminal cancers.
- *Triple-negative breast cancer*: These cancers are typically characterized by ER/PR/HER2-neu–negative expressions. Based on the triple-negative expressions, they are further sub-classified into:
  - *Basal subtype*: They express the basal cytokeratin markers and are associated with high levels of proliferation-associated gene expression.
  - *Claudin low group*: Claudins are transmembrane proteins which maintain tight inter-cellular junctions. If the claudin level is low, the tight junctions weaken. These tumors have primitive stem cell characteristics and show marked epithelial mesenchymal transition (EMT) and therefore show increased chances of metastasis. They have higher stromal invasion and are associated with tumor-infiltrating lymphocytes (TILs). Studies have shown a higher proportion of T-regulatory cells, which makes these cancers resistant to immune checkpoint therapy.
  - Interferon-rich subtype.
  - Mesenchymal.
  - Mesenchymal stem cell–like.
  - Luminal androgen receptor subtypes.

- **Prognostication of BC using molecular signatures** (Figure 6.3)

It is evident that the amplicons, proliferating genes, antiapoptotic genes, and angiogenic genes play a major role in shaping the outcome of BC.

There is strong evidence in favor of using these molecular models in establishing the risk categories of a cancer. Its role is maximum in node-negative early breast cancers (mostly ER-positive cancers) (9).

It helps in predicting the subset of patients who are expected to benefit from chemotherapy. It also spares the subset in whom chemotherapy is unlikely to be of any help and thus spares the patient of its side effects.

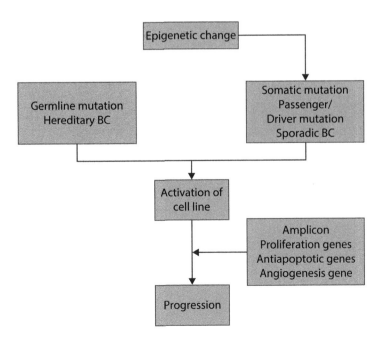

FIGURE 6.3   Flowchart for the initiation and progression of breast cancer.

Certain genes can effectively predict drug resistance of a particular tumor. Thus, a second-line therapy can be initiated without delay.

Molecular signatures, therefore, are essential not only for understanding the biological behavior of cancer but also to implement precision therapy.

REFERENCES

1. Malvia S, Bagadi SA, Dubey US, Saxena S. Epidemiology of breast cancer in Indian women. *Asia Pac J Clin Oncol.* 2017 Aug;13(4):289–295. doi: 10.1111/ajco.12661.
2. McCormack VA, dos Santos Silva I. Breast density and parenchymal patterns as markers of breast cancer risk: a meta-analysis. *Cancer Epidemiol Biomarkers Prev.* 2006;15(6):1159–1169.
3. Collaborate Group on Hormonal Study. Breast cancer and breastfeeding: Collaborative reanalysis of individual data from 47 epidemiological studies in 30 countries, including 50302 women with breast cancer and 96973 women without the disease. *Lancet.* 2002 Jul 20;360(9328):187–195.
4. *Devita Text Book of Oncology*, Edition 11.
5. Nora M. H, Editor. *Management of the Patient at High Risk for Breast Cancer:* Springer Science, 2013.
6. https://www.cancer.gov
7. Sarkar et al. Decreased expression of BRCA2 accelarates sporadic breast cancer progression. *Indian J Surg Oncol.* 2015 Dec;6(4):378–383.
8. Sarkar et al. Decreased expression of BRCA2 accelarates sporadic breast cancer progression. *Eur J Surg Oncol.* 2017 May;43(5)
9. Saprino JA et al. Prospective validation of a 21-gene expression assay in breast cancer. *N Engl J Med.* 2015;373:2005–2014.

Management of the High-Risk Patient

7

Sumohan Chatterjee and Hannah L. Bromley

INTRODUCTION

Breast cancer is the most common cancer diagnosed in women worldwide (1). Around 1 in 10 women will develop the disease during their lifetime (2), but the incidence is higher in North America and Western Europe and is rapidly increasing in the developing world (3).

It is common for women to volunteer a family history as the incidence of breast cancer increases (4, 5). A family history does not necessarily negate shared causality, and most women are safely reassured that they are not at increased risk of breast cancer (6). Breast cancer risk is multifactorial and comprises environmental, lifestyle, hormonal, and genetic factors (7).

About 5%–10% of breast cancers may be attributed to inherited mutations in cancer susceptibility genes (8-10). Breast cancer risk among women with an inherited predisposition is significantly higher compared with the general population. A woman with a germline breast cancer susceptibility gene (*BRCA1*) has a 65% (95% confidence interval [CI]: 0.44–0.78) increased lifetime risk of developing breast cancer compared with an average woman in same population (10, 11).

Individuals may be classified into low (population level), moderate (2–3 times population level), or high (>3 times population level) risk of developing breast cancer (12). There is evidence to suggest that women who are at high risk of breast cancer have a worse prognosis (12). It is therefore important to identify high-risk individuals so that they may be offered early intervention, either by screening, lifestyle changes, or preventive therapy.

Traditionally, high-risk individuals were identified though family history alone or epidemiological algorithms (13). Studies examining familial correlation as early as the 1940s have demonstrated a hereditary predisposition among different generations (14). As technology has advanced, the identification of high-risk breast cancer genes and assessment of mammographic density, when combined with established risk factors (15), has trebled the number of women reaching the high-risk threshold (Europe: >10% lifetime risk, USA: >20% lifetime risk) (4, 16, 17).

This chapter focuses on the assessment and management of women at high risk of breast cancer.

DOI: 10.1201/9780367821982-7

Risk Factors

Family history

Initial assessment of an individual with concern because of an affected relative but with no personal history should include a detailed medical, gynecological, and family history; review of lifestyle factors; and clinical breast examination.

The presence of a significant family history is the most important risk factor in high-risk individuals. Around 5% of all women with breast cancer have an inherited predisposition, and incidence is higher among women with early-onset or aggressive tumors (18). Certain gene mutations may also confer increased susceptibility to other cancers such as bowel, ovarian, and sarcoma (19).

Typically, there are no phenotypic traits that help to identify those who carry a pathological inherited mutation. Thorough evaluation of family pedigree is therefore critical to identify the presence of a predisposing oncogene within the family. Multiple primary cancers or early-onset breast cancer increases the likelihood of an inherited predisposition (20).

Important features in a family history include age at onset (< 50 years), bilateral or male disease, presence of other related early-onset cancers, and the number of affected relatives, including first-degree (mother, sister, daughter) and second-degree (grandmother, aunt, niece) relatives on both sides of the family. Ascertaining relevant family descent, in particular Ashkenazi Jewish and Icelandic ancestry (*BRCA* carriers), may also raise clinical suspicion (21).

Lifestyle factors

Hormonal, reproductive, and changes in lifestyle factors have long been recognized to be important in the development of breast cancer. Increased exogenous hormone use and an aging demographic may in part be related to the increasing incidence of breast cancer in the general population (1).

Prolonged estrogen exposure, either through the combined oral contraceptive (COC) or hormone replacement therapy (HRT), is associated with stimulation of breast cells and increased breast cancer risk. Early menarche (< 12 years), nulliparity, late menopause, and other lifestyle factors (e.g., obesity, alcohol, and smoking intake; childhood chest irradiation) all increase breast cancer risk (22).

DETERMINING BREAST CANCER RISK

There are few families where it is possible to be certain of inherited dominance. Risk assessment tools are used to identify the degree of family history at which genetic assessment is required. These include models that quantify individual breast cancer risk (e.g., 10-year versus lifetime risk) (23) and those that provide the probability of harboring a deleterious mutation. The Gail (24), Claus (18), and Tyrer-Cuzick (25) models estimate breast cancer risk using family history and other risk factors. The Manchester scoring (26) and BOADICEA (27) algorithms estimate *BRCA1/2* carrier probability.

Individuals presenting with a history suggestive of a high breast cancer risk should undergo formal assessment using a validated tool to ascertain their risk, carrier probability, and potential screening requirement (17). Women may be classified as having low, moderate, or high risk of breast cancer (Table 7.1) (28).

Low risk (lifetime risk < 17%)

- No significant family history.
- Near general population risk.
- Reassure and discharge to primary care (reassess if risk changes).

TABLE 7.1   Breast cancer risk categorization (4)

BREAST CANCER RISK CATEGORY	10-YEAR RISK OF BREAST CANCER	LIFETIME RISK OF BREAST CANCER	MANAGEMENT SETTING
Low risk	<3%	<17%	Primary care +/– national screening program
Moderate risk	3%–8%	17%–30%	Secondary care (breast family history clinic)
High risk	>8%	>30%	Tertiary care and genetic assessment +/– testing

Moderate risk (lifetime risk 17%–30%)

- One first-degree relative with breast cancer < 40 years.
- One first-degree male relative with breast cancer (any age).
- One first-plus one second-degree relative with breast cancer (any age).
- Two first-degree relatives with breast cancer (any age).
- Consider additional surveillance in secondary care (Figure 7.1).

High risk (lifetime risk > 30%)

- Four first-degree relatives (any age), three < 60 years, two < 50 years.
- One breast cancer < 50 years plus one ovarian cancer.
- One male plus one female breast cancer < 50 years.
- Two ovarian cancers (any age).
- Breast cancer with Jewish ancestry.
- Refer to tertiary center for potential genetic testing, enhanced surveillance, and risk-reducing treatment.

GENETIC MUTATIONS AND TESTING

In most breast cancers, the cause is unknown (19). Somatic (noninheritable) genetic changes arise *de novo* from both genetic and environmental factors due to a failure of DNA repair mechanisms. Germline (inheritable) mutations account for 5%–10% of breast cancers. They exhibit an autosomal dominant pattern whereby one abnormal copy and one normal copy are inherited from either parent.

Several susceptibility genes predisposing to a high risk of breast cancer have been identified (19) (Table 7.2). The breast cancer susceptibility genes (*BRCA1* and *BRCA2*) are the most well-known of the high-risk genes and account for a fifth of all familial breast cancers (29, 30). *BRCA* mutation carriers have a higher lifetime risk of both breast and ovarian cancer. Incidence is highest in Europe and America, in particular the Ashkenazi Jewish population (1 in 800) (21), although global incidence is increasing as genetic testing is more widely implemented (31, 32).

Partial genetic changes, termed single-nucleotide polymorphisms (SNPs), account for approximately 8% of familial breast cancer risk (33, 34). Germline mutations in other low-penetrance breast cancer susceptibility genes (*ATM, CHEK2, PALB2, BRIP1,* and *NF1*) are reported but carry a low-to-moderate lifetime breast cancer risk (35).

Genetic testing is only routinely offered to individuals with >10% likelihood of carrying a high-risk breast cancer mutation based on family history criteria or a risk assessment model, or in those with a known family member with a breast cancer mutation (4, 36). Genetic blood testing carries a high false-negative

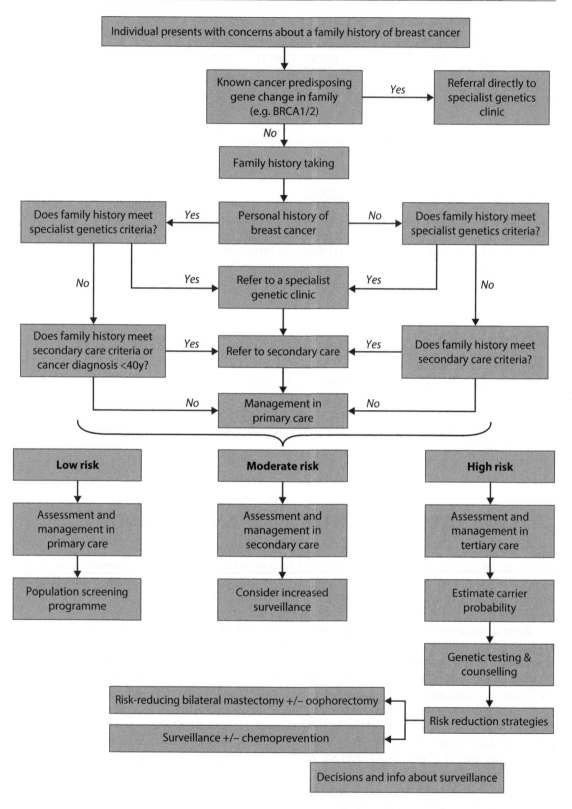

FIGURE 7.1   Algorithm for the management of the high-risk breast cancer patient.

TABLE 7.2 High-risk breast cancer–associated susceptibility genes

GENE	LOCATION	TUMORS	RISK OF BREAST CANCER (%)	INCIDENCE
BRCA1	17q	Breast, ovary	60–90	1 in 1,000
BRCA2	13q	Breast, ovary, prostate, pancreas	40–60	1 in 800
TP53 (Li–Fraumeni)	17p	Breast, sarcoma, glioma	95	1 in 30,000
PTEN (Cowden)	10q	Breast, thyroid, endometrial, colorectal	60	1 in 200,000
STK11 (Peutz–Jeghers)	19p	Breast, gastrointestinal	40	1 in 25,000
CDH1 (E-cadherin)	16q	Breast, gastric	20–40	Rare

Source: From Reference (19).

risk, and failure to identify a mutation in an individual with a known family mutation does not necessarily reduce an individual's lifetime risk estimate (6).

Patients with a family history of breast cancer have complex issues that are best dealt with by a specialist in genetics and tertiary multidisciplinary service. The likelihood of finding a mutation should be estimated prior to testing (37). Individuals should be given time to contemplate the likely risks and benefits of treatment and the potential implications of genetic testing on other family members (38).

Management of High-Risk Women

Surveillance

Screening facilitates the early detection of breast cancer and confers a survival benefit through timely therapeutic intervention (39). Early surveillance should be offered to high-risk individuals for breast cancer who have not had risk-reducing surgery. Screening may include annual digital mammographic surveillance, with or without magnetic resonance imaging (MRI), in women with a known genetic mutation (Table 7.3). Women carrying a *TP53* mutation should *only* be offered MRI surveillance due to an increased susceptibility to genetic damage from irradiation (40).

TABLE 7.3 Recommended screening strategy for women at high risk of breast cancer

RISK	AGES	SURVEILLANCE	FREQUENCY	NOTES
BRCA1 carrier	20–29	N/A	N/A	Review MRI annually on basis of breast density
BRCA2 carrier	30–39	MRI	Annual	
Not tested equivalent	40–49	MRI + Mammography	Annual	
high-risk group	50+	Mammography +/– MRI	Annual	
TP53 (Li–Fraumeni)	20+	MRI*	Annual	No mammography
A-T homozygote	25+	MRI	Annual	No mammography
A-T heterozygote	40–49	Mammography	Annual	Routine population screening from 50
	50+	Mammography	Routine screening	
Supradiaphragmatic radiation < age 30	30–39	MRI	Annual	Surveillance to start at age 30 or 8 years after first irradiation
	40–49	MRI +/– Mammography	Annual	
	50+	Mammography +/– MRI	Annual	Review MRI annually in basis of breast density

* Mammography is *not* recommended in women with a known *TP53* mutation due to the risk of ionizing radiation.

Data comparing screening modalities suggest that both the sensitivity and specificity of MRI is higher than that of mammography in *BRCA1/2* mutation carriers (41). MRI is recommended for only the very high-risk group (i.e., *BRCA1/2* and *TP53* carriers), however, due to the high cost and limited capacity.

Ultrasound is not routinely used in screening but may be used as an adjunct in the diagnosis of a palpable breast lump. Breast self-examination has improved symptomatic breast cancer detection, and women of all risk groups should practice breast awareness in addition to breast cancer screening (17). Ovarian cancer screening has not demonstrated a significant and cost-effective mortality reduction.

Risk factor reduction

Modification of hormonal and reproductive risk factors may reduce the risk of breast cancer (4).

Although some risk factors, such as age and family history, cannot be altered, other behaviors can be modified (Table 7.4), and the potential benefit of lifestyle modification should be discussed.

Chemoprevention

Removing the effect of estrogen on the breast via exogenous hormonal manipulation can be utilized in high-risk women, particularly where risk-reducing surgery is unsuitable or unacceptable.

Options include estrogen receptor modulators (tamoxifen and raloxifene) or aromatase inhibitors (anastrozole or exemestane), provided there are no thromboembolic or endometrial cancer contraindications (42). Women taking tamoxifen demonstrated a 38% reduction in estrogen receptor–positive breast cancer, although uptake is low due to associated side effect toxicity (43, 44).

Novel targeted chemoprevention, including RANKL inhibitors, antiprogestins, retinoic acid derivatives, bisphosphonates, and metformin, are under investigation (15).

Risk-reducing surgery

Bilateral risk-reducing mastectomy (BRRM) is the most effective method for reducing breast cancer risk, provided the risks from surgery are not outweighed by other comorbidities or contraindications. Meta-analyses of patients with *BRCA1/2* mutations found surgery reduced the risk of breast cancer by 90%–95% (45). The level of risk reduction achieved is directly proportional to the amount of breast tissue removed during surgery; a nipple-sparing approach will improve cosmesis but slightly increase breast cancer risk (2%–5%) as the nipple–areolar complex is left behind (46). Occult breast cancer diagnosis is reported in < 5% (47). Evidence from a Dutch multicenter cohort study of 1,712 *BRCA1* mutation carriers also demonstrated lower overall and breast cancer–specific mortality following BRRM (48).

TABLE 7.4   Risk-modifying behaviors to reduce breast cancer risk

RISK FACTOR	MODIFICATION
Alcohol	Excess alcohol increases breast cancer risk
Smoking	Smoking cessation advice
Weight and physical exercise	Encourage maintenance of a healthy body mass index Increased exercise may reduce breast cancer risk
Exogenous estrogen	Avoidance of HRT or short-term use only Advise women over 35 years of the increased risk of breast cancer (versus decreased ovarian cancer risk) from taking combined hormonal contraception
Breastfeeding	Reduces future breast cancer risk

BRCA mutation carriers may be offered risk-reducing salpingo-oophorectomy after childbearing is complete. Women will be rendered postmenopausal following oophorectomy and may further reduce the risk of breast cancer up to 50% (49). The risk of ovarian cancer is negligible before the age of 40 (*BRCA1*) or 50 (*BRCA2*), and so surgery is usually delayed (4).

Long-term studies of the physical and psychological impact of risk-reducing surgery suggest most high-risk women who undergo BRRM exhibit lower levels of anxiety and cancer-related worry compared to those who do not, although some are affected by the cosmetic and sexual implications (38, 50).

FUTURE DIRECTIONS

There has been rapid improvement in understanding the mechanisms of hereditary breast cancer predisposition in the last 30 years, including the discovery of germline mutations and breast cancer syndromes. More recently, over 300 partial genetic changes or SNPs have been linked to breast cancer (15). Further research to ascertain how family history and SNPs can be used alongside other known risk factors to predict breast cancer risk is necessary. Several studies have shown promising results utilizing SNPs and mammographic density in developing personalized screening and prevention in familial breast cancer clinics (34, 51).

CONCLUSION

Demand for genetic services in women with a family history of breast cancer has increased significantly. It is important to differentiate individuals at a high risk of breast cancer so that they may be assessed and counseled in the appropriate care setting. Management of high-risk women should include a discussion of screening, lifestyle modification, chemoprevention, and preventative surgery. Future research is likely to facilitate more personalized breast cancer screening and management of high-risk individuals.

CHAPTER SUMMARY

- Preliminary assessment of the high-risk individual should include a detail medical, gynecological, and family history.
- Individuals at high risk of breast cancer should undergo formal breast cancer risk assessment using a validated carrier probability and breast cancer risk calculator.
- High-risk patients should be referred for formal assessment and discussion of genetic testing, enhanced surveillance, and risk-reducing treatment if appropriate.
- Risk-reducing surgery is the most effective method for reducing breast cancer risk in *BRCA* mutation carriers.
- Psychological counseling should be offered to all women and their families who have ongoing concerns about a family history or an increased risk of breast cancer.

REFERENCES

1. Ferlay J, Colombet M, Soerjomataram I, Mathers C, Parkin D, Piñeros M, et al. Estimating the global cancer incidence and mortality in 2018: GLOBOCAN sources and methods. *International Journal of Cancer.* 2019;144(8):1941–53.

2. IARC Working Group on the Evaluation of Cancer-Preventive Interventions. *Handbooks of Cancer Prevention: Breast Cancer Screening.* Lyon, France: International Agency for Research on Cancer; 2014.

3. Coleman MP, Quaresma M, Berrino F, Lutz J-M, De Angelis R, Capocaccia R, et al. Cancer survival in five continents: a worldwide population-based study (CONCORD). *Lancet Oncology.* 2008;9(8):730–56.

4. National Collaborating Centre for Cancer. *Classification and care of people at risk of familial breast cancer and management of breast cancer and related risks in people with a family history of breast cancer.* London (UK): National Institute for Health and Care Excellence (NICE); 2013.

5. Hill A, Doyle J, McDermott E, O'higgins N. Hereditary breast cancer. *British Journal of Surgery.* 1997;84(10):1334–9.

6. Harvey J, Down S, Bright-Thomas R, Winstanley J, Bishop H. *Breast disease management: a multidisciplinary manual.* OUP Oxford; 2013.

7. Turkoz FP, Solak M, Petekkaya I, Keskin O, Kertmen N, Sarici F, et al. Association between common risk factors and molecular subtypes in breast cancer patients. *Breast.* 2013;22(3):344–50.

8. Olivier M, Goldgar DE, Sodha N, Ohgaki H, Kleihues P, Hainaut P, et al. Li-Fraumeni and related syndromes: correlation between tumor type, family structure, and TP53 genotype. *Cancer Research.* 2003;63(20):6643–50.

9. Walsh T, Casadei S, Coats KH, Swisher E, Stray SM, Higgins J, et al. Spectrum of mutations in BRCA1, BRCA2, CHEK2, and TP53 in families at high risk of breast cancer. *JAMA.* 2006;295(12):1379–88.

10. Antoniou A, Pharoah PD, Narod S, Risch HA, Eyfjord JE, Hopper JL, et al. Average risks of breast and ovarian cancer associated with BRCA1 or BRCA2 mutations detected in case series unselected for family history: a combined analysis of 22 studies. *American Journal of Human Genetics.* 2003;72(5):1117–30.

11. Saslow D, Boetes C, Burke W, Harms S, Leach MO, Lehman CD, et al. American Cancer Society guidelines for breast screening with MRI as an adjunct to mammography. *CA Cancer Journal for Clinicians.* 2007;57(2):75–89.

12. Evans D, Lalloo F. Risk assessment and management of high risk familial breast cancer. *Journal of Medical Genetics.* 2002;39(12):865–71.

13. Easton DF, Bishop D, Ford D, Crockford G. Genetic linkage analysis in familial breast and ovarian cancer: results from 214 families. Breast Cancer Linkage Consortium. *American Journal of Human Genetics.* 1993;52(4):678.

14. Collaborative Group on Hormonal Factors in Breast Cancer. Familial breast cancer: collaborative reanalysis of individual data from 52 epidemiological studies including 58 209 women with breast cancer and 101 986 women without the disease. *Lancet.* 2001;358(9291):1389–99.

15. Evans DG, Howell SJ, Howell A. Personalized prevention in high risk individuals: Managing hormones and beyond. *Breast.* 2018;39:139–47.

16. Owens DK, Davidson KW, Krist AH, Barry MJ, Cabana M, Caughey AB, et al. Risk assessment, genetic counseling, and genetic testing for BRCA-related cancer: US Preventive Services Task Force recommendation statement. *JAMA.* 2019;322(7):652–65.

17. Paluch-Shimon S, Cardoso F, Sessa C, Balmana J, Cardoso M, Gilbert F, et al. Prevention and screening in BRCA mutation carriers and other breast/ovarian hereditary cancer syndromes: ESMO Clinical Practice Guidelines for cancer prevention and screening. *Annals of Oncology.* 2016;27(suppl_5):v103–v10.

18. Claus EB, Risch N, Thompson WD. Autosomal dominant inheritance of early-onset breast cancer. Implications for risk prediction. *Cancer.* 1994;73(3):643–51.

19. Armstrong AC, Evans GD. Management of women at high risk of breast cancer. *BMJ.* 2014;348:g2756.

20. Malkin D, Li FP, Strong LC, Fraumeni JF, Jr., Nelson CE, Kim DH, et al. Germ line p53 mutations in a familial syndrome of breast cancer, sarcomas, and other neoplasms. *Science.* 1990;250(4985):1233–8.

21. Manchanda R, Loggenberg K, Sanderson S, Burnell M, Wardle J, Gessler S, et al. Population testing for cancer predisposing BRCA1/BRCA2 mutations in the Ashkenazi-Jewish community: a randomized controlled trial. *JNCI: Journal of the National Cancer Institute.* 2015;107(1).

22. van Veen EM, Brentnall AR, Byers H, Harkness EF, Astley SM, Sampson S, et al. Use of single-nucleotide polymorphisms and mammographic density plus classic risk factors for breast cancer risk prediction. *JAMA Oncology.* 2018;4(4):476–82.

23. Evans DGR, Howell A. Breast cancer risk-assessment models. *Breast Cancer Research: BCR*. 2007;9(5):213.
24. Gail M, Benichou J. Validation studies on a model for breast cancer risk. *Journal of the National Cancer Institute*. 1994;86(8):573.
25. Tyrer J, Duffy SW, Cuzick J. A breast cancer prediction model incorporating familial and personal risk factors. *Statistics in Medicine*. 2004;23(7):1111–30.
26. Evans D, Eccles D, Rahman N, Young K, Bulman M, Amir E, et al. A new scoring system for the chances of identifying a BRCA1/2 mutation outperforms existing models including BRCAPRO. *Journal of Medical Genetics*. 2004;41(6):474–80.
27. Antoniou AC, Pharoah P, Smith P, Easton DF. The BOADICEA model of genetic susceptibility to breast and ovarian cancer. *British Journal of Cancer*. 2004;91(8):1580–90.
28. Antoniou AC, Hardy R, Walker L, Evans DG, Shenton A, Eeles R, et al. Predicting the likelihood of carrying a BRCA1 or BRCA2 mutation: validation of BOADICEA, BRCAPRO, IBIS, Myriad and the Manchester scoring system using data from UK genetics clinics. *Journal of Medical Genetics*. 2008;45(7):425–31.
29. Claus EB, Petruzella S, Matloff E, Carter D. Prevalence of BRCA1 and BRCA2 mutations in women diagnosed with ductal carcinoma in situ. *JAMA*. 2005;293(8):964–9.
30. Miki Y, Swensen J, Shattuck-Eidens D, Futreal PA, Harshman K, Tavtigian S, et al. A strong candidate for the breast and ovarian cancer susceptibility gene BRCA1. *Science*. 1994;266(5182):66–71.
31. Nakamura S, Kwong A, Kim S-W, Iau P, Patmasiriwat P, Dofitas R, et al. Current status of the management of hereditary breast and ovarian cancer in Asia: first report by the Asian BRCA consortium. *Public Health Genomics*. 2016;19(1):53–60.
32. Fackenthal JD, Zhang J, Zhang B, Zheng Y, Hagos F, Burrill DR, et al. High prevalence of BRCA1 and BRCA2 mutations in unselected Nigerian breast cancer patients. *International Journal of Cancer*. 2012;131(5):1114–23.
33. Michailidou K, Lindström S, Dennis J, Beesley J, Hui S, Kar S, et al. Association analysis identifies 65 new breast cancer risk loci. *Nature*. 2017;551(7678):92.
34. Evans DG, Brentnall A, Byers H, Harkness E, Stavrinos P, Howell A, et al. The impact of a panel of 18 SNPs on breast cancer risk in women attending a UK familial screening clinic: a case–control study. *Journal of Medical Genetics*. 2017;54(2):111–3.
35. Coppa A, Nicolussi A, D'Inzeo S, Capalbo C, Belardinilli F, Colicchia V, et al. Optimizing the identification of risk-relevant mutations by multigene panel testing in selected hereditary breast/ovarian cancer families. *Cancer Medicine*. 2018;7(1):46–55.
36. Daly MB, Axilbund JE, Buys S, Crawford B, Farrell CD, Friedman S, et al. Genetic/familial high-risk assessment: breast and ovarian. *Journal of the National Comprehensive Cancer Network*. 2010;8(5):562–94.
37. Basu NN, Ross GL, Evans DG, Barr L. The Manchester guidelines for contralateral risk-reducing mastectomy. *World Journal of Surgical Oncology*. 2015;13:237.
38. French DP, Southworth J, Howell A, Harvie M, Stavrinos P, Watterson D, et al. Psychological impact of providing women with personalised 10-year breast cancer risk estimates. *British Journal of Cancer*. 2018;118(12):1648–57.
39. Elmore JG, Armstrong K, Lehman CD, Fletcher SW. Screening for breast cancer. *JAMA*. 2005;293(10):1245–56.
40. Kratz CP, Achatz MI, Brugieres L, Frebourg T, Garber JE, Greer M-LC, et al. Cancer screening recommendations for individuals with Li-Fraumeni syndrome. *Clinical Cancer Research*. 2017;23(11):e38–e45.
41. Warner E, Plewes DB, Shumak RS, Catzavelos GC, Di Prospero LS, Yaffe MJ, et al. Comparison of breast magnetic resonance imaging, mammography, and ultrasound for surveillance of women at high risk for hereditary breast cancer. *Journal of Clinical Oncology*. 2001;19(15):3524–31.
42. Cuzick J, Sestak I, Bonanni B, Costantino JP, Cummings S, DeCensi A, et al. Selective oestrogen receptor modulators in prevention of breast cancer: an updated meta-analysis of individual participant data. *Lancet*. 2013;381(9880):1827–34.
43. Ropka ME, Keim J, Philbrick JT. Patient decisions about breast cancer chemoprevention: a systematic review and meta-analysis. *Journal of Clinical Oncology*. 2010;28(18):3090–5.
44. Metcalfe KA, Birenbaum-Carmeli D, Lubinski J, Gronwald J, Lynch H, Moller P, et al. International variation in rates of uptake of preventive options in BRCA1 and BRCA2 mutation carriers. *International Journal of Cancer*. 2008;122(9):2017–22.
45. Hartmann LC, Lindor NM. The role of risk-reducing surgery in hereditary breast and ovarian cancer. *New England Journal of Medicine*. 2016;374(5):454–68.
46. Carbine NE, Lostumbo L, Wallace J, Ko H. Risk-reducing mastectomy for the prevention of primary breast cancer. *Cochrane Database of Systematic Reviews*. 2018;4(4):Cd002748.

47. Heemskerk-Gerritsen BA, Menke-Pluijmers MB, Jager A, Tilanus-Linthorst MM, Koppert LB, Obdeijn IM, et al. Substantial breast cancer risk reduction and potential survival benefit after bilateral mastectomy when compared with surveillance in healthy BRCA1 and BRCA2 mutation carriers: a prospective analysis. *Annals of Oncology.* 2013;24(8):2029–35.

48. Heemskerk-Gerritsen BAM, Jager A, Koppert LB, Obdeijn AI-M, Collée M, Meijers-Heijboer HEJ, et al. Survival after bilateral risk-reducing mastectomy in healthy BRCA1 and BRCA2 mutation carriers. *Breast Cancer Research and Treatment.* 2019;177(3):723–33.

49. Rebbeck TR, Kauff ND, Domchek SM. Meta-analysis of risk reduction estimates associated with risk-reducing salpingo-oophorectomy in BRCA1 or BRCA2 mutation carriers. *JNCI: Journal of the National Cancer Institute.* 2009;101(2):80–7.

50. Hopwood P, Lee A, Shenton A, Baildam A, Brain A, Lalloo F, et al. Clinical follow-up after bilateral risk reducing ('prophylactic') mastectomy: mental health and body image outcomes. *Psycho-Oncology: Journal of the Psychological, Social and Behavioral Dimensions of Cancer.* 2000;9(6):462–72.

51. Brentnall AR, Harkness EF, Astley SM, Donnelly LS, Stavrinos P, Sampson S, et al. Mammographic density adds accuracy to both the Tyrer-Cuzick and Gail breast cancer risk models in a prospective UK screening cohort. *Breast Cancer Research.* 2015;17(1):147.

Breast Cancer Screening

8

A Need for Comparative Effectiveness Research

Ismail Jatoi, Nikita Shorokhov, and
Somasundaram Subramanian

Worldwide, there is considerable interest in screening as a means of reducing the burden of breast cancer mortality, and screening mammography has generally been accepted as the standard breast cancer screening method (1, 2). However, there is harm associated with mammography screening: High rates of false-positives, radiation exposure, cost, and overdiagnosis (which will be discussed further in the paragraphs that follow) (3). It is important to recognize that screening mammography programs target large numbers of healthy, asymptomatic women. The vast majority of these women will never develop breast cancer and therefore will derive absolutely no benefit from screening, but many might be harmed. In fact, the number of women who are harmed from mammography screening very likely far exceeds those who derive a benefit. It was recently estimated that for every 1,000 women in the United States who undergo biennial screening mammography between the ages of 40 and 74, approximately 8 breast cancer deaths will be prevented, 1,529 will have a false-positive result, 213 unnecessary biopsies will be performed, and 21 will be overdiagnosed with breast cancer (4). In light of the potential adverse effects of mammography screening, we should now consider alternative forms of screening with less risk of harm and undertake trials comparing screening mammography with alternative screening strategies (i.e., comparative effectiveness research). Such trials might be particularly relevant in low- and middle-income countries, where the harms of mammography screening may create an unnecessary burden on health care resources. In this chapter, we provide an argument for a trial comparing screening mammography versus screening clinical breast examination (CBE).

Female breast cancer is now the most commonly diagnosed cancer in the world, with an estimated 2.3 million new cases reported annually, representing 11.7% of the total number of new cancer cases diagnosed worldwide (1). Breast cancer incidence is increasing throughout the world, and this has been reported in Eurasia as well (2). For example, in the Russian Federation alone, during the period 1980–2013, breast cancer incidence climbed from about 33 to 47 cases per 100,000 women, although mortality rates declined from 17.6 to 15.7 (5). In many parts of Russia, mammography screening is available to women aged 35 and older, though no randomized trials have specifically assessed its efficacy for women below age 40, and the Canadian National Breast Screening Study II and the United Kingdom Age Trial found no mortality benefit for women aged 40–49 (6–8).

DOI: 10.1201/9780367821982-8

61

The greatest harm associated with mammography screening is overdiagnosis, which refers to detection of cancers that pose no threat to life and would never have been detected in the absence of screening (3, 9). Overdiagnosis is easier to conceptualize if we consider four possible implications for patients with screen-detected cancers (10). First, the patient may survive the cancer diagnosis if it is diagnosed with screening, but would have died had the cancer been diagnosed clinically. Second, the patient would have survived, irrespective of whether the cancer had been diagnosed with screening or usual clinical detection. Third, the patient may die of the cancer, irrespective of whether it is detected by screening or the usual means of clinical detection. Finally, the patient may survive the screen-detected cancer but would have lived just as long and never have known that she had cancer had she never undergone screening (i.e., the cancer was overdiagnosed as a consequence of screening).

The proportion of cancers that are overdiagnosed in mammography screening programs may be as high as 30%–50% in some geographical areas, and a recent evidence-based review from the U.S. Preventive Services Task Force (USPSTF) concluded that approximately 11%–22% of all breast cancers (*in situ* and invasive) in the United States are overdiagnosed as a consequence of mammography screening (3, 11). Indeed, in the United States, the widespread use of mammography screening between the years 1975 and 2004 led to a dramatic increase in the age-adjusted incidence of ductal carcinoma *in situ* (DCIS), from 5.8 to 32.5 cases per 100,000 women (12). If, as commonly assumed, DCIS generally progresses to invasive breast cancer, then such a sharp increase in the detection and expiration of DCIS during the years 1975–2004 should have resulted in a substantial decline in the incidence of invasive breast cancer. Yet rates of invasive breast cancer climbed from 100.0 to 124.3 cases per 100,000 women during the same period of time, suggesting that most cases of DCIS detected as a consequence of mammography are overdiagnosed and have no propensity to progress to invasive cancer (12, 13). Moreover, it is worth noting that screening mammography also substantially increases detection rates of early-stage invasive cancers, but it has only a marginal effect in reducing the incidence of metastatic breast cancer, suggesting that even invasive cancers are overdiagnosed as a consequence of mammography screening (14). Overdiagnosis results in unnecessary treatments, with the potential for an excess in morbidity and mortality from those unnecessary treatments. Overdiagnosis also has a very adverse effect on quality of life. Indeed, patients are unnecessarily labeled "cancer patients" due to overdiagnosis, and this may result in some patients being denied employment, denied life insurance, or having to pay higher premiums for health care insurance coverage (13). Furthermore, overdiagnosis wastes precious health care resources that might be better utilized addressing more urgent health care needs, and this is a particular concern when one considers implementation of mammography screening programs in developing countries (15).

Worldwide, at least 13 randomized trials have assessed the effects of various breast cancer screening methods on breast cancer–specific mortality as the primary endpoint (3). Nine trials examined the efficacy of mammography screening, two trials (undertaken in St. Petersburg, Russia and Shanghai, China) examined the efficacy of screening breast self-examination (BSE), and two trials in India (undertaken in Mumbai and Trivandrum) examined the efficacy of screening CBE on breast cancer–specific mortality (3). The mammography screening trials showed that screening may reduce breast cancer–specific mortality by as much as 20%, but there appears to be an age interaction (16). Specifically, a mortality benefit is evident for women who undergo screening from age 50 and above, but a mortality benefit is not readily evident for women below that age. The underlying reason for this age interaction is not clear. However, it is worth noting that screening preferentially detects more indolent cancers that spend a greater length of time in the preclinical phase (i.e., length bias) (3). Thus, estrogen receptor (ER)–positive cancers are preferentially detected with mammography screening and ER-negative are less likely to be screen-detected. As younger (premenopausal) women have a higher proportion of ER-negative cancers, one might therefore speculate that they may derive less benefit from mammography screening. In developing countries, a higher proportion of breast cancers are diagnosed in premenopausal women, and these women would not be expected to derive much benefit from screening mammography. For younger women, the harms of screening mammography may far outweigh any potential benefits.

In addition to the age interaction, there is also a treatment interaction with respect to the efficacy of mammography screening, with recent improvements in breast cancer therapy potentially reducing the benefit of screening (17, 18). This might be better understood if we consider three categories of breast cancer with relevance to screening: (1) Cancers that are curable only if detected by screening; (2) cancers that are incurable, irrespective of whether detected by screening or usual clinical means; and (3) cancers that are readily curable, whether detected clinically or by screening. If we consider these three categories of breast cancers, it should be evident that as treatments improve over time, fewer patients will require screening to achieve a breast cancer cure. Thus, with improvements in therapy, many cancers will no longer require screening to achieve a cure and will be readily curable even if detected clinically.

The St. Petersburg and Shanghai trials failed to demonstrate any mortality benefit for screening BSE, and screening BSE may unnecessarily increase patient anxiety and lead to unnecessary breast biopsies (3, 19, 20). Thus, there is no clear evidence to support the use of BSE as a screening strategy. It is important to recognize the distinction between screening BSE and screening CBE. In screening BSE, women are taught how to examine their own breasts to detect cancers earlier, while in screening CBE, trained professionals undertake the breast examinations (21). Two trials in India (undertaken in Mumbai and Trivandrum) indicate that screening CBE can produce a substantial downstaging of disease (3, 22, 23). Recently, Mittra et al. reported results of the Mumbai trial. A total of 151,538 women aged 35–64 with no history of breast cancer were randomized to either screening CBE or no screening (23). After 20 years of follow-up, there was an overall nonsignificant 15% reduction in breast cancer mortality in the screening CBE arm versus the control arm, but a post hoc subset analysis demonstrated a statistically significant 30% relative reduction in mortality attributable to screening women over the age of 50. Although the results of the Mumbai trial are encouraging, it should be pointed out that this was a cluster randomized controlled trial, only 20 clusters, and this may have created imbalances between the study and control arms of the trial.

Currently, a large randomized trial in Japan is comparing screening mammography versus mammography + breast ultrasound (24). Early results of the Japanese trial indicate that breast cancer detection rates are significantly greater for women screened with mammography + breast ultrasound versus mammography alone, but the effects on mortality are not yet known, and it will be several more years before any potential mortality effects are discernable (3).

Clearly, there is a need for comparative effectiveness research, whereby screening methods are compared to discern strategies that provide the greatest mortality advantage and the least adverse effects on quality of life (25). It might be easier to launch such trials in Eurasian countries, where large segments of the population have not yet readily embraced screening mammography. However, such trials should only recruit patients from regions where standard treatments are readily available, as any potential benefit of screening will be derived from early treatment and not simply early detection. Also, it is important to again emphasize that substantial improvements in breast cancer treatment will ultimately reduce the benefit of screening.

The Eurasian Federation of Oncology (EAFO) and Eurasian Cancer Research Council (ECRC) convened the II EAFO Breast Cancer Forum from October 11–13, 2019 in Moscow, Russian Federation. Prior to the forum, a questionnaire was sent to the EAFO and ECRC contact list, and 81 oncologists from nine countries responded. Fifty-three of the respondents were from Russia, and the remainder from other countries of the former Soviet Union. The vast majority (94%) believe that breast cancer screening is an effective means of reducing breast cancer mortality and recommend it for women with an average breast cancer risk. Forty-three percent recommend initiation of screening mammography for women starting at age 35, 37% recommend starting at age 40, 12% starting at age 45, and only 7% recommend screening only for women aged 50 and above. Among the respondents, 30% consider false-positives to be the greatest drawback of screening mammography, while cost, radiation exposure, and overdiagnosis received 28%, 26%, and 16% of the votes, respectively. When asked if they would be willing to randomize women to a trial comparing mammography versus CBE, 43 indicated "yes" and 38 indicated "no." Additionally, when asked if they would be willing to recruit to a trial randomizing women to screening mammography versus screening automated breast ultrasound (ABUS), 64 indicated "yes" and 17 indicated "no." Thus, there is a perhaps a window of opportunity for a Eurasian trial comparing screening mammography with an alternative screening modality. The EAFO and ECRC are committed to further exploring this opportunity.

Clearly, there is now an urgent need to compare technology-based screening (i.e., mammography) with screening CBE. Such a trial should, ideally, not only compare the mortality effects of these two screening strategies but also assess quality of life outcomes, perhaps with a composite endpoint incorporating both mortality and quality of life (26). It is important that we now realize that screening has enormous implications on quality of life that may impact large numbers of asymptomatic women. In this era of effective adjuvant systemic therapies, technology-based screening may not necessarily be the best screening option, as the same mortality benefit may now perhaps be achieved with screening CBE, with better quality of life outcomes (27). Thus, screening CBE merits closer scrutiny, particularly for low- and middle-income countries, and a randomized trial comparing screening mammography versus screening CBE is needed.

REFERENCES

1. Sung H, Ferlay J, Siegel RL, Laversanne M, Soerjomataram I, Jemal A, et al. Global Cancer Statistics 2020: GLOBOCAN estimates of incidence and mortality worldwide for 36 cancers in 185 countries. *CA Cancer J Clin*. 2021;71(3):209–49.
2. Goss PE, Strasser-Weippl K, Lee-Bychkovsky BL, Fan L, Li J, Chavarri-Guerra Y, et al. Challenges to effective cancer control in China, India, and Russia. *Lancet Oncol*. 2014;15(5):489–538.
3. Jatoi I, Anderson WF, Miller AB, Brawley OW. The history of cancer screening. *Curr Probl Surg*. 2019; 56(4):138–63.
4. Qaseem A, Lin JS, Mustafa RA, Horwitch CA, Wilt TJ, Clinical Guidelines Committee of the American College of Physicians. Screening for breast cancer in average-risk women: A guidance statement from the American College of Physicians. *Ann Intern Med*. 2019;170(8):547–60.
5. Barchuk A, Bespalov A, Huhtala H, Chimed T, Laricheva I, Belyaev A, et al. Breast and cervical cancer incidence and mortality trends in Russia 1980–2013. *Cancer Epidemiol*. 2018;55:73–80.
6. Moss SM, Wale C, Smith R, Evans A, Cuckle H, Duffy SW. Effect of mammographic screening from age 40 years on breast cancer mortality in the UK Age trial at 17 years' follow-up: a randomised controlled trial. *Lancet Oncol*. 2015;16(9):1123–32.
7. Miller AB, Wall C, Baines CJ, Sun P, To T, Narod SA. Twenty five year follow-up for breast cancer incidence and mortality of the Canadian National Breast Screening Study: randomised screening trial. BMJ. 2014;348:g366.
8. Duffy SW, Vulkan D, Cuckle H, Parmar D, Sheikh S, Smith RA, et al. Effect of mammographic screening from age 40 years on breast cancer mortality (UK Age trial): final results of a randomised, controlled trial. *Lancet Oncol*. 2020;21(9):1165–72.
9. Peeters PH, Verbeek AL, Straatman H, Holland R, Hendriks JH, Mravunac M, et al. Evaluation of overdiagnosis of breast cancer in screening with mammography: results of the Nijmegen programme. *Int J Epidemiol*. 1989;18(2):295–9.
10. Marcus PM, Prorok PC, Miller AB, DeVoto EJ, Kramer BS. Conceptualizing overdiagnosis in cancer screening. *J Natl Cancer Inst*. 2015;107(4):1–4.
11. Nelson HD, Pappas M, Cantor A, Griffin J, Daeges M, Humphrey L. Harms of breast cancer screening: systematic review to update the 2009 U.S. Preventive Services Task Force recommendation. *Ann Intern Med*. 2016;164(4):256–67.
12. Virnig BA, Tuttle TM, Shamliyan T, Kane RL. Ductal carcinoma in situ of the breast: a systematic review of incidence, treatment, and outcomes. *J Natl Cancer Inst*. 2010;102(3):170–8.
13. Jatoi I, Baum M. Mammographically detected ductal carcinoma in situ: are we over diagnosing breast cancer? *Surgery*. 1995;118(1):118–20.
14. Jatoi I, Anderson WF. Breast-cancer tumor size and screening effectiveness. *N Engl J Med*. 2017;376(1):93.
15. Shrank WH, Rogstad TL, Parekh N. Waste in the US health care system: estimated costs and potential for savings. *JAMA*. 2019;322(15):1501–9.

16. Nelson HD, Fu R, Cantor A, Pappas M, Daeges M, Humphrey L. Effectiveness of breast cancer screening: systematic review and meta-analysis to update the 2009 U.S. Preventive Services Task Force recommendation. *Ann Intern Med.* 2016;164(4):244–55.

17. Jatoi I. The impact of advances in treatment on the efficacy of mammography screening. *Prev Med.* 2011;53(3):103–4.

18. Jatoi I, Miller AB. Why is breast-cancer mortality declining? *Lancet Oncol.* 2003;4(4):251–4.

19. Thomas DB, Gao DL, Ray RM, Wang WW, Allison CJ, Chen FL, et al. Randomized trial of breast self-examination in Shanghai: final results. *J Natl Cancer Inst.* 2002;94(19):1445–57.

20. Semiglazov VF, Manikhas AG, Moiseenko VM, Protsenko SA, Kharikova RS, Seleznev IK, et al. Results of a prospective randomized investigation [Russia (St.Petersburg)/WHO] to evaluate the significance of self-examination for the early detection of breast cancer. *Vopr Onkol.* 2003;49(4):434–41.

21. Mittra I. Breast screening: the case for physical examination without mammography. *Lancet.* 1994;343(8893):342–4.

22. Sankaranarayanan R, Ramadas K, Thara S, Muwonge R, Prabhakar J, Augustine P, et al. Clinical breast examination: preliminary results from a cluster randomized controlled trial in India. *J Natl Cancer Inst.* 2011; 103(19):1476–80.

23. Mittra I, Mishra GA, Dikshit RP, Gupta S, Kulkarni VY, Shaikh HKA, et al. Effect of screening by clinical breast examination on breast cancer incidence and mortality after 20 years: prospective, cluster randomised controlled trial in Mumbai. *BMJ.* 2021;372:n256.

24. Ohuchi N, Suzuki A, Sobue T, Kawai M, Yamamoto S, Zheng YF, et al. Sensitivity and specificity of mammography and adjunctive ultrasonography to screen for breast cancer in the Japan Strategic Anti-cancer Randomized Trial (J-START): a randomised controlled trial. *Lancet.* 2016;387(10016):341–8.

25. Fiore LD, Lavori PW. Integrating randomized comparative effectiveness research with patient care. *N Engl J Med.* 2016;374(22):2152–8.

26. Jatoi I, Gail MH. The need for combined assessment of multiple outcomes in noninferiority trials in oncology. *JAMA Oncol.* 2020;6(3):420–4.

27. Jatoi I, Pinsky PF. Breast cancer screening trials: endpoints and over-diagnosis. *J Natl Cancer Inst.* 2021;113((9):11311135.

Management of High-Risk Lesions and *In Situ* Cancers

9

Amanda L. Amin and Amy C. Degnim

FLAT EPITHELIAL ATYPIA

Flat epithelial atypia (FEA) was defined in 2003 by the World Health Organization (WHO) as a presumably neoplastic intraductal alteration characterized by enlarged acini and terminal ducts lined by layers of monotonous epithelial cells with low-grade cytologic atypia but lacking architectural atypia required for the diagnosis of atypical hyperplasia (3, 4). FEA is thought to be a possible precursor lesion in the pathway for development of breast cancer based on molecular data (5, 6), and it is frequently found in close proximity to other high-risk lesions such as atypical ductal hyperplasia (ADH), atypical lobular hyperplasia (ALH), and lobular carcinoma *in situ* (LCIS) (7). FEA is identified in approximately 0.7%–12.2% of benign breast biopsies, usually presenting as screen-detected calcifications on mammogram (8–12). There is no current consensus on whether FEA identified on CNB without the presence of additional high-risk lesions warrants surgical excision (13), but the data support a decision process that includes the patient context and specifically whether a finding of atypical hyperplasia at excision would alter that patient's management in light of other preexisting comorbidities.

When CNB identifies FEA, National Comprehensive Cancer Center (NCCN) recommendations suggest select patients may be suitable for monitoring in the absence of surgical excision, but does not provide guidance as to patient specifics (14). Historically, there has been a wide range in upgrade rate to underlying malignancy, from 0% to 42% (9–12, 15–42). In a meta-analysis of studies evaluating pure FEA on CNB by Rudin and colleagues, there was significant heterogeneity across studies, so when restricting to higher-quality studies with stricter criteria, upgrade to malignancy was 7.5% (either invasive or ductal carcinoma insitu [DCIS]), with upgrade to invasive cancer in only 3% (13). Upgrade to ADH was more common, with ADH identified in 18.6% of surgical excisions for pure FEA. While not a malignancy itself, ADH carries a higher risk for future malignancy and warrants a discussion on more frequent screening and chemoprevention (provided later). As excision of pure FEA upgrades to malignancy or higher-risk atypia for at least 25% of patients, which may alter treatment recommendations, the general recommendation would be that patients be considered for excision, while also taking into account preferences and patient comorbidities (13). More recent studies citing lower malignancy upgrade rates of <3% describe better lesion sampling with larger gauge needles (9–11g) with vacuum assistance and radiographic-pathologic

DOI: 10.1201/9780367821982-9

concordance (43–49). This rate is on par with the Breast Imaging–Reporting and Data System (BI-RADS 3) lesions, which are typically recommended for surveillance over excision (50). However, the risk of upgrade to ADH and whether that would impact an individual patient's management may remain a reason to consider surgical excision.

The long-term future risk of malignancy does not appear to be significantly affected by the presence of FEA. In Said and colleagues' study of 282 women with FEA with a median follow-up of 17 years, nearly half of women had coexisting atypical hyperplasia (AH) with FEA. When comparing future risk of breast cancer for those with FEA alone to those with FEA + AH, risk with FEA alone was on par with women with proliferative breast disease, and those with FEA + AH had an elevated risk on par with women with AH alone (4). As the presence of FEA does not appear to be an independent risk factor for future breast cancer beyond that of any proliferative lesion, increased surveillance and chemoprevention do not appear necessary for FEA alone.

ATYPICAL HYPERPLASIA

AH is a high-risk lesion found in approximately 10% of benign breast biopsies (51). Histologically, AH is classified by dysplastic, monotonous epithelial cell populations occupying a transitional zone between benign and malignant breast disease (6, 52–54). AH can be subclassified into ALH and ADH based on microscopic appearance, and they occur with similar frequency and carry similar long-term malignancy risk (Table 9.1) (55–59).

The long-term risk of breast cancer is affected by many factors including lifetime estrogen exposure (age at menarche and menopause, parity, breastfeeding, hormone replacement therapy use), family history genetics, chest wall radiation at a young age, obesity, alcohol consumption, and physical activity, in addition to breast-specific features such as mammographic density and benign breast disease. Multiple large cohort studies have investigated future breast cancer risk after benign biopsies (Nashville Breast Cohort, Partners Cohort, Nurses' Health Study, Breast Cancer Surveillance Consortium, Mayo Clinic Benign Breast Disease [BBD] Cohort). AH is recognized across multiple studies as a significant marker of future breast cancer risk, approximately four-fold higher than the general population, which translates into 1%–2% absolute risk/year (Table 9.1) (55, 60, 61). With the Mayo BBD Cohort, Hartmann and colleagues have further stratified risk by the number of atypical foci, demonstrating that increasing foci of atypia increases the future risk of breast cancer, with women with three or more foci having a 25-year risk of malignancy close to 50% (55). In most studies, ADH and ALH carry similar long-term risk, whereas in some studies ALH appears to have a slightly higher risk than ADH. In women with AH, future breast cancer risk persists beyond 15 years and affects both breasts similarly, with 40% of later cancers being contralateral (55, 60, 62).

TABLE 9.1 Benign breast disease and long-term risk

NONPROLIFERATIVE	PROLIFERATIVE	ATYPICAL HYPERPLASIA	LCIS
Fibroadenoma	Radial scar	ADH	LCIS
Cysts, fibrosis	CCH & FEA	ALH	
UDH	Papilloma		
Aprocrine metaplasia	Sclerosing adenosis		
	Florid duct hyperplasia		
~ Population	0.5% per year	1%–2% per year	2% per year

ADH: Atypical ductal hyperplasia, ALH: Atypical lobular hyperplasia, LCIS: Lobular carcinoma *in situ*, UDH: Usual ductal hyperplasia.

Atypical Lobular Hyperplasia and Upgrade after Core Needle Biopsy

Page and colleagues established criteria for the diagnosis of ALH in 1985 to include expanded acini of the lobule, filled with small, monotonous, round, or polygonal cells lacking cohesion and loss of acinar lumens (58, 63). ALH is frequently an incidental finding on CNB (2, 49). There is large variability in the studies attempting to define upgrade rate after needle biopsy, many with a small sample size, and ALH is frequently grouped with LCIS as lobular neoplasia (LN). The historical upgrade risk ranges from 0% to 67% for LN (55). Many of these studies also did not exclude additional high-risk lesions, such as papillomas or radial sclerosing lesions, or discordant lesions, which would presumably contribute to the higher upgrade rate. In contemporary studies that have controlled for all of those factors, upgrade rate is consistently <3% (8, 64–71). Because of the low incidence of malignancy at a site of pure ALH, surgical excision is not required for incidental ALH with concordant radiology and pathology (14, 72–74).

Atypical Ductal Hyperplasia and Upgrade after Core Needle Biopsy

ADH, like DCIS, frequently presents as calcifications on screening mammogram (70, 75). Unfortunately, ADH and DCIS are histologically virtually identical, with the distinction being quantity of atypia, creating challenges in accurate diagnosis by core biopsy. A lesion is characterized as ADH if low-grade cytologic atypia and monomorphism combined with epithelial architectural complexity involves two or more membrane-bound spaces but measures less than 2 mm in linear extent (58). Because the amount of sampling of the lesion can be the distinction between ADH and DCIS, surgical excision is typically recommended for ADH to rule out underlying malignancy (14, 70, 76).

Contemporary studies report an upgrade rate of 15%–25% to DCIS or invasive cancer and approximately 3% risk of invasive breast cancer alone (8, 77–94). As such, 75%–85% do not have any cancer and nearly 97% do not have invasive cancer, which has resulted in additional studies focused on identifying those patients at lowest risk of upgrade who could be successfully managed with observation over surgical excision.

The earliest studies investigating the feasibility of selecting a low risk for upgrade group for observation incorporated patient factors such as younger age (<50 years) and only screen-detected lesions (no palpable masses or nipple discharge); radiographic features such as small lesion size (<1.5 cm) and imaging presentation of calcifications without a mass; and pathologic features including low burden of atypical foci (only one focus), which resulted in an upgrade rate of 5.6% (95). Subsequent studies restricted observation to radiographic calcifications without a mass while incorporating pathologic features of no individual cell necrosis and the extent of lesion removal by biopsy (>95%), which carries an upgrade rate of 6% (81). This is further refined to allow observation when there is no necrosis and using a combination of volume of atypia with the degree of sampling (only one focus and >50% removed or three or fewer foci and >90% removed), with a resulting upgrade rate of 4.9% (86). In general, the lowest risk seems to be in concordant lesions without a mass, small lesions, and complete or near-complete removal (well sampled) (96). When these criteria are not met, surgical excision should be performed (76, 97, 98). Since most upgrades are to DCIS and the surgical management of DCIS is being called into question (see DCIS section later), the surgical excision of ADH should also be questioned. Menen and colleagues demonstrated patients with ADH meeting the previous low-risk criteria can be safely offered observation over excision, with the subsequent breast cancer rate of 5.6% over a median 3-year follow-up, with the majority not being at the ADH biopsy site (99).

LOBULAR CARCINOMA *IN SITU*

Foote and Stewart first described LCIS in 1941 (100). LCIS is part of the LN spectrum that also includes ALH, with the two differentiated by the quantity of atypia, with distension and filling of >50% of the acini in a terminal duct lobular unit in LCIS and <50% for ALH (101–103). Both LCIS and ALH are monomorphic epithelial cell populations with minimal nuclear atypia that lack cellular cohesion and contain frequent intracytoplasmic vacuoles negative for E-cadherin because of somatic alterations of the *CDH1* gene on the long arm of chromosome 16 (104). LCIS, similar to ALH, is typically an incidental finding on percutaneous biopsy performed for an imaging finding that yields other concordant pathology, but LCIS may occasionally be associated with microcalcifications on screening mammogram (8, 49, 70, 84, 105).

Reports in the literature of upgrade rate after surgical excision for LN, as discussed in the ALH subsection, have been 15%–33% (8, 66, 67, 94). There are several histologic subtypes of LCIS, the most common being the classic type, which typically has an incidental presentation. Additional subtypes such as pleomorphic LCIS and LCIS with comedo-necrosis are typically associated with calcifications and may be misclassified as DCIS. Less is known about these nonclassic variants, as most reports are from a single institution with small numbers, but reported upgrade rates to underlying malignancy are up to 70% (106–114). Therefore, surgical excision is recommended for all nonclassic-type LCIS (49, 115–118). However, classic-type LCIS with radiographic-pathologic correlation has a low upgrade rate (1%–3%) (49, 72) and can be observed mammographically (74). Taylor and colleagues used the National Cancer Database (NCDB) to investigate the surgical practices for patients with LCIS. Nearly 85% of the 30,105 women with LCIS underwent excision, including 4% with unilateral mastectomy and 5.1% with bilateral mastectomy, which was reported as overtreatment for this entity (119).

However, women with LCIS do have a substantially elevated future risk of breast cancer, approximately an eight-fold relative risk and a 2%/year absolute risk (Table 9.1) (120). Other contributing factors are age at diagnosis and number of atypical foci (74, 120). Based on a large Surveillance, Epidemiology, and End Results (SEER) study, it also appears that race and ethnicity play a role in future breast cancer risk, with black women with LCIS having a 1.3 times higher risk of future breast cancer than white women with LCIS (121). Therefore, risk stratification should be performed considering these factors, allowing high-risk screening and offering chemoprevention to be considered when appropriate.

DUCTAL CARCINOMA *IN SITU*

DCIS is usually an asymptomatic neoplastic process confined to the ductal system of the breast, although more unique presentations include nipple discharge, palpable masses, or nipple skin changes consistent with Paget's disease. With lack of invasion, DCIS lacks the ability to metastasize (stage 0 on American Joint Committee on Cancer [AJCC] 8th Edition staging) (122). DCIS accounts for approximately 10% of all breast cancer diagnoses and 20% of all screen-detected cancers, with 48,100 women being diagnosed with DCIS in 2019 in the United States (123).

Although the classification of DCIS as a cancer has been recently called into question, including changing the name to indolent lesion of epithelial origin (IDLE) and removing the word carcinoma entirely (124), standard of care is to proceed with surgical excision with either lumpectomy or mastectomy, depending on the extent of the abnormality and patient preference. Although DCIS lacks the ability to metastasize, axillary staging is appropriate in a certain subset of patients. DCIS on CNB is upgraded to invasive cancer in 21% and to microinvasive (DCIS-M) cancer in 5.5%, resulting in approximately 25% ultimately requiring axillary staging (125). Therefore, patients having planned mastectomy or those with a high risk to be upgraded to invasive disease on final pathology include patients with a large area of DCIS

(>5 cm) mass on exam or imaging, DCIS-M, or when the lumpectomy location will inhibit the ability to obtain accurate axillary staging with sentinel lymph node dissection in the future (126, 127).

Because DCIS is a nonobligate precursor to the development of invasive carcinoma, the goals of therapy include prevention of local progression to invasive cancer or recurrence, all while minimizing the toxicity of treatment (128). The surgical options for DCIS are similar to invasive cancer, including lumpectomy plus whole-breast irradiation (WBI) or mastectomy (129). Regardless of the surgical treatment, there is strong evidence that local recurrence (LR) outcomes are best when the margin after excision is negative. There has been much deliberation about the appropriate margin width for lowest recurrence risk after lumpectomy. Society of Surgical Oncology (SSO)/American Society for Radiation Oncology (ASTRO)/American Society of Surgical Oncology (ASCO) consensus guidelines, published in 2016, recommend a surgical margin width of 2 mm for DCIS undergoing lumpectomy and WBI and that trying to achieve wider margins may decrease cosmesis without LR improvement (130).

There is strong evidence that WBI after lumpectomy reduces local recurrence, but there has been significant interest in identifying the patients with low enough local recurrence risk who may be able to avoid radiation after lumpectomy (131). There have been four randomized controlled trials evaluating the omission of WBI for DCIS with more than 10 years of follow-up. Meta-analysis of these trials still demonstrates that WBI decreases the rates of locoregional events by half (relative risk [RR] 0.53) resulting in a 15% absolute risk reduction, but there are no changes in distant recurrence, contralateral breast events, or overall survival (132–136). To assist in identification of who meets criteria for low-risk DCIS, commercially available multigene assay OncotypeDx DCIS Score (Genomic Health, Redwood City, CA) can be used to help predict recurrence risk without radiation (137). DCIS is a cautionary group for accelerated partial breast irradiation (APBI) (130).

There are several actively accruing trials worldwide that are challenging traditional management of DCIS with excision and additional adjuvant treatments: LOw Risk DCIS (LORD, NCT02492607) in the Netherlands, the LOw RISk (LORIS) DCIS Trial in the UK, and Comparison of Operative to Monitoring and Endocrine Therapy for Low Risk DCIS (COMET, NCT02926911) in the United States (138–142). All are enrolling women with screen-detected, grade I–II, ER+ DCIS and randomizing participants to either standard-of-care treatment or active surveillance with a primary outcome to determine who progresses to invasive cancer on active surveillance.

PREVENTION THERAPY

For all women who have AH, LCIS, or DCIS, future breast cancer risk is elevated to varying degrees. NCCN management recommendations include clinical encounters every 6–12 months, annual mammogram after age 30, consider annual MRI after age 25, risk reduction strategies, and breast awareness (14). American Society of Clinical Oncology (ASCO) guidelines recommend discussion of prevention therapy with women who have a 5-year absolute risk of breast cancer of 1.7% or higher (143, 144). Prevention with tamoxifen, raloxifene, anastrazole, or exemestane generally has a 50% reduction in risk (145–147), with an even greater risk reduction in women with AH and LCIS (~65%–70%) (Figure 9.1) (55, 60, 120).

Acceptance of prevention therapy has been low for women with DCIS and even more so for those with AH or LCIS (148–151). Reasons for this low rate include clinicians and women underestimating their future risk of breast cancer and women's fear of adverse effects from this therapy. Tamoxifen is associated with elevated RR of endometrial cancer (RR 2.25), cataracts (RR 1.22), and thromboembolic events (RR 1.93); and anastrazole and exemestane are associated with bone loss, although absolute risks are low. Future directions for prevention include low-dose oral tamoxifen or a topical tamoxifen formulation. A study of tamoxifen 5 mg orally per day in high-risk women showed a similar risk reduction benefit (52% reduction of ipsilateral breast cancer events and 76% reduction in contralateral breast cancer events) with minimal side effects compared with the traditional dosage of 20 mg oral daily (152). Because the systemic

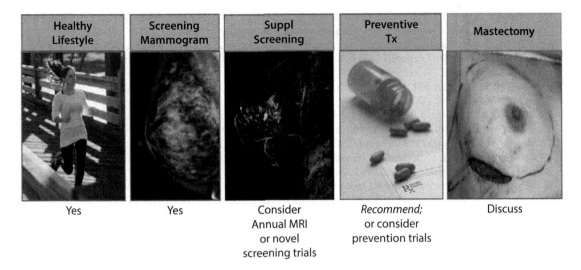

Healthy Lifestyle	Screening Mammogram	Suppl Screening	Preventive Tx	Mastectomy
Yes	Yes	Consider Annual MRI or novel screening trials	*Recommend;* or consider prevention trials	Discuss

FIGURE 9.1   Management based upon risk: ADH/ALH.

side effects of oral medication are a large reason for lack of adherence or acceptance for chemoprevention, a topical formulation of tamoxifen (4-OHT) that can be applied to the breast skin is also under investigation in DCIS (153, 154).

REFERENCES

1. Gutwein LG, Ang DN, Liu H, Marshall JK, Hochwald SN, Copeland EM, et al. Utilization of minimally invasive breast biopsy for the evaluation of suspicious breast lesions. *Am J Surg.* 2011;202(2):127–32.
2. Racz JM, Carter JM, Degnim AC. Challenging atypical breast lesions including flat epithelial atypia, radial scar, and intraductal papilloma. *Ann Surg Oncol.* 2017;24(10):2842–7.
3. Tavassoli FA, Hoefler H; Rosai J. Intraductal proliferative lesions. In: Tavassoli FA, Devilee P, editors. *Pathology and Genetic Tumours of the Breast and Female Genital Organs.* Lyon, France: IARC Press; 2003. pp. 65–6.
4. Said SM, Visscher DW, Nassar A, Frank RD, Vierkant RA, Frost MH, et al. Flat epithelial atypia and risk of breast cancer: A Mayo cohort study. *Cancer.* 2015;121(10):1548–55.
5. Reis-Filho JS, Simpson PT, Gale T, Lakhani SR. The molecular genetics of breast cancer: The contribution of comparative genomic hybridization. *Pathol Res Pract.* 2005;201(11):713–25.
6. Bombonati A, Sgroi DC. The molecular pathology of breast cancer progression. *J Pathol.* 2011;223(2):307–17.
7. Schnitt SJ, Vincent-Salomon A. Columnar cell lesions of the breast. *Adv Anat Pathol.* 2003;10(3):113–24.
8. Mooney KL, Bassett LW, Apple SK. Upgrade rates of high-risk breast lesions diagnosed on core needle biopsy: A single-institution experience and literature review. *Mod Pathol.* 2016;29(12):1471–84.
9. Becker AK, Gordon PB, Harrison DA, Hassell PR, Hayes MM, van Niekerk D, et al. Flat ductal intraepithelial neoplasia 1A diagnosed at stereotactic core needle biopsy: Is excisional biopsy indicated? *AJR Am J Roentgenol.* 2013;200(3):682–8.
10. Martel M, Barron-Rodriguez P, Tolgay Ocal I, Dotto J, Tavassoli FA. Flat DIN 1 (flat epithelial atypia) on core needle biopsy: 63 cases identified retrospectively among 1,751 core biopsies performed over an 8-year period (1992–1999). *Virchows Arch.* 2007;451(5):883–91.
11. Kunju LP, Kleer CG. Significance of flat epithelial atypia on mammotome core needle biopsy: Should it be excised? *Hum Pathol.* 2007;38(1):35–41.
12. Piubello Q, Parisi A, Eccher A, Barbazeni G, Franchini Z, Iannucci A. Flat epithelial atypia on core needle biopsy: Which is the right management? *Am J Surg Pathol.* 2009;33(7):1078–84.

13. Rudin AV, Hoskin TL, Fahy A, Farrell AM, Nassar A, Ghosh K, et al. Flat epithelial atypia on core biopsy and upgrade to cancer: A systematic review and meta-analysis. *Ann Surg Oncol.* 2017;24(12):3549–58.
14. National Comprehensive Cancer Center. National Comprehensive Cancer Network Clinical Guidelines. Breast Cancer Screening and Diagnosis 2019 [Available from: https://www.nccn.org/professionals/physician_gls/pdf/breast-screening.pdf.] Accessed 9 May 2020.
15. Lim CN, Ho BC, Bay BH, Yip G, Tan PH. Nuclear morphometry in columnar cell lesions of the breast: Is it useful? *J Clin Pathol.* 2006;59(12):1283–6.
16. Chivukula M, Bhargava R, Tseng G, Dabbs DJ. Clinicopathologic implications of "flat epithelial atypia" in core needle biopsy specimens of the breast. *Am J Clin Pathol.* 2009;131(6):802–8.
17. Senetta R, Campanino PP, Mariscotti G, Garberoglio S, Daniele L, Pennecchi F, et al. Columnar cell lesions associated with breast calcifications on vacuum-assisted core biopsies: Clinical, radiographic, and histological correlations. *Mod Pathol.* 2009;22(6):762–9.
18. Hayes B, Quinn C. Pathology of B3 lesions of the breast. *Diagn Histopathol.* 2009(15):459–69.
19. Darvishian F, Singh B, Simsir A, Ye W, Cangiarella JF. Atypia on breast core needle biopsies: Reproducibility and significance. *Ann Clin Lab Sci.* 2009;39(3):270–6.
20. Tomasino RM, Morello V, Gullo A, Pompei G, Agnese V, Russo A, et al. Assessment of "grading" with Ki-67 and c-kit immunohistochemical expressions may be a helpful tool in management of patients with flat epithelial atypia (FEA) and columnar cell lesions (CCLs) on core breast biopsy. *J Cell Physiol.* 2009;221(2):343–9.
21. Noske A, Pahl S, Fallenberg E, Richter-Ehrenstein C, Buckendahl AC, Weichert W, et al. Flat epithelial atypia is a common subtype of B3 breast lesions and is associated with noninvasive cancer but not with invasive cancer in final excision histology. *Hum Pathol.* 2010;41(4):522–7.
22. Lee TY, Macintosh RF, Rayson D, Barnes PJ. Flat epithelial atypia on breast needle core biopsy: A retrospective study with clinical-pathological correlation. *Breast J.* 2010;16(4):377–83.
23. Ingegnoli A, d'Aloia C, Frattaruolo A, Pallavera L, Martella E, Crisi G, et al. Flat epithelial atypia and atypical ductal hyperplasia: Carcinoma underestimation rate. *Breast J.* 2010;16(1):55–9.
24. Noel JC, Buxant F, Engohan-Aloghe C. Immediate surgical resection of residual microcalcifications after a diagnosis of pure flat epithelial atypia on core biopsy: A word of caution. *Surg Oncol.* 2010;19(4):243–6.
25. Flegg KM, Flaherty JJ, Bicknell AM, Jain S. Surgical outcomes of borderline breast lesions detected by needle biopsy in a breast screening program. *World J Surg Oncol.* 2010;8:78.
26. Sohn V, Porta R, Brown T. Flat epithelial atypia of the breast on core needle biopsy: An indication for surgical excision. *Mil Med.* 2011;176(11):1347–50.
27. Lavoue V, Roger CM, Poilblanc M, Proust N, Monghal-Verge C, Sagan C, et al. Pure flat epithelial atypia (DIN 1a) on core needle biopsy: Study of 60 biopsies with follow-up surgical excision. *Breast Cancer Res Treat.* 2011;125(1):121–6.
28. Rakha EA, Lee AH, Jenkins JA, Murphy AE, Hamilton LJ, Ellis IO. Characterization and outcome of breast needle core biopsy diagnoses of lesions of uncertain malignant potential (B3) in abnormalities detected by mammographic screening. *Int J Cancer.* 2011;129(6):1417–24.
29. Solorzano S, Mesurolle B, Omeroglu A, El Khoury M, Kao E, Aldis A, et al. Flat epithelial atypia of the breast: Pathological-radiological correlation. *AJR Am J Roentgenol.* 2011;197(3):740–6.
30. Verschuur-Maes AH, Witkamp AJ, de Bruin PC, van der Wall E, van Diest PJ. Progression risk of columnar cell lesions of the breast diagnosed in core needle biopsies. *Int J Cancer.* 2011;129(11):2674–80.
31. Peres A, Barranger E, Becette V, Boudinet A, Guinebretiere JM, Cherel P. Rates of upgrade to malignancy for 271 cases of flat epithelial atypia (FEA) diagnosed by breast core biopsy. *Breast Cancer Res Treat.* 2012;133(2):659–66.
32. Uzoaru I, Morgan BR, Liu ZG, Bellafiore FJ, Gaudier FS, Lo JV, et al. Flat epithelial atypia with and without atypical ductal hyperplasia: To re-excise or not. Results of a 5-year prospective study. *Virchows Arch.* 2012;461(4):419–23.
33. Bianchi S, Bendinelli B, Castellano I, Piubello Q, Renne G, Cattani MG, et al. Morphological parameters of flat epithelial atypia (FEA) in stereotactic vacuum-assisted needle core biopsies do not predict the presence of malignancy on subsequent surgical excision. *Virchows Arch.* 2012;461(4):405–17.
34. Biggar MA, Kerr KM, Erzetich LM, Bennett IC. Columnar cell change with atypia (flat epithelial atypia) on breast core biopsy-outcomes following open excision. *Breast J.* 2012;18(6):578–81.
35. Yamaguchi R, Tanaka M, Tse GM, Yamaguchi M, Terasaki H, Akiba J, et al. Pure flat epithelial atypia is uncommon in subsequent breast excisions for atypical epithelial proliferation. *Cancer Sci.* 2012;103(8):1580–5.
36. Polom K, Murawa D, Murawa P. Flat epithelial atypia diagnosed on core needle biopsy—Clinical challenge. *Rep Pract Oncol Radiother.* 2012;17(2):93–6.

37. Khoumais NA, Scaranelo AM, Moshonov H, Kulkarni SR, Miller N, McCready DR, et al. Incidence of breast cancer in patients with pure flat epithelial atypia diagnosed at core-needle biopsy of the breast. *Ann Surg Oncol.* 2013;20(1):133–8.

38. Villa A, Chiesa F, Massa T, Friedman D, Canavese G, Baccini P, et al. Flat epithelial atypia: Comparison between 9-gauge and 11-gauge devices. *Clin Breast Cancer.* 2013;13(6):450–4.

39. Ceugnart L, Doualliez V, Chauvet MP, Robin YM, Bachelle F, Chaveron C, et al. Pure flat epithelial atypia: Is there a place for routine surgery? *Diagn Interv Imaging.* 2013;94(9):861–9.

40. Uzan C, Mazouni C, Ferchiou M, Ciolovan L, Balleyguier C, Mathieu MC, et al. A model to predict the risk of upgrade to malignancy at surgery in atypical breast lesions discovered on percutaneous biopsy specimens. *Ann Surg Oncol.* 2013;20(9):2850–7.

41. Dialani V, Venkataraman S, Frieling G, Schnitt SJ, Mehta TS. Does isolated flat epithelial atypia on vacuum-assisted breast core biopsy require surgical excision? *Breast J.* 2014;20(6):606–14.

42. Calhoun BC, Sobel A, White RL, Gromet M, Flippo T, Sarantou T, et al. Management of flat epithelial atypia on breast core biopsy may be individualized based on correlation with imaging studies. *Mod Pathol.* 2015;28(5):670–6.

43. Lamb LR, Bahl M, Gadd MA, Lehman CD. Flat epithelial atypia: upgrade rates and risk-stratification approach to support informed decision making. *J Am Coll Surg.* 2017;225(6):696–701.

44. Hugar SB, Bhargava R, Dabbs DJ, Davis KM, Zuley M, Clark BZ. Isolated flat epithelial atypia on core biopsy specimens is associated with a low risk of upgrade at excision. *Am J Clin Pathol.* 2019;151(5):511–5.

45. Alencherry E, Goel R, Gore S, Thompson C, Dubchuk C, Bomeisl P, et al. Clinical, imaging, and intervention factors associated with the upgrade of isolated flat epithelial atypia. *Clin Imaging.* 2019;54:21–4.

46. McCroskey Z, Sneige N, Herman CR, Miller RA, Venta LA, Ro JY, et al. Flat epithelial atypia in directional vacuum-assisted biopsy of breast microcalcifications: Surgical excision may not be necessary. *Mod Pathol.* 2018;31(7):1097–106.

47. Schiaffino S, Gristina L, Villa A, Tosto S, Monetti F, Carli F, et al. Flat epithelial atypia: Conservative management of patients without residual microcalcifications post-vacuum-assisted breast biopsy. *Br J Radiol.* 2018;91(1081):20170484.

48. Chan PMY, Chotai N, Lai ES, Sin PY, Chen J, Lu SQ, et al. Majority of flat epithelial atypia diagnosed on biopsy do not require surgical excision. *Breast.* 2018;37:13–7.

49. Calhoun BC. Core needle biopsy of the breast: An evaluation of contemporary data. *Surg Pathol Clin.* 2018;11(1):1–16.

50. Baum JK, Hanna LG, Acharyya S, Mahoney MC, Conant EF, Bassett LW, et al. Use of BI-RADS 3-probably benign category in the American College of Radiology Imaging Network Digital Mammographic Imaging Screening Trial. *Radiology.* 2011;260(1):61–7.

51. Simpson JF. Update on atypical epithelial hyperplasia and ductal carcinoma in situ. *Pathology.* 2009;41(1):36–9.

52. Ellis IO. Intraductal proliferative lesions of the breast: morphology, associated risk and molecular biology. *Mod Pathol.* 2010;23(Suppl 2):S1–S7.

53. Allred DC, Mohsin SK, Fuqua SA. Histological and biological evolution of human premalignant breast disease. *Endocr Relat Cancer.* 2001;8(1):47–61.

54. Santen RJ, Mansel R. Benign breast disorders. *N Engl J Med.* 2005;353(3):275–85.

55. Hartmann LC, Degnim AC, Santen RJ, Dupont WD, Ghosh K. Atypical hyperplasia of the breast–risk assessment and management options. *N Engl J Med.* 2015;372(1):78–89.

56. Dupont WD, Page DL. Risk factors for breast cancer in women with proliferative breast disease. *N Engl J Med.* 1985;312(3):146–51.

57. Hartmann LC, Sellers TA, Frost MH, Lingle WL, Degnim AC, Ghosh K, et al. Benign breast disease and the risk of breast cancer. *N Engl J Med.* 2005;353(3):229–37.

58. Page DL, Dupont WD, Rogers LW, Rados MS. Atypical hyperplastic lesions of the female breast. A long-term follow-up study. *Cancer.* 1985;55(11):2698–708.

59. Degnim AC, Visscher DW, Berman HK, Frost MH, Sellers TA, Vierkant RA, et al. Stratification of breast cancer risk in women with atypia: A Mayo cohort study. *J Clin Oncol.* 2007;25(19):2671–7.

60. Coopey SB, Mazzola E, Buckley JM, Sharko J, Belli AK, Kim EM, et al. The role of chemoprevention in modifying the risk of breast cancer in women with atypical breast lesions. *Breast Cancer Res Treat.* 2012;136(3):627–33.

61. Donaldson AR, McCarthy C, Goraya S, Pederson HJ, Sturgis CD, Grobmyer SR, et al. Breast cancer risk associated with atypical hyperplasia and lobular carcinoma in situ initially diagnosed on core-needle biopsy. *Cancer.* 2018;124(3):459–65.

62. Hartmann LC, Radisky DC, Frost MH, Santen RJ, Vierkant RA, Benetti LL, et al. Understanding the premalignant potential of atypical hyperplasia through its natural history: A longitudinal cohort study. *Cancer Prev Res (Phila).* 2014;7(2):211–7.

63. No author listed. Is 'fibrocystic disease' of the breast precancerous? *Arch Pathol Lab Med.* 1986;110(3):171–3.

64. Shah-Khan MG, Geiger XJ, Reynolds C, Jakub JW, Deperi ER, Glazebrook KN. Long-term follow-up of lobular neoplasia (atypical lobular hyperplasia/lobular carcinoma in situ) diagnosed on core needle biopsy. *Ann Surg Oncol.* 2012;19(10):3131–8.

65. Allen S, Levine EA, Lesko N, Howard-Mcnatt M. Is excisional biopsy and chemoprevention warranted in patients with atypical lobular hyperplasia on core biopsy? *Am Surg.* 2015;81(9):876–8.

66. Sen LQ, Berg WA, Hooley RJ, Carter GJ, Desouki MM, Sumkin JH. Core breast biopsies showing lobular carcinoma in situ should be excised and surveillance is reasonable for atypical lobular hyperplasia. *AJR Am J Roentgenol.* 2016;207(5):1132–45.

67. Nakhlis F, Gilmore L, Gelman R, Bedrosian I, Ludwig K, Hwang ES, et al. Incidence of adjacent synchronous invasive carcinoma and/or ductal carcinoma in-situ in patients with lobular neoplasia on core biopsy: Results from a prospective multi-institutional registry (TBCRC 020). *Ann Surg Oncol.* 2016;23(3):722–8.

68. Bahl M, Lamb LR, Lehman CD. Pathologic outcomes of architectural distortion on digital 2D versus tomosynthesis mammography. *AJR Am J Roentgenol.* 2017;209(5):1162–7.

69. Muller KE, Roberts E, Zhao L, Jorns JM. Isolated atypical lobular hyperplasia diagnosed on breast biopsy: Low upgrade rate on subsequent excision with long-term follow-up. *Arch Pathol Lab Med.* 2018;142(3):391–5.

70. Lewin AA, Mercado CL. Atypical ductal hyperplasia and lobular neoplasia: Update and easing of guidelines. *AJR Am J Roentgenol.* 2020;214(2):265–75.

71. Genco IS, Tugertimur B, Chang Q, Cassell L, Hajiyeva S. Outcomes of classic lobular neoplasia diagnosed on breast core needle biopsy: A retrospective multi-center study. *Virchows Arch.* 2020;476(2):209–17.

72. Schmidt H, Arditi B, Wooster M, Weltz C, Margolies L, Bleiweiss I, et al. Observation versus excision of lobular neoplasia on core needle biopsy of the breast. *Breast Cancer Res Treat.* 2018;168(3):649–54.

73. Nakhlis F. How do we approach benign proliferative lesions? *Curr Oncol Rep.* 2018;20(4):34.

74. Thomas PS. Diagnosis and management of high-risk breast lesions. *J Natl Compr Canc Netw.* 2018;16(11):1391–6.

75. Collins LC. Precursor lesions of the low-grade breast neoplasia pathway. *Surg Pathol Clin.* 2018;11(1):177–97.

76. Schiaffino S, Calabrese M, Melani EF, Trimboli RM, Cozzi A, Carbonaro LA, et al. Upgrade rate of percutaneously diagnosed pure atypical ductal hyperplasia: Systematic review and meta-analysis of 6458 lesions. *Radiology.* 2020;294(1):76–86.

77. Eby PR, Ochsner JE, DeMartini WB, Allison KH, Peacock S, Lehman CD. Is surgical excision necessary for focal atypical ductal hyperplasia found at stereotactic vacuum-assisted breast biopsy? *Ann Surg Oncol.* 2008;15(11):3232–8.

78. Forgeard C, Benchaib M, Guerin N, Thiesse P, Mignotte H, Faure C, et al. Is surgical biopsy mandatory in case of atypical ductal hyperplasia on 11-gauge core needle biopsy? A retrospective study of 300 patients. *Am J Surg.* 2008;196(3):339–45.

79. Wagoner MJ, Laronga C, Acs G. Extent and histologic pattern of atypical ductal hyperplasia present on core needle biopsy specimens of the breast can predict ductal carcinoma in situ in subsequent excision. *Am J Clin Pathol.* 2009;131(1):112–21.

80. Kohr JR, Eby PR, Allison KH, DeMartini WB, Gutierrez RL, Peacock S, et al. Risk of upgrade of atypical ductal hyperplasia after stereotactic breast biopsy: Effects of number of foci and complete removal of calcifications. *Radiology.* 2010;255(3):723–30.

81. Nguyen CV, Albarracin CT, Whitman GJ, Lopez A, Sneige N. Atypical ductal hyperplasia in directional vacuum-assisted biopsy of breast microcalcifications: Considerations for surgical excision. *Ann Surg Oncol.* 2011;18(3):752–61.

82. McGhan LJ, Pockaj BA, Wasif N, Giurescu ME, McCullough AE, Gray RJ. Atypical ductal hyperplasia on core biopsy: An automatic trigger for excisional biopsy? *Ann Surg Oncol.* 2012;19(10):3264–9.

83. McLaughlin CT, Neal CH, Helvie MA. Is the upgrade rate of atypical ductal hyperplasia diagnosed by core needle biopsy of calcifications different for digital and film-screen mammography? *AJR Am J Roentgenol.* 2014;203(4):917–22.

84. Menes TS, Rosenberg R, Balch S, Jaffer S, Kerlikowske K, Miglioretti DL. Upgrade of high-risk breast lesions detected on mammography in the Breast Cancer Surveillance Consortium. *Am J Surg.* 2014;207(1):24–31.

85. Khoury T, Chen X, Wang D, Kumar P, Qin M, Liu S, et al. Nomogram to predict the likelihood of upgrade of atypical ductal hyperplasia diagnosed on a core needle biopsy in mammographically detected lesions. *Histopathology.* 2015;67(1):106–20.

86. Pena A, Shah SS, Fazzio RT, Hoskin TL, Brahmbhatt RD, Hieken TJ, et al. Multivariate model to identify women at low risk of cancer upgrade after a core needle biopsy diagnosis of atypical ductal hyperplasia. *Breast Cancer Res Treat.* 2017;164(2):295–304.
87. Lamb LR, Bahl M, Hughes KS, Lehman CD. Pathologic upgrade rates of high-risk breast lesions on digital two-dimensional vs tomosynthesis mammography. *J Am Coll Surg.* 2018;226(5):858–67.
88. Tozbikian G, George M, Zynger DL. Diagnostic terminology used to describe atypia on breast core needle biopsy: Correlation with excision and upgrade rates. *Diagn Pathol.* 2019;14(1):69.
89. Sutton T, Farinola M, Johnson N, Garreau JR. Atypical ductal hyperplasia: Clinicopathologic factors are not predictive of upgrade after excisional biopsy. *Am J Surg.* 2019;217(5):848–50.
90. Rageth CJ, Rubenov R, Bronz C, Dietrich D, Tausch C, Rodewald AK, et al. Atypical ductal hyperplasia and the risk of underestimation: Tissue sampling method, multifocality, and associated calcification significantly influence the diagnostic upgrade rate based on subsequent surgical specimens. *Breast Cancer.* 2019;26(4):452–8.
91. Williams KE, Amin A, Hill J, Walter C, Inciardi M, Gatewood J, et al. Radiologic and pathologic features associated with upgrade of atypical ductal hyperplasia at surgical excision. *Acad Radiol.* 2019;26(7):893–9.
92. Weiss JB, Do WS, Forte DM, Sheldon RR, Childers CK, Sohn VY. Is bigger better? Twenty-year institutional experience of atypical ductal hyperplasia discovered by core needle biopsy. *Am J Surg.* 2019;217(5):906–9.
93. Sergesketter AR, Thomas SM, Fayanju OM, Menendez CS, Rosenberger LH, Greenup RA, et al. The influence of age on the histopathology and prognosis of atypical breast lesions. *J Surg Res.* 2019;241:188–98.
94. Bahl M, Barzilay R, Yedidia AB, Locascio NJ, Yu L, Lehman CD. High-risk breast lesions: A machine learning model to predict pathologic upgrade and reduce unnecessary surgical excision. *Radiology.* 2018;286(3):810–8.
95. Ko E, Han W, Lee JW, Cho J, Kim EK, Jung SY, et al. Scoring system for predicting malignancy in patients diagnosed with atypical ductal hyperplasia at ultrasound-guided core needle biopsy. *Breast Cancer Res Treat.* 2008;112(1):189–95.
96. Schiaffino S, Massone E, Gristina L, Fregatti P, Rescinito G, Villa A, et al. Vacuum assisted breast biopsy (VAB) excision of subcentimeter microcalcifications as an alternative to open biopsy for atypical ductal hyperplasia. *Br J Radiol.* 2018;91(1085):20180003.
97. American Society of Breast Surgeons. Consensus guidelines on concordance assessment of image-guided breast biopsies and management of borderline or high-risk lesions. 2016. Available from: https://www.breastsurgeons.org/docs/statements/Consensus-Guideline-on-Concordance-Assessment-of-Image-Guided-Breast-Biopsies.pdf.
98. Racz JM, Degnim AC. When does atypical ductal hyperplasia require surgical excision? *Surg Oncol Clin N Am.* 2018;27(1):23–32.
99. Menen RS, Ganesan N, Bevers T, Ying J, Coyne R, Lane D, et al. Long-term safety of observation in selected women following core biopsy diagnosis of atypical ductal hyperplasia. *Ann Surg Oncol.* 2017;24(1):70–6.
100. Foote FW, Stewart FW. Lobular carcinoma in situ: A rare form of mammary cancer. *Am J Pathol.* 1941;17(4):491–6.3.
101. Page DL. Atypical hyperplasia, narrowly and broadly defined. *Hum Pathol.* 1991;22(7):631–2.
102. Tavassoli FA. Lobular neoplasia: Evolution of its significance and morphologic spectrum. *Int J Surg Pathol.* 2010;18(3 Suppl):174S–7S.
103. Rosen PP, Kosloff C, Lieberman PH, Adair F, Braun DW, Jr. Lobular carcinoma in situ of the breast. Detailed analysis of 99 patients with average follow-up of 24 years. *Am J Surg Pathol.* 1978;2(3):225–51.
104. Wen HY, Brogi E. Lobular carcinoma in situ. *Surg Pathol Clin.* 2018;11(1):123–45.
105. Racz JM, Carter JM, Degnim AC. Lobular neoplasia and atypical ductal hyperplasia on core biopsy: Current surgical management recommendations. *Ann Surg Oncol.* 2017;24(10):2848–54.
106. Wazir U, Wazir A, Wells C, Mokbel K. Pleomorphic lobular carcinoma in situ: Current evidence and a systemic review. *Oncol Lett.* 2016;12(6):4863–8.
107. Singh K, Paquette C, Kalife ET, Wang Y, Mangray S, Quddus MR, et al. Evaluating agreement, histological features, and relevance of separating pleomorphic and florid lobular carcinoma in situ subtypes. *Hum Pathol.* 2018;78:163–70.
108. Shamir ER, Chen YY, Chu T, Pekmezci M, Rabban JT, Krings G. Pleomorphic and florid lobular carcinoma in situ variants of the breast: A clinicopathologic study of 85 cases with and without invasive carcinoma from a single academic center. *Am J Surg Pathol.* 2019;43(3):399–408.
109. Masannat YA, Husain E, Roylance R, Heys SD, Carder PJ, Ali H, et al. Pleomorphic LCIS what do we know? A UK multicenter audit of pleomorphic lobular carcinoma in situ. *Breast.* 2018;38:120–4.
110. Hoffman DI, Zhang PJ, Tchou J. Breast-conserving surgery for pure non-classic lobular carcinoma in situ: A single institution's experience. *Surg Oncol.* 2019;28:190–4.
111. Desai AA, Jimenez RE, Hoskin TL, Day CN, Boughey JC, Hieken TJ. Treatment outcomes for pleomorphic lobular carcinoma in situ of the breast. *Ann Surg Oncol.* 2018;25(10):3064–8.

112. Savage JL, Jeffries DO, Noroozian M, Sabel MS, Jorns JM, Helvie MA. Pleomorphic lobular carcinoma in situ: Imaging features, upgrade rate, and clinical outcomes. *AJR Am J Roentgenol.* 2018;211(2):462–7.
113. Guo T, Wang Y, Shapiro N, Fineberg S. Pleomorphic lobular carcinoma in situ diagnosed by breast core biopsy: Clinicopathologic features and correlation with subsequent excision. *Clin Breast Cancer.* 2018;18(4):e449–e54.
114. Fasola CE, Chen JJ, Jensen KC, Allison KH, Horst KC. Characteristics and clinical outcomes of pleomorphic lobular carcinoma in situ of the breast. *Breast J.* 2018;24(1):66–9.
115. Chivukula M, Haynik DM, Brufsky A, Carter G, Dabbs DJ. Pleomorphic lobular carcinoma in situ (PLCIS) on breast core needle biopsies: Clinical significance and immunoprofile. *Am J Surg Pathol.* 2008;32(11):1721–6.
116. Flanagan MR, Rendi MH, Calhoun KE, Anderson BO, Javid SH. Pleomorphic lobular carcinoma in situ: Radiologic-pathologic features and clinical management. *Ann Surg Oncol.* 2015;22(13):4263–9.
117. Carder PJ, Shaaban A, Alizadeh Y, Kumarasuwamy V, Liston JC, Sharma N. Screen-detected pleomorphic lobular carcinoma in situ (PLCIS): Risk of concurrent invasive malignancy following a core biopsy diagnosis. *Histopathology.* 2010;57(3):472–8.
118. Bagaria SP, Shamonki J, Kinnaird M, Ray PS, Giuliano AE. The florid subtype of lobular carcinoma in situ: Marker or precursor for invasive lobular carcinoma? *Ann Surg Oncol.* 2011;18(7):1845–51.
119. Taylor LJ, Steiman J, Schumacher JR, Wilke LG, Greenberg CC, Neuman HB. Surgical management of lobular carcinoma in situ: Analysis of the National Cancer Database. *Ann Surg Oncol.* 2018;25(8):2229–34.
120. King TA, Pilewskie M, Muhsen S, Patil S, Mautner SK, Park A, et al. Lobular carcinoma in situ: A 29-year longitudinal experience evaluating clinicopathologic features and breast cancer risk. *J Clin Oncol.* 2015;33(33):3945–52.
121. Dania V, Liu Y, Ademuyiwa F, Weber JD, Colditz GA. Associations of race and ethnicity with risk of developing invasive breast cancer after lobular carcinoma in situ. *Breast Cancer Res.* 2019;21(1):120.
122. Hortobagyi GC, JL; D'Orsi CJ; Edge SB; Mittendorf EA; Rugo HS; Solin LJ; Weaver DL; Winchester DJ; Giuliano A. Breast. In: Amin ME, SB; Greene, F; Byrd, DR; Brookland, RK, Washington, MK; Gershenwald, JE; Compton, CC; Hess, KR; Sullivan, DC; Jessup, JM; Brierley, JD; Gaspar, LE; Schilsky, RL; Balch, CM; Winchester, DP; Asare, EA; Madera, M; Gress, DM; Meyer, LR, editor. *AJCC Cancer Staging Manual.* 8th ed. New York, NY: Springer; 2017, pp. 589–628.
123. American Cancer Society. *Breast Cancer Facts and Figures* 2019–2020. Atlanta, GA: American Cancer Society; 2020 [Available from: https://www.cancer.org/content/dam/cancer-org/research/cancer-facts-and-statistics/breast-cancer-facts-and-figures/breast-cancer-facts-and-figures-2019-2020.pdf. Accessed 20 May 2020.
124. Esserman LJ, Thompson IM, Reid B, Nelson P, Ransohoff DF, Welch HG, et al. Addressing overdiagnosis and overtreatment in cancer: A prescription for change. *Lancet Oncol.* 2014;15(6):e234–42.
125. Francis AM, Haugen CE, Grimes LM, Crow JR, Yi M, Mittendorf EA, et al. Is sentinel lymph node dissection warranted for patients with a diagnosis of ductal carcinoma in situ? *Ann Surg Oncol.* 2015;22(13):4270–9.
126. Lyman GH, Temin S, Edge SB, Newman LA, Turner RR, Weaver DL, et al. Sentinel lymph node biopsy for patients with early-stage breast cancer: American Society of Clinical Oncology clinical practice guideline update. *J Clin Oncol.* 2014;32(13):1365–83.
127. National Comprehensive Cander Network. NCCN Clinical Practice Guidelines in Oncology: National Comprehensive Cancer Network; 2020 [Version 4]. Available from: https://www.nccn.org/professionals/physician_gls/pdf/breast.pdf. Accessed 30 May 2020.
128. DeVaux RS, Herschkowitz JI. Beyond DNA: The role of epigenetics in the premalignant progression of breast cancer. *J Mammary Gland Biol Neoplasia.* 2018;23(4):223–35.
129. Fisher ER, Dignam J, Tan-Chiu E, Costantino J, Fisher B, Paik S, et al. Pathologic findings form the National Surgical Adjuvant Breast Project (NSABP) eight-year update of Protocol B-17: Intraductal carcinoma. *Cancer.* 1999;86(3):429–38.
130. Morrow M, Van Zee KJ, Solin LJ, Houssami N, Chavez-MacGregor M, Harris JR, et al. Society of Surgical Oncology–American Society for Radiation Oncology–American Society of Clinical Oncology Consensus Guideline on Margins for Breast-Conserving Surgery with Whole-Breast Irradiation in Ductal Carcinoma in Situ. *Ann Surg Oncol.* 2016;23(12):3801–10.
131. McCormick B, Winter K, Hudis C, Kuerer HM, Rakovitch E, Smith BL, et al. RTOG 9804: A prospective randomized trial for good-risk ductal carcinoma in situ comparing radiotherapy with observation. *J Clin Oncol.* 2015;33(7):709–15.
132. Garg PK, Jakhetiya A, Pandey R, Chishi N, Pandey D. Adjuvant radiotherapy versus observation following lumpectomy in ductal carcinoma in-situ: A meta-analysis of randomized controlled trials. *Breast J.* 2018;24(3):233–9.
133. Wapnir IL, Dignam JJ, Fisher B, Mamounas EP, Anderson SJ, Julian TB, et al. Long-term outcomes of invasive ipsilateral breast tumor recurrences after lumpectomy in NSABP B-17 and B-24 randomized clinical trials for DCIS. *J Natl Cancer Inst.* 2011;103(6):478–88.

134. Donker M, Litiere S, Werutsky G, Julien JP, Fentiman IS, Agresti R, et al. Breast-conserving treatment with or without radiotherapy in ductal carcinoma in situ: 15-year recurrence rates and outcome after a recurrence, from the EORTC 10853 randomized phase III trial. *J Clin Oncol.* 2013;31(32):4054–9.
135. Warnberg F, Garmo H, Emdin S, Hedberg V, Adwall L, Sandelin K, et al. Effect of radiotherapy after breast-conserving surgery for ductal carcinoma in situ: 20 years follow-up in the randomized SweDCIS Trial. J Clin Oncol. 2014;32(32):3613–8.
136. Cuzick J, Sestak I, Pinder SE, Ellis IO, Forsyth S, Bundred NJ, et al. Effect of tamoxifen and radiotherapy in women with locally excised ductal carcinoma in situ: Long-term results from the UK/ANZ DCIS trial. *Lancet Oncol.* 2011;12(1):21–9.
137. Nofech-Mozes S, Hanna W, Rakovitch E. Molecular evaluation of breast ductal carcinoma in situ with Oncotype DX DCIS. *Am J Pathol.* 2019;189(5):975–80.
138. Borstkanker Onderzoek Groep, European Organisation for Research and Treatment of Cancer–EORTC. Management of Low-Risk DCIS (LORD). Netherlands: The Netherlands Cancer Institute; 2015. https://clini-caltrials.gov/ct2/show/NCt02492607. Accessed 1 June 2020.
139. Elshof LE, Tryfonidis K, Slaets L, van Leeuwen-Stok AE, Skinner VP, Dif N, et al. Feasibility of a prospective, randomised, open-label, international multicentre, phase III, non-inferiority trial to assess the safety of active surveillance for low risk ductal carcinoma in situ—The LORD study. Eur J Cancer. 2015;51(12):1497–510.
140. Birmingham University, UK. Surgery versus active monitoring for low risk ductal carcinoma in situ (DCIS). Birmingham, United Kingdom: Institute for Cancer Studies; 2014, http://www.isrctn.com/ISRCTN27544579. Accessed 1 June 2020
141. Francis A, Thomas J, Fallowfield L, Wallis M, Bartlett JM, Brookes C, et al. Addressing overtreatment of screen detected DCIS: The LORIS trial. *Eur J Cancer.* 2015;51(16):2296–303.
142. Hwang SP, A; Thompson, A. Comparison of operative to monitoring and endocrine therapy (COMET) trial for low risk DCIS Alliance Foundation Trials. LLC; 2017, https://clinicaltrials.gov/ct2/show/NCT0292691. Accessed 1 June 2020.
143. Visvanathan K, Hurley P, Bantug E, Brown P, Col NF, Cuzick J, et al. Use of pharmacologic interventions for breast cancer risk reduction: American Society of Clinical Oncology clinical practice guideline. *J Clin Oncol.* 2013;31(23):2942–62.
144. Brewster AM, Thomas P, Brown P, Coyne R, Yan Y, Checka C, et al. A system-level approach to improve the uptake of antiestrogen preventive therapy among women with atypical hyperplasia and lobular cancer in situ. *Cancer Prev Res (Phila).* 2018;11(5):295–302.
145. Cuzick J, Sestak I, Forbes JF, Dowsett M, Cawthorn S, Mansel RE, et al. Use of anastrozole for breast cancer prevention (IBIS-II): Long-term results of a randomised controlled trial. *Lancet.* 2020;395(10218):117–22.
146. Nelson HD, Fu R, Zakher B, Pappas M, McDonagh M. Medication use for the risk reduction of primary breast cancer in women: Updated evidence report and systematic review for the US Preventive Services Task Force. *JAMA.* 2019;322(9):868–86.
147. U.S. Preventive Services task Force, Owens DK, Davidson KW, Krist AH, Barry MJ, Cabana M, et al. Medication use to reduce risk of breast cancer: US Preventive Services Task Force Recommendation Statement. *JAMA.* 2019;322(9):857–67.
148. Karavites LC, Kane AK, Zaveri S, Xu Y, Helenowski I, Hansen N, et al. Tamoxifen acceptance and adherence among patients with ductal carcinoma in situ (DCIS) treated in a multidisciplinary setting. *Cancer Prev Res (Phila).* 2017;10(7):389–97.
149. Roche CA, Tang R, Coopey SB, Hughes KS. Chemoprevention acceptance and adherence in women with high-risk breast lesions. *Breast J.* 2019;25(2):190–5.
150. Roetzheim RG, Lee JH, Fulp W, Matos Gomez E, Clayton E, Tollin S, et al. Acceptance and adherence to chemoprevention among women at increased risk of breast cancer. *Breast.* 2015;24(1):51–6.
151. Flanagan MR, Zabor EC, Stempel M, Mangino DA, Morrow M, Pilewskie ML. Chemoprevention uptake for breast cancer risk reduction varies by risk factor. *Ann Surg Oncol.* 2019;26(7):2127–35.
152. DeCensi A, Puntoni M, Guerrieri-Gonzaga A, Caviglia S, Avino F, Cortesi L, et al. Randomized Placebo Controlled Trial of Low-Dose Tamoxifen to Prevent Local and Contralateral Recurrence in Breast Intraepithelial Neoplasia. *J Clin Oncol.* 2019;37(19):1629–37.
153. Lee O, Ivancic D, Allu S, Shidfar A, Kenney K, Helenowski I, et al. Local transdermal therapy to the breast for breast cancer prevention and DCIS therapy: Preclinical and clinical evaluation. *Cancer Chemother Pharmacol.* 2015;76(6):1235–46.
154. Lee O, Khan SA. Novel routes for administering chemoprevention: Local transdermal therapy to the breasts. *Semin Oncol.* 2016;43(1):107–15.

Staging of Breast Cancer

10

Ayush Keshav Singhal and Diptendra Kumar Sarkar

Staging of cancer is based on clinical or pathological findings, which imply the extent of the disease itself.

The American Joint Committee on Cancer (AJCC) staging system is based on the TNM system, where T refers to tumor, N to nodes, and M to metastasis.

PRIMARY TUMOR (T)

- Primary tumor refers to the size of the invasive component of the cancer in which the maximum size of the tumor focus is taken into consideration.
- In cases of post-neoadjuvant therapy, dense fibrosis is not included in pathological measurements.
- Clinical measurement can be assessed by:
  - Physical examination (measurement by Vernier calipers)
  - Imaging modalities:
    – Ultrasound
    – Mammography
    – Magnetic resonance imaging
- Pathological measurements can be assessed by:
  - Gross measurements
  - Microscopic measurements

T Staging

- *Tx*: Tumor is not assessed in size.
- *T0*: There is no evidence of tumor.
- *Tis*: Ductal carcinoma *in situ*.
  - Paget's disease of the nipple (not associated with carcinoma or carcinoma *in situ*).
- *T1*: Tumor less than 2 cm in size.
  - *T1mi*: Tumor is less than 1 mm.
  - *T1a*: Tumor is more than 1 mm but not more than 5 mm.
  - *T1b*: Tumor is more than 5 mm but not more than 10 mm.
  - *T1c*: Tumor is more than 10 mm but not more than 20 mm.

DOI: 10.1201/9780367821982-10

- *T2*: Tumor is more than 20 mm but no more than 50 mm.
- *T3*: Tumor is more than 50 mm.
- *T4*: Any size tumor with direct extension to the chest wall and/or to the skin (ulceration or nodules).
    - *T4a*: Tumor has spread into the chest wall.
    - *T4b*: Tumor has spread into the skin and there may be edema.
    - *T4c*: Tumor has spread to both the skin and the chest wall.
    - *T4d*: Inflammatory carcinoma.

Nodal Staging (N)

Nodal staging describes the spread to axillary lymph nodes.

Clinical

- Clinical assessment
- Ultrasonography
    - *cNX*: Lymph node could not be assessed.
    - *cN0*: No lymph nodal metastasis.
    - *cN1*: Metastasis to ipsilateral level I, II axillary lymph nodes.
    - *cN1mi*: Micrometastases larger than 0.2 mm, but not more than 2 mm.
    - **cN2**:
        - *cN2a*: Metastasis in ipsilateral level I, II axillary lymph node fixed to one another or to other structures.
        - *cN2b*: Metastasis only in ipsilateral internal mammary lymph node in absence of axillary lymph node metastasis.
    - **cN3**:
        - *cN3a*: Metastasis in infraclavicular lymph node.
        - *cN3b*: Metastasis in ipsilateral internal mammary lymph node and axillary lymph node.
        - *cN3c*: Metastasis in ipsilateral supraclavicular lymph node.

Pathologic

- *pNX*: Lymph nodes can't be assessed.
- *pN0*: No regional lymph node metastasis or only isolated tumor cells (ITCs).
- **pN1**:
    - *pN1mi*: Micrometastases (200 cancer cells but are less than 2 mm and larger than 0.2 mm).
    - *pN1a*: Metastasis to one to three lymph nodes and at least one is larger than 2 mm.
    - *pN1b*: Metastasis in ipsilateral internal mammary sentinel node excluding isolated tumor cell.
    - *pN1c*: pN1a and pN2b combined.
- **pN2**:
    - *pN2a*: Metastasis in four to nine axillary lymph nodes (at least one greater than 2.0 mm).
    - *pN2b*: Metastasis in clinically detected internal mammary lymph node with or without microscopic confirmation; with pathologically negative axillary lymph nodes.
- **pN3**:
    - *pN3a*: Metastasis in 10 or more lymph nodes and at least one is larger than 2 mm, or to infraclavicular area.
        pN3b: pN1a or pN2a in presence of cN2b or pN2a in presence of P1Nb.
        pN3c: Metastasis in ipsilateral supraclavicular lymph node.

Distant Metastasis (M)

Metastasis (M) describes if the cancer has spread to a different part of the body.

- *M0*: No clinical or radiological evidence of distant metastasis.
- *cMo(i+)*: No clinical or radiological evidence of distant metastasis in the presence of tumor cells or deposit no larger than 0.2 mm detected microscopically or by molecular techniques.
- *cM1*: Distant metastasis detected by clinical or radiological means.
- *pM1*: Histologically proven distant metastasis or nonregional lymph nodes; deposits greater than 0.2 mm.

Histologic grade

All invasive breast carcinomas should be assigned histologic grade by using the Scarff–Bloom–Richardson grading system, which includes tubule formation, nuclear pleomorphism, and calibrated mitotic count, which are assigned a value from 1 to 3 for each feature.

Invasive cancer

- *GX*: Grade cannot be assessed.
- *G1*: Low combined histologic grade (3–5 points).
- *G2*: Intermediate (6–7 points).
- *G3*: High combined histologic grade (8–9 points).

TABLE 10.1   AJCC anatomic staging

STAGE	T	N	M
0	TIS	N0	M0
1A	T1	N0	M0
1B	T0	N1Mi	M0
	T1	N1Mi	M0
IIA	T0	N1	M0
	T1	N1	M0
	T2	N0	M0
IIB	T2	N1	M0
	T3	N0	M0
IIIA	T0	N2	M0
	T1	N2	M0
	T2	N2	M0
	T3	N1	M0
	T3	N2	M0
IIIB	T4	N0	M0
	T4	N1	M0
	T4	N2	M0
IIIC	ANY T	N3	M0
IV	ANY T	ANY N	M1

Ductal carcinoma in situ

- *GX*: Grade cannot be assessed.
- *G1*: Low nuclear grade.
- *G2*: Intermediate nuclear grade.
- *G3*: High nuclear grade.

CLINICAL PROGNOSTIC STAGING

This is based on clinical tumor, node, and metastasis information obtained from the history, physical examination, imaging performed, and relevant biopsies (ER/PR/HER2-neu), see Table 10.2.

TABLE 10.2 Clinical prognostic stage group

TNM	GRADE	HER2 STATUS	ER STATUS	PR STATUS	STAGE GROUP
Tis N0 M0	Any	Any	Any	Any	0
T1b N0 M0	G1	Positive	Positive / Negative	Positive / Negative	IA
T0 N1mi M0		Negative	Positive	Positive / Negative	IA
T1b N1mi M0			Negative	Positive	IA
				Negative	IB
	G2	Positive	Positive / Negative	Positive / Negative	IA
		Negative	Positive	Positive / Negative	IA
			Negative	Positive	IA
				Negative	IB
	G3	Positive	Positive/ Negative	Positive / Negative	IA
		Negative	Positive	Positive	IA
				Negative	IB
			Negative	Positive	IB
				Negative	IB
T0 N1c M0	G1	Positive	Positive	Positive	IB
T1 N1c M0				Negative	IIA
T2 N0 M0			Negative	Positive	IA
				Negative	IIA
		Negative	Positive	Positive	IB
				Negative	IIA
			Negative	Positive	IIA
				Negative	IIA
	G2	Positive	Positive	Positive	IB
				Negative	IIA
			Negative	Positive	IIA
				Negative	IIA
		Negative	Positive	Positive	IB
				Negative	IIA
			Negative	Positive	IIA
				Negative	IIB

(Continued)

TABLE 10.2   Clinical prognostic stage group *(Continued)*

TNM	GRADE	HER2 STATUS	ER STATUS	PR STATUS	STAGE GROUP
	G3	Positive	Positive	Positive	IB
				Negative	IIA
			Negative	Positive	IIA
				Negative	IIA
		Negative	Positive	Positive	IIA
				Negative	IIB
			Negative	Positive	IIB
				Negative	IIB
T2 N1^d M0	G1	Positive	Positive	Positive	IB
T3 N0 M0				Negative	IIA
			Negative	Positive	IIA
				Negative	IIB
		Negative	Positive	Positive	IIA
				Negative	IIB
			Negative	Positive	IIB
				Negative	IIB
	G2	Positive	Positive	Positive	IB
				Negative	IIA
			Negative	Positive	IIA
				Negative	IIB
		Negative	Positive	Positive	IIA
				Negative	IIB
			Negative	Positive	IIB
				Negative	IIIB
	G3	Positive	Positive	Positive	IB
				Negative	IIB
			Negative	Positive	IIB
				Negative	IIB
		Negative	Positive	Positive	IIB
				Negative	IIIA
			Negative	Positive	IIIA
				Negative	IIIB
T0 N2 M0	G1	Positive	Positive	Positive	IIA
T1^b N2 M0				Negative	IIIA
T2 N2 M0			Negative	Positive	IIIA
T3 N1^d M0				Negative	IIIA
T3 N2 M0		Negative	Positive	Positive	IIA
				Negative	IIIA
			Negative	Positive	IIIA
				Negative	IIIB

(Continued)

TABLE 10.2   Clinical prognostic stage group *(Continued)*

TNM	GRADE	HER2 STATUS	ER STATUS	PR STATUS	STAGE GROUP
	G2	Positive	Positive	Positive	IIA
				Negative	IIIA
			Negative	Positive	IIIA
				Negative	IIIA
		Negative	Positive	Positive	IIA
				Negative	IIIA
			Negative	Positive	IIIA
				Negative	IIIB
	G3	Positive	Positive	Positive	IIB
				Negative	IIIA
			Negative	Positive	IIIA
				Negative	IIIA
		Negative	Positive	Positive	IIIA
				Negative	IIIB
			Negative	Positive	IIIB
				Negative	IIIC
T4 N0 M0	G1	Positive	Positive	Positive	IIIA
T4 N1[d] M0				Negative	IIIB
T4 N2 M0			Negative	Positive	IIIB
AnyTN3 M0				Negative	IIIB
		Negative	Positive	Positive	IIIB
				Negative	IIIB
			Negative	Positive	IIIB
				Negative	IIIC
	G2	Positive	Positive	Positive	IIIA
				Negative	IIIB
			Negative	Positive	IIIB
				Negative	IIIB
		Negative	Positive	Positive	IIIB
				Negative	IIIB
			Negative	Positive	IIIB
				Negative	IIIC
	G3	Positive	Positive	Positive	IIIB
				Negative	IIIB
			Negative	Positive	IIIB
				Negative	IIIB
		Negative	Positive	Positive	IIIB
				Negative	IIIC
			Negative	Positive	IIIC
				Negative	IIIC
Any T, Any N, M1	Any	Any	Any	Any	IV

PATHOLOGICAL PROGNOSTIC STAGING

This applies to breast cancer patients treated with surgery as the initial treatment. It includes information used for clinical staging plus findings at surgery and pathological findings from surgical resection. It doesn't apply to patients treated with systemic therapy or radiation prior to surgical resection, see Table 10.3.

TABLE 10.3 Pathological prognostic stage groups

TNM	GRADE	HER2 STATUS	ER STATUS	PR STATUS	STAGE GROUP
Tis N0 M0	Any	Any	Any	Any	0
T1b N0 M0	G1	Positive	Positive / Negative	Positive / Negative	IA
T0 N1mi M0		Negative	Positive / Negative	Positive / Negative	IA
T1b N1mi M0	G2	Positive	Positive / Negative	Positive / Negative	IA
		Negative	Positive	Positive / Negative	IA
			Negative	Positive	IA
				Negative	IB
	G3	Positive	Positive / Negative	Positive / Negative	IA
		Negative	Positive	Positive	IA
				Negative	IA
			Negative	Positive	IA
				Negative	IB
T0 N1c M0	G1	Positive	Positive	Positive	IA
T1b N1c M0				Negative	IB
T2 N0 M0			Negative	Positive	IB
				Negative	IIA
		Negative	Positive	Positive	IA
				Negative	IB
			Negative	Positive	IB
				Negative	IIA
	G2	Positive	Positive	Positive	IA
				Negative	IB
			Negative	Positive	IB
				Negative	IIA
		Negative	Positive	Positive	IA
				Negative	IIA
			Negative	Positive	IIA
				Negative	IIA
	G3	Positive	Positive	Positive	IA
				Negative	IIA
			Negative	Positive	IIA
				Negative	IIA
		Negative	Positive	Positive	IB
				Negative	IIA
			Negative	Positive	IIA
				Negative	IIA

(Continued)

TABLE 10.3   Pathological prognostic stage groups *(Continued)*

TNM	GRADE	HER2 STATUS	ER STATUS	PR STATUS	STAGE GROUP
T2 N1^c M0	G1	Positive	Positive	Positive	IA
T3 N0 M0				Negative	IIB
			Negative	Positive	IIB
				Negative	IIB
		Negative	Positive	Positive	IA
				Negative	IIB
			Negative	Positive	IIB
				Negative	IIB
	G2	Positive	Positive	Positive	IB
				Negative	IIB
			Negative	Positive	IIB
				Negative	IIB
		Negative	Positive	Positive	IB
				Negative	IIB
			Negative	Positive	IIB
				Negative	IIB
	G3	Positive	Positive	Positive	IB
				Negative	IIB
			Negative	Positive	IIB
				Negative	IIB
		Negative	Positive	Positive	IIA
				Negative	IIB
			Negative	Positive	IIB
				Negative	IIIA
T0 N2 M0	G1	Positive	Positive	Positive	IB
T1^b N2 M0				Negative	IIIA
T2 N2 M0			Negative	Positive	IIIA
T3 N1^d M0				Negative	IIIA
T3 N2 M0		Negative	Positive	Positive	IB
				Negative	IIIA
			Negative	Positive	IIIA
				Negative	IIIA
	G2	Positive	Positive	Positive	IB
				Negative	IIIA
			Negative	Positive	IIIA
				Negative	IIIA
		Negative	Positive	Positive	IB
				Negative	IIIA
			Negative	Positive	IIIA
				Negative	IIIB

(Continued)

TABLE 10.3   Pathological prognostic stage groups *(Continued)*

TNM	GRADE	HER2 STATUS	ER STATUS	PR STATUS	STAGE GROUP
	G3	Positive	Positive	Positive	IIA
				Negative	IIIA
			Negative	Positive	IIIA
				Negative	IIIA
		Negative	Positive	Positive	IIB
				Negative	IIIA
			Negative	Positive	IIIA
				Negative	IIIC
T4 N0 M0	G1	Positive	Positive	Positive	IIIA
T4 N1^d M0				Negative	IIIB
T4 N2 M0			Negative	Positive	IIIB
AnyTN3 M0				Negative	IIIB
		Negative	Positive	Positive	IIIA
				Negative	IIIB
			Negative	Positive	IIIB
				Negative	IIIB
T4 N0 M0	G2	Positive	Positive	Positive	IIIA
T4 N1 M0				Negative	IIIB
T4 N2 M0			Negative	Positive	IIIB
AnyTN3 M0				Negative	IIIB
		Negative	Positive	Positive	IIIA
				Negative	IIIB
			Negative	Positive	IIIB
				Negative	IIIC
T4 N0 M0	G3	Positive	Positive	Positive	IIIB
T4 N1 M0				Negative	IIIB
T4 N2 M0			Negative	Positive	IIIB
AnyTN3 M0				Negative	IIIB
		Negative	Positive	Positive	IIIB
				Negative	IIIC
			Negative	Positive	IIIC
				Negative	IIIC
Any T, Any N, M1	Any	Any	Any	Any	IV

GENOMIC PROFILE FOR PATHOLOGICAL PROGNOSTIC STAGING

Obtaining genomic profiles is not needed for Pathological Prognostic staging. Genomic profiles may be done for appropriate treatment. If the Oncotype DX test is performed in T1N0M0 and T2N0M0 with ER positive HER2-neu–negative breast cancer and recurrence score is less than 11, then it is assigned pathological prognostic stage IA. If Oncotype DX is not performed or score more than 11 then classified based on above tables. Oncotype DX is the only multigene panel included in Pathological prognostic staging.

When Oncotype DX score < 11, see Table 10.4.

TABLE 10.4 Genomic profile for pathological prognostic stage

TNM	GRADE	HER2 STATUS	ER STATUS	PR STATUS	PATHOLOGICAL PROGNOSTIC STAGE GROUP
T1N0M0 T2N0M0	ANY	Negative	Positive	Any	IA

POST-NEOADJUVANT STAGING

- The largest single focus of residual invasive tumor determines ypT, with a modifier (m) indicating multiple foci of the residual tumor and does not include areas of fibrosis within the tumor bed.
- In cases of only residual cancer that is intravascular or intralymphatic (LVI), the ypT0 category is assigned but not classified as complete pathologic response.
- ypN categories are the same as those used for pN.

Treatment Response Categories

No response (NR)

No apparent change in either the T or N categories compared to clinical (pretreatment) assignment or an increase in the T or N category at the time of pathologic evaluation.

Partial response (cPR and pPR)

A decrease in either or both T or N category compared to clinical (pretreatment) assignment and with no increase in either T or N.

Complete response (cCR and pCR)

Clinical response is based on history, physical exam, and available imaging studies.

BIBLIOGRAPHY

1. Giuliano AE, Edge SB, Hortobagyi GN. Eighth Edition of the AJCC Cancer Staging Manual: Breast Cancer. *Ann Surg Oncol [Internet]*. 2018 Jul [cited 9 Nov 2023];25(7):1783–5. Available from: http://link.springer.com/10.1245/s10434-018-6486-6
2. Breast Cancer Treatment (PDQ®) - NCI [Internet]. 2023 [cited 9 Nov 2023]. Available from: https://www.cancer.gov/types/breast/hp/breast-treatment-pdq

CORE AREA V: MANAGEMENT OF BREAST CANCER

The Management of Impalpable Breast Lesions

11

Leena S. Chagla and Bahaty Riogi

INTRODUCTION

Impalpable breast lesions are defined as incidental lesions detected on imaging that cannot be felt clinically. With an increase in imaging, these lesions are becoming more common in clinical practice, and may be encountered in the following scenarios:

- In a population-based screening program or on family history screening in a high-risk population.
- On surveillance mammography or MRI in patients treated for breast cancer.
- Patients being investigated for non-breast-related ailments (for instance, CT scan or an MRI detects an abnormality in the breast).
- Patients presenting with a breast symptom and a second incidental ipsilateral or contralateral lesion is picked up on breast imaging.
- Palpable lesions can become impalpable following neoadjuvant chemotherapy (NAC) or endocrine therapy, and this group of patients will be discussed separately.

ASSESSMENT

The first step in managing impalpable lesions is assessment.

DOI: 10.1201/9780367821982-11

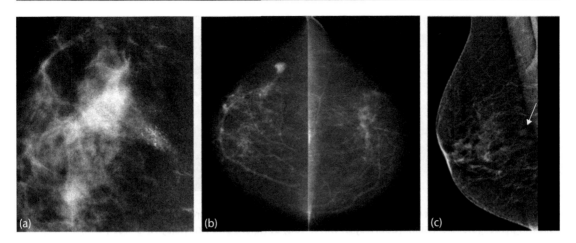

FIGURE 11.1 Some impalpable lesions on mammogram. (a) Microcalcification, (b) craniocaudal views with mass lesion on right breast, and (c) asymmetrical density (*arrow*) on oblique view of right breast. (Courtesy Dr. Olga Harris, St Helens and Knowsley NHS Trust, UK.)

The mammographic abnormalities that are recalled for assessment are mass lesions, microcalcification, asymmetrical density (Figure 11.1), and stromal deformities. The assessment would consist of a focal ultrasound scan, paddle views if indicated, and a tissue biopsy (core biopsy or vacuum-assisted biopsy is done if a bigger sample is required).

Lesions picked up on CT and MRI scans need to be evaluated by mammograms and an ultrasound scan to see if they can be biopsied under traditional imaging. If not, MRI-guided biopsies can be done in centers with the appropriate equipment.

Once these lesions are biopsied, the histology (B1–B5) will guide the management, similar to palpable lesions, which may range from reassurance, to surveillance, to therapeutic excision. Excision may be either through conventional open surgical or minimally invasive techniques. Accurate preoperative localization of these lesions is essential to enable adequate surgical excision and an acceptable cosmetic result.

We now discuss the various localization techniques available for surgical excision of these lesions. Patients with extensive ductal carcinoma *in situ* (DCIS) or multifocal impalpable disease, where the decision to offer mastectomy has already been made, do not require localization, but the pathologist may wish to X-ray the cut-up specimen to help locate the tumor.

LOCALIZATION TECHNIQUES

Wire-guided localization (WGL): The first localization using a fine wire was first described by Dodd et al. in 1965 (1). Later, the Frank–Hall hookwire, invented by a chest surgeon (Dr. Frank) and a radiologist (Dr. Hall) in 1976, gained popularity (2). In the early days, the wire was inserted blindly, roughly in the vicinity of the lesion. Post-insertion mammograms were taken, and if the wire was within 2 cm of the lesion, it was deemed a successful localization. Over the years, the wires became more sophisticated, as did the insertion techniques. Now most wires are inserted within 10 mm of the lesion in any given plane (3).

Though wires were first discovered over 40 years ago, even today, the majority of all localizations are still done with a wire, which is referred to by many as the gold standard (4). Multiple wires can be used to bracket diffuse lesions (Figure 11.2).

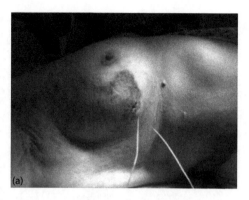
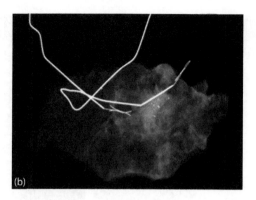

FIGURE 11.2   Localization with wires. (a) Bracketing wires in the right breast and (b) specimen mammogram following wire-guided excision. (Courtesy of Mr. R. Jois, St Helens and Knowsley NHS Trust, UK.)

However, wires are fraught with problems, which include difficult placement in a dense breast, difficult repositioning, trauma and patient discomfort due to a foreign body protruding from the breast, displacement of the wire, pneumothorax, transection or loss of the wire, and injury to the surgeon and pathologist (associated with the barbs), to mention a few. So, the hunt for the perfect localization technique continues.

IOUS: In 1988, Schwartz et al. reported the use of intraoperative ultrasound (IOUS) in the localization of an impalpable breast lesion (5). High identification rates (>95%) have been reported with IOUS, but lesions less than 5 mm in obese patients can be missed (6–9). Carbon marking may be utilized by injecting sterile charcoal suspension into the lesion under ultrasound guidance. Methylene blue may also be used, but it disperses faster than charcoal in the breast (10). IOUS cannot detect mammographic lesions that are not visible on US such as microcalcifications.

ROLL: In 1996, radioisotope occult lesion localization (ROLL) was first used in the European Institute of Oncology, Milan. Here, the breast lesion is localized with 0.2 mL of 99mTc macro-aggregates of albumin (MAA) injected into the lesion (Figure 11.3). The lesion is then detected intraoperatively with the help of a gamma probe (Figure 11.5a), like the one used for the detection of sentinel lymph nodes. Similar retrieval rates have been reported between WGL and ROLL, with a shorter operating time and less specimen weight in favor of ROLL (11). We introduced this technique in our unit in the UK in 2002, and have written extensively on its use (12–14).

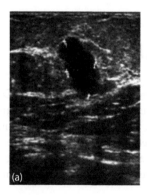
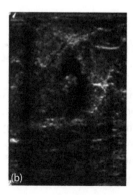
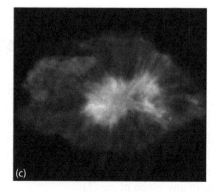

FIGURE 11.3   Radioisotope occult lesion localization (ROLL). (a) Ultrasound image of lesion before injection. (b) Ultrasound after injection of radioisotope, and (c) specimen mammogram following ROLL-guided excision. (Courtesy Miss L. Chagla, St Helens and Knowsley NHS Trust, UK.)

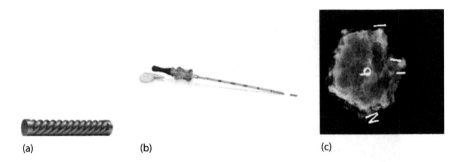

(a)   (b)   (c)

FIGURE 11.4 (a) Magseed approximately 5 mm in size, (b) seed introducer, and (c) specimen mammogram following Magseed-guided excision with seed and coil located centrally and clips on the edges for orientation. (Used with permission from Endomagnetics Limited. Image [c] courtesy of Miss L. Chagla, St Helens and Knowsley NHS Trust, UK.)

Today numerous other techniques are available, discussed next.

Radioiodine seed: This technique was first described by Gray et al. in 2001 (15). Here, iodine-125 seeds are inserted up to 2 weeks before the date of surgery. The same gamma probe can be used in the ROLL technique described above is used to detect the radio-iodine seed. This probe can also be used for sentinel lymph node biopsy (SLNB), so the capital investment could be worthwhile. The only issue with this technique is the safety regarding handling of the seed, its retrieval, and disposal (16).

Magseed: First described in 2007, this technique uses a metal seed the size of a grain of rice (Figure 11.4), which can be inserted into the lesion months prior to surgery. This seed is magnetized by the probe (Figure 11.5) when it approaches the seed and emits an audible sound, which facilitates localization. The counts from the probe tell you how far you are from the lesion. The main advantages are it is easy to use, no radiation is involved, and it can be inserted at the time of diagnosis, thus saving the patient an additional trip to the hospital and uncoupling the localization from the surgery. Like the other techniques, this can be used for both US-guided and stereo-guided localizations. The only disadvantage is that it currently costs a lot more than the cost of the wire or radioisotope. One needs to be aware of the fact that the seed only becomes magnetized when it is within 3–4 cm of the probe, which may be an issue in posterior lesions in a large breast. The company is also marketing iron filings to use with this probe for SLNB (Magtrace), so radioactivity is not necessary.

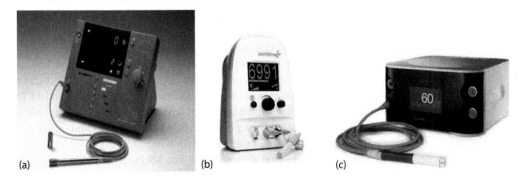

(a)   (b)   (c)

FIGURE 11.5 Different localization probes. (a) Gamma probe, (b) Sentimag probe, and (c) Savi Scout® console. (Used with permission from Endomagnetics Limited.)

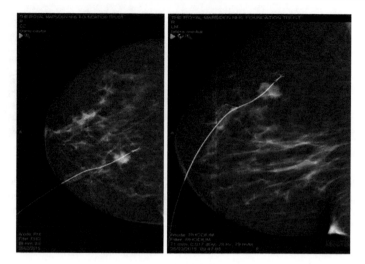

FIGURE 11.6   Post-localization mammogram films showing a wire, clip, and lesion. Craniocaudal view on the left and lateromedial view on the right. (Courtesy of Miss Ricky Roche, Royal Marsden Hospital, UK.)

Savi Scout: This nonwire localization technique was invented in 2014. It uses a nonradioactive tiny reflector the size of a rice grain. This is placed in the breast, and it emits electromagnetic signals picked up by the console (Figure 11.5). The reflector does not interfere with MRI and can stay in the breast permanently (17, 18).

These are just some of the available localization techniques. The authors only have personal experience with the use of wires, ROLL, and Magseed. Whatever technique is used, it is the responsibility of the surgeon to remove the lesion accurately without removing large areas of the breast. The following are some tips for surgeons for the management of impalpable lesions:

- Ideally try to get histology prior to surgery as benign lesions (B2) do not need excision.
- Not all B3 lesions need excision (follow local B3 protocol).
- B4 and B5 lesions need excision following localization, so work with your radiologist and use a localization technique that you are both comfortable with.
- Always ask for post-localization images (craniocaudal [CC] and true lateral) if the technique used deploys a radio-opaque marker in the breast (not for ROLL or US skin marking) (Figure 11.6).
- Study the images yourself and measure the distance of the lesion/marker from the nipple in both planes (CC and true lateral). This will give you a rough idea about the location of the impalpable lesion. Also measure the distance between the localization device (for example, the wire) and the lesion if the device is not in the lesion.
- Always obtain a specimen X-ray to confirm that the lesion and the localization device are in the excised specimen. It is important to orient the specimen with the use of clips that are visible on the X-ray, so, if required, cavity shaves can be taken from the appropriate margin. Most teams will have their own protocol for the orientation of excised specimens (Figures 11.5c and 11.7).
- Aim to have the lesion in the center of the excised specimen with only the required amount of normal breast tissue around it. The newer localization methods make this easier and do not give the comet-shaped excised specimens that were often seen with wires.
- With experience, the incisions can be placed remotely and not necessarily directly over the lesion for the use of oncoplastic incisions and techniques.
- You must mark the cavity of the excised lesion with clips for radiotherapy and future mammograms.

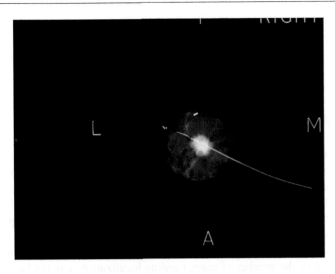

FIGURE 11.7   Specimen orientation; specimen mammogram following wire-guided excision. L, lateral; M, medial; A, anterior. (Courtesy of Miss Ricky Roche, Royal Marsden Hospital, UK.)

Management of Missed Lesions

Sometimes the excised specimen does not contain the lesion, causing a lot of upset and anxiety both to the patient and the surgeon. Every attempt at prevention by careful planning and following the tips provided earlier should make this a rare occurrence. Causes could be either because the localization failed or because you have not retrieved the localization device. Sometimes it is easy to rectify on the table but resist the temptation of doing a large wide local excision (WLE) or quadrantectomy to find the lesion.

You may only realize that the lesion is missed at final histology, which should always be discussed with images at a multidisciplinary team (MDT) meeting. In either case, one needs to be entirely honest with the patient (duty of candor), repeat imaging (mammograms and US) in 6–8 weeks, and relocalize the lesion. Sometimes, it is useful to use two modalities of localization techniques (for example, ROLL and wire).

Minimally Invasive Techniques

Today, it is possible to achieve minimally invasive excision of small breast lesions in the radiology department under local anesthesia. The Breast Lesion Excision System (BLES) is an example. It uses a calibrated, image-guided, single-pass biopsy system with a radiofrequency cutting mechanism. Through a small incision (<10 mm), lesions up to 30 mm can be excised as an intact specimen without distorting the morphology to allow histological assessment. This technology has been used for excision of some B3 lesions (19). Complications include hematoma, skin burn, delayed healing, and infection (20, 21).

Localization Following Neoadjuvant Therapy

High rates of response following NAC have increased the rate of breast-conserving surgery (BCS). It is therefore important to place a marker or the localization device (if licensed to stay in for the duration of the treatment) prior to starting treatment. It is also important to document where in the lesion this device is deployed (for example, lateral edge or center), as the lesion may completely disappear following treatment. (The specimen X-ray in Figure 11.4c shows an initial coil placed which is then localized with a Magseed when there was a complete response.) The actual surgical technique of excision remains the same.

Low-Resource Centers

In low-resource centers, the level of skill and availability of expensive technology may vary. Nonetheless, once a suspicious impalpable lesion is detected, a mammogram, ultrasound, and biopsy should be done to further evaluate the breast. In lesions that are detected on ultrasound, IOUS, skin marking or tattooing of the lesion has been used as described earlier. Personal communication with colleagues working in low-resource countries has confirmed that the wire-guided localization technique is most frequently used. This method can be adopted in new units, as it is relatively affordable and easy to set up, as no fancy probes or access to radioisotope is required. Most low-income countries do not have a population screening program, and so the number of cases needing localization may not be great. However, NAC is often available, and these localization techniques can be used following NAC when breast conservation is being contemplated and palpable lesions have now become impalpable. If breast conservation is offered to the patient, it is important to place a coil within the lesion before starting chemotherapy as explained earlier.

In conclusion, whatever the technique or setting, multidisciplinary involvement cannot be overemphasized, as accurate localization and adequate excision are dependent on input from the radiologist, pathologist, and surgeon.

REFERENCES

1. Dodd GD, Fry K, Delany W. Pre-operative localization of occult carcinoma in the breast. In: Neaton TF, editor. *Management of the patient with cancer*. Philadelphia: WB Saunders; 1966. pp. 88–133.
2. Hall FM, Kopans DB, Sadowsky NL, et al. Development of wire localization for occult breast lesions: Boston remembrances. *Radiology [Internet]*. 2013 Sep [cited 2020 May 31];268(3):622–7. Available from: http://www.ncbi.nlm.nih.gov/pubmed/23970507
3. Watkins R, Winstanley J, Patnick J. Quality Assurance Guidelines for Surgeons in Breast Cancer Screening. Edited by Mark Sibbering Roger Watkins, John Winstanley, and Julietta Patnick. [Internet]. 2009 [cited 2020 May 31]. Available from: https://assets.publishing.service.gov.uk/government/uploads/system/uploads/attachment_data/file/465694/nhsbsp20.pdf
4. Chan BK, Wiseberg-Firtell JA, Jois RH, et al. Localization techniques for guided surgical excision of non-palpable breast lesions. *Cochrane Database Syst Rev [Internet]*. 2015 Dec 31 [cited 2020 Jun 8];(12). Available from: http://doi.wiley.com/10.1002/14651858.CD009206.pub2
5. Schwartz GF, Goldberg BB, Rifkin MD, et al. Ultrasonographic localization of non-palpable breast masses. *Ultrasound Med Biol [Internet]*. 1988 Jan [cited 2020 Jun 8];14(Suppl 1):23–5. Available from: https://linkinghub.elsevier.com/retrieve/pii/0301562988900439
6. Kaufman CS, Jacobson L, Bachman B, et al. Intraoperative ultrasonography guidance is accurate and efficient according to results in 100 breast cancer patients. *Am J Surg [Internet]*. 2003 Oct [cited 2020 Jun 8]; 186(4):378–82. Available from: http://www.ncbi.nlm.nih.gov/pubmed/14553854
7. Bennett I, Greenslade J, Chiam H. Intraoperative ultrasound-guided excision of nonpalpable breast lesions. *World J Surg [Internet]*. 2005 [cited 2020 Jun 8];29(3). Available from: https://pubmed.ncbi.nlm.nih.gov/15706446/
8. Ngô C, Pollet AG, Laperrelle J, et al. Intraoperative ultrasound localization of nonpalpable breast cancers. *Ann Surg Oncol [Internet]*. 2007 Sep [cited 2020 Jun 8];14(9):2485–9. Available from: http://www.ncbi.nlm.nih.gov/pubmed/17541694

9. Ramos M, Díaz JC, Ramos T, et al. Ultrasound-guided excision combined with intraoperative assessment of gross macroscopic margins decreases the rate of reoperations for non-palpable invasive breast cancer. *Breast [Internet]*. 2013 Aug [cited 2020 Jun 8];22(4):520–4. Available from: http://www.ncbi.nlm.nih.gov/pubmed/23110817

10. Canavese G, Catturich A, Vecchio C, et al. Pre-operative localization of non-palpable lesions in breast cancer by charcoal suspension. *Eur J Surg Oncol [Internet]*. 1995 [cited 2020 Jun 8];21(1). Available from: https://pubmed.ncbi.nlm.nih.gov/7851552/

11. Ocal K, Dag A, Turkmenoglu O, et al. Radioguided occult lesion localization versus wire-guided localization for non-palpable breast lesions: Randomized controlled trial. *Clinics (Sao Paulo) [Internet]*. 2011 [cited 2020 Jun 1];66(6):1003–7. Available from: http://www.ncbi.nlm.nih.gov/pubmed/21808866

12. Audisio RA, Nadeem R, Harris O, et al. Radioguided occult lesion localisation (ROLL) is available in the UK for impalpable breast lesions. *Ann R Coll Surg Engl [Internet]*. 2005 Mar [cited 2020 May 31];87(2):92–5. Available from: http://www.ncbi.nlm.nih.gov/pubmed/15826415

13. Nadeem R, Chagla LS, Harris O, et al. Occult breast lesions: A comparison between radioguided occult lesion localisation (ROLL) vs. wire-guided lumpectomy (WGL). *Breast [Internet]*. 2005 Aug [cited 2020 May 31];14(4):283–9. Available from: http://www.ncbi.nlm.nih.gov/pubmed/15985370

14. Ramesh HSJ, Anguille S, Chagla LS, et al. Recurrence after ROLL lumpectomy for invasive breast cancer. *Breast [Internet]*. 2008 Dec [cited 2020 May 31];17(6):637–9. Available from: http://www.ncbi.nlm.nih.gov/pubmed/18595701

15. Gray RJ, Salud C, Nguyen K, et al. Randomized prospective evaluation of a novel technique for biopsy or lumpectomy of nonpalpable breast lesions: Radioactive seed versus wire localization. *Ann Surg Oncol [Internet]*. 2001 Oct [cited 2020 May 31];8(9):711–5. Available from: http://www.ncbi.nlm.nih.gov/pubmed/11597011

16. Milligan R, Pieri A, Critchley A, et al. Radioactive seed localization compared with wire-guided localization of non-palpable breast carcinoma in breast conservation surgery – the first experience in the United Kingdom. *Br J Radiol [Internet]*. 2018 [cited 2020 Jun 13];91(1081). Available from: https://pubmed.ncbi.nlm.nih.gov/29076748/

17. SCOUT® Radar Localization to Reduce Radiology and Surgical Delays [Internet]. [cited 2020 May 26]. Available from: https://www.ciannamedical.com/savi-scout/how-it-works/

18. FDA Expands Indication for Savi Scout Reflector I 2018-08-07 I FDANews [Internet]. [cited 2020 May 26]. Available from: https://www.fdanews.com/articles/187914-fda-expands-indication-for-savi-scout-reflector

19. Whitworth P, Schonholz S, Phillips R, et al. Minimally invasive intact excision of high-risk breast lesions and small breast cancers: The Intact Percutaneous Excision (IPEX) Registry. *Ann Surg Oncol [Internet]*. 2019 Apr 12 [cited 2020 May 26];26(4):954–60. Available from: http://link.springer.com/10.1245/s10434-019-07212-2

20. Graham C. Evaluation of percutaneous vacuum assisted intact specimen breast biopsy device for ultrasound visualized breast lesions: Upstage rates and long term follow-up for high risk lesions and DCIS. *Breast [Internet]*. 2017 [cited 2020 May 26];33. Available from: https://pubmed.ncbi.nlm.nih.gov/28279887/

21. Al-Harethee W, Theodoropoulos G, Filippakis GM, et al. Complications of percutaneous stereotactic vacuum assisted breast biopsy system utilizing radio frequency. *Eur J Radiol [Internet]*. 2013 [cited 2020 May 26]; 82(4). Available from: https://pubmed.ncbi.nlm.nih.gov/22227260/

Paget's Disease of the Breast

12

Ronit Roy and Diptendra Kumar Sarkar

Paget's disease of the breast, a disorder of the nipple–areola complex, causes eczema-like changes in the nipple and areola.

It is almost always associated with an underlying invasive or noninvasive carcinoma (1).

EPIDEMIOLOGY

It is an uncommon disease, accounting for 1%–4.3% of all the breast carcinomas. It can also affect men, but is extremely rare (2).

It is often associated with underlying ductal carcinoma *in situ* (DCIS) and/or invasive ductal cancer. It occurs most commonly in postmenopausal women. The average age at diagnosis is 57 years, but the disease has been found in adolescents and in people in their late 80s (3).

CLINICAL FEATURES

Paget's disease usually presents with a thickened, eczematoid, erythematous, sometimes, crusted lesion with irregular borders in the nipple–areola complex. Pain and itching are generally associated with these lesions. The lesion may be mistaken for eczema or some other inflammatory conditions. Paget's disease always starts in the nipple and may extend to the areola. The lesions are almost unilateral, but very rarely can be bilateral. These can help in distinguishing Paget's from eczema.

Serous and bloody discharge may occur. Paget's disease may result in ulceration and destruction of the nipple–areola complex. It is associated with an underlying breast cancer in 92%–100% of cases (4). Approximately 50% of patients present with an associated palpable mass. Patients presenting without a clinical mass more likely have DCIS (5). Lymph node enlargement may be found commonly in cases with a palpable tumor.

DOI: 10.1201/9780367821982-12

PATHOGENESIS

The exact pathogenesis of Paget's disease of the breast is not well understood.

One of the accepted theories is the epidermotropic theory, which suggests that the Paget cells originate from ductal cancer cells, which migrate along the basal membrane of the nipple (6).

The other theory considers Paget's disease of the breast to be an *in situ* carcinoma. In the disease, *in situ* malignant transformation occurs and the Paget cells are malignant keratinocytes appearing *in situ* and, therefore, independent of any underlying carcinoma (7).

RADIOLOGICAL FEATURES

The diagnosis is generally based on clinical findings, but radiologic findings are important to determine further management. Mammographic findings include skin thickening, nipple retraction, subareolar or more diffuse microcalcifications, a discrete mass, or architectural distortion. Due to the multicentricity of Paget's disease, it is important to evaluate the entire breast.

Ultrasound (US) examination may be helpful, but mostly the findings are nonspecific.

Breast magnetic resonance imaging (MRI) is known to be highly sensitive, especially in patients whose mammographic or US findings are normal or nonspecific. MRI may show abnormal nipple enhancement, thickening of the nipple–areola complex, an associated enhancing DCIS or invasive tumor, or a combination of all these (8).

DIAGNOSIS

The diagnosis of Paget's disease is not different from other breast diseases. Triple assessment is the key. The diagnosis can be made from a wedge biopsy or punch biopsy. But as the sensitivity is less, it is sometimes necessary to take a second biopsy (4). When a patient has nipple–areola skin changes, a full-thickness biopsy is important to establish the diagnosis.

HISTOPATHOLOGY

It is characterized by invasion of the epidermis by Paget cells, which are large pleomorphic cells with hyperchromatic nuclei and discernible nucleoli, with abundant pale, clear cytoplasm, which often contains mucin. Paget cells are more often located in the basal region of the epidermis either as single layers or as clusters of cells.

IMMUNOHISTOCHEMISTRY

Paget cells show a similar immunohistochemical staining pattern as that of adenocarcinomas growing within the breast. Paget cells are positive for CK7 in almost all cases and are not reactive for CK20.

Paget's disease often is estrogen receptor (ER) and progesterone receptor negative (4). Paget cells also express p53 (9), p21, Ki67, cyclin D1, and oncoprotein HER2 (10).

DIFFERENTIAL DIAGNOSIS

The differential diagnoses of Paget's disease include inflammatory changes like atopic or contact dermatitis of the nipple, chronic eczema, psoriasis, mammary ductal ectasia with chronic nipple discharge, Bowen's disease, basal cell carcinoma, superficial spreading malignant melanoma, etc. Because of the close similarity to skin lesions, the diagnosis may be delayed or misdiagnosed.

TREATMENT

The surgical treatment of Paget's disease is still controversial. Mastectomy with or without axillary lymph node dissection was regarded as the standard therapy for Paget's disease in the past (11).

Central quadrantectomy with or without radiation is a treatment option (12, 13). Data suggest that local control may be achieved with breast conservation surgery with negative margins followed by whole-breast radiation therapy (14). For Paget's disease with an associated cancer, the surgery includes removal of the nipple–areola complex with removal of peripheral cancer with a negative margin (14). Mastectomy should be reserved when relapse occurs or if the disease is multicentric (15).

Axillary staging surgery is not necessary when breast-conserving therapy is used to treat Paget's disease with underlying DCIS without evidence of invasive cancer. In the presence of an underlying invasive breast cancer treated with breast-conserving surgery (BCS), sentinel lymph node biopsy (SLNB) should be performed. In cases treated by total mastectomy, axillary staging is recommended for patients with invasive disease and should also be considered for patients with underlying DCIS without evidence of invasive disease because the final pathology may reveal an invasive cancer in the mastectomy specimen and the mastectomy precludes subsequent SLNB (14).

Adjuvant systemic therapy is administered according to the stage of the cancer. Patients treated with BCS and without an associated cancer or those with associated ER-positive DCIS should consider tamoxifen for risk reduction (14). Patients with invasive cancer should receive adjuvant systemic therapy based on the stage and hormone receptor status.

PROGNOSIS

Factors of an unfavorable prognosis include the presence of a palpable breast tumor, lymph node enlargement, histological type of breast cancer, and age (16). Patients with a palpable mass are mostly associated with underlying invasive carcinoma and a high rate of axillary lymph node metastasis (10). Overall survival has been shown to correlate with lymph node status and is reported to be 75%–95% in patients with negative lymph nodes and as low as 20%–25% in those with positive lymph nodal status (10). The 10-year disease-specific survival rate is 47% in patients with positive nodes and 93% in those with negative nodes (16). These results show that adjuvant treatment is recommended on the basis of lymph node status and features of the primary tumor.

REFERENCES

1. Caliskan, M., Gatti, G., Sosnovskikh, I, et al. Paget's disease of the breast: the experience of the European institute of oncology and review of the literature. *Breast Cancer Res Treat.* 2008;112:513–21. https://doi.org/10.1007/s10549-007-9880-5
2. Tavassoli FA. Norwalk, Connecticut: Appleton and Lange. *Pathology of the breast.* Norwalk, Connecticut: Appleton & Lange; 1999; pp. 731–60. [Google Scholar].
3. Kanitakis J. Mammary and extramammary Paget's disease. *J Eur Acad Dermatol Venereol.* 2007;21:581–90.
4. Rosen PP. *Rosen's breast pathology.* 2nd ed. Philadelphia: Lippincott-Raven; 2001. *Paget's disease of the nipple*; pp. 565–80.
5. Franceschini G, Masetti R, D'Ugo D, Palumbo F, D'Alba P, Mulè A, et al. Synchronous bilateral Paget's disease of the nipple associated with bilateral breast carcinoma. *Breast J.* 2005;11:355–6.
6. Muir R. The pathogenesis of Paget's disease of the nipple and associated lesions. *Br J Surg.* 1935;22:728–37.
7. Sagami S. Electron microscopic studies in Paget's disease. *Med J Osaka Univ.* 1963;14:173–88.
8. Frei KA, Bonel HM, Pelte MF, Hylton NM, Kinkel K. Paget disease of the breast: findings at magnetic resonance imaging and histopathologic correlation. *Invest Radiol.* 2005;40:363–7.
9. Ellis PE, Fong LF, Rolfe KJ, Crow JC, Reid WM, Davidson T, et al. The role of p53 and Ki67 in Paget's disease of the vulva and the breast. *Gynecol Oncol.* 2002;86:150–6.
10. Fu W, Lobocki CA, Silberberg BK, Chelladurai M, Young SC. Molecular markers in Paget disease of the breast. *J Surg Oncol.* 2001;77:171–8.
11. Paone JF, Baker RR. Pathogenesis and treatment of Paget's disease of the breast. *Cancer.* 1981;48:825–9.
12. Dixon AR, Galea MH, Ellis IO, Elston CW, Blamey RW. Paget's disease of the nipple. *Br J Surg.* 1991; 78:722–3.
13. Bulens P, Vanuytsel L, Rijnders A, van der Chueren E. Breast conserving treatment of Paget's disease. *Radiother Oncol.* 1990;17:305–9.
14. NCCN Guidelines, Version 4.2023: Paget Disease. https://www.nccn.org/professionals/physician_gls/pdf/breast.pdf
15. Stockdale AD, Brierley JD, White WF, Folkes A, Rostom AY. Radiotherapy for Paget's disease of the nipple: a conservative alternative. *Lancet.* 1989;2:664–6.
16. Kawase K, Dimaio DJ, Tucker SL, Buchholz TA, Ross MI, Feig BW, et al. Paget's disease of the breast: there is a role for breast-conserving therapy. *Ann Surg Oncol.* 2005;12:391–7.

Management of Early Breast Cancer

13

Deo SVS and Ashutosh Mishra

INTRODUCTION

Breast cancer is the most commonly diagnosed cancer and the leading cause of death in women. As per GLOBOCAN 2020, breast cancer represents one in four cancers diagnosed among women globally, and there were almost 2.26 million new cases worldwide, which contributes 24.5% of total cancer cases in women (1). However, in most of the Western world, the mortality rate has decreased in recent years because of earlier detection and improved treatment (2, 3).

From a management point of view, breast cancer can be broadly grouped into early, locally advanced, and metastatic breast cancer. Early breast cancer (EBC) is defined as disease that is confined to the breast with or without limited regional lymph node involvement and absence of distant metastasis. EBCs are potentially curable, and currently we are in the era of treatment optimization and de-escalation of conventional therapies.

There is an obvious disparity in the proportion of EBCS in high-income and low- and middle-income countries. In high-income countries, 70%–80% of patients present with EBC; while in low-income countries, EBC constitutes 30%–40% of cases.

STAGING

Currently, breast cancer is staged as per the 8th Edition of the American Joint Committee on Cancer (AJCC) TNM staging system. This updated staging system is a bit different and cumbersome in comparison to the traditional TNM system. In addition to traditional TNM staging, breast cancer staging comprises biomarker testing for estrogen receptor (ER), progesteron receptor (PR), and HER2 expression; tumor grade; and, in the instance of node-negative, ER-positive, HER2-negative cancers, incorporation of the Oncotype DX genomic assay (4, 5). As per the AJCC staging system, stage 0, I–IIB are classified as EBC. This includes ductal carcinoma *in situ* (DCIS), IA–T1N0, IB–T0N1mic or T1N1mic, IIA–T0N1, T1N1, T2N0, IIB–T2N1, and T3N0. There is some controversy pertaining to T3N0 as a type of EBC.

In EBC, staging assessment and evaluation are usually targeted at locoregional spread. Distant or occult metastasis is unlikely, and comprehensive metastatic workup is not recommended.

DOI: 10.1201/9780367821982-13

WORKUP

The EBC workup can be divided into general assessment of patient performance status and primary tumor–related workup. Any suspicious breast lump should be assessed by means of *triple assessment*, i.e., clinical, radiological, and histopathological examination.

Assessment of general performance status

- *History*: A detailed history of etiological factors should be enquired of, including age, sex, family history, prior breast biopsy or any intervention, personal history of breast cancer, prior history of DCIS/lobular carcinoma *in situ* (LCIS)/atypical hyperplasia, history of smoking, and alcohol intake, lifestyle, and dietary patterns.
- Menarche, menopause, parity.
- General physical examination.
- Basic blood workup (full blood count, liver function test [LFT], kidney function test [KFT], alkaline phosphatase, and calcium).
- Cardiac evaluation (if planned for anthracycline or trastuzumab therapy).

Assessment of the breast

- Breast size, shape, ptosis.
- Skin changes (ulceration, edema or peau d'orange, tethering, dimpling, erythema, dilated veins, previous surgical or nonsurgical scar marks).
- *Nipple status*: Inversion, ulceration, retraction, or bloody discharge.
- *Examination of the breast lump*: Location, size, consistency, borders, nodularity, mobility, fixation to skin or muscle, multifocality.
- Tumor versus breast ratio assessment.
- Status of axillary lymph nodes.
- Supraclavicular lymph node assessment.
- Assessment of contralateral breast and axilla.

IMAGING

Imaging includes bilateral mammography and ultrasonography of the breast and regional lymph nodes (6). An MRI of the breast is not routinely recommended.

Mammography

Mammography is the basic investigation for a symptomatic breast lump in women older than 35 years. It is a good modality for fatty and less dense breasts. Mammography can specifically detect the lesion characteristics, size, presence of microcalcification, and presence of multifocal disease. The sensitivity and specificity of mammograms vary from 67% to 97% and 65% to 80%, respectively (7). The Breast Imaging–Reporting and Data System (BI-RADS) and American College of Radiology (ACR) grading system are used for standardized reporting of mammography findings and breast density, respectively.

Ultrasonography

Ultrasonography (USG) is the initial investigation of choice for any palpable breast lump in women younger than 35 years of age. It is a good imaging modality for dense breasts and characterization of the axillary lymph node. The sensitivity of USG varies from 68% to 97% and specificity from 74% to 94%for diagnosing various benign and malignant breast pathologies (7).

MRI

MRI is not a modality of choice for routine EBC staging, although it is reserved for special situations and as a problem-solving tool. The sensitivity and specificity of contrast enhanced (CE)-MRI range between 90%–100% and 70%–80%, respectively (8–12). Breast MRI, on one hand, has high sensitivity for evaluation of the extent of disease, particularly in invasive breast cancer in patients with dense breasts, while on other hand, it has shown more false positives and high pickup of occult disease, which leads to overtreatment and more mastectomies.

Two prospective randomized controlled trials (RCTs) have assessed the utility of breast MRI in determining disease extent, but none of them demonstrated any improvement in post-lumpectomy re-excision rates (13, 14). In a systematic review (15), preoperative MRI breast evaluation has documented alteration of treatment in 7.8%–33.3% of women despite no difference having been noted in local recurrence or survival. There is also no conclusive evidence that the preoperative breast MRI increases the margin negative resection rate (16, 17).

Current indications of MRI include (18):

- Familial breast cancer associated with *BRCA* mutations.
- Lobular cancers.
- Dense breasts.
- Suspicion of multifocality/multicentricity (particularly in lobular breast cancer).
- Large discrepancies between conventional imaging and clinical examination.
  - Before neoadjuvant systemic therapy and to evaluate the response to this therapy.
  - When the findings of conventional imaging are inconclusive (such as a positive axillary lymph node status with an occult primary tumor in the breast).
- It may also be considered in the case of breast implants.

Other Imaging Modalities

Several new techniques are being tested for screening and diagnostic imaging, such as three-dimensional (3D) mammography (digital breast tomosynthesis), 3D ultrasound, shear wave elastography, and CE mammography/spectral mammography. None of these are yet routinely implemented, but they have the potential to increase diagnostic accuracy, especially in women with dense breasts.

Histopathological Confirmation

Core needle biopsy is mandatory to confirm the diagnosis, including assessment of histology, grade, ER, PgR, HER2, and Ki67. It should be attempted preferably under stereotactic guidance. As per updated AJCC 8th Edition TNM staging guidelines, it has become important to keep all information related to biomarkers (ER, PR, HER2) and proliferative markers (ki67) beforehand. In multifocal and multicentric tumors, all lesions should be biopsied.

TABLE 13.1 Molecular subtypes of breast cancer

INTRINSIC SUBTYPE	CLINICOPATHOLOGICAL SURROGATE DEFINITION
Luminal A	Luminal A–like • ER-positive • HER2-negative • Ki67 low • PR high • Low-risk molecular signature (if available)
Luminal B	Luminal B–like (HER2-negative) • ER-positive • HER2-negative • Either Ki67 high or PR low • High-risk molecular signature (if available) Luminal B–like (HER2-positive) • ER-positive • HER2-positive • Any Ki67 • Any PR
HER2 enriched	HER2-positive (nonluminal) • HER2-positive • ER and PR absent
Basal-like	Triple-negative • ER and PR absent • HER2-negative

Source: Adapted from the 2013 St Gallen Consensus Conference (13).

Assessment of regional lymph nodes

Regional lymph node assessment is an integral part of breast cancer staging. It should include a combination of:

- Clinical examination.
- Ultrasound or ultrasound-guided fine needle aspiration cytology (FNAC) or biopsy of suspicious nodes.

Traditionally, axillary nodal assessment and staging are performed by clinical examination only. However, physical examination is neither a sensitive nor reliable method to ascertain the status of the axillary lymph nodes, especially in patients with low-volume disease burden. The positive predictive value of clinical palpation ranges from 60% to 80%, while the negative predictive value ranges between 50 % and 60% (20, 21). To overcome the significant morbidity associated with axial lymph node dissection (ALND), sentinel lymph node biopsy (SLNB) has been introduced as a minimally invasive staging tool in patients with clinically negative axilla. Subsequently, for clinically palpable or suspicious axillary nodes, axillary ultrasonography (AUSG) along with fine needle aspiration cytology/core biopsy (FNAB) was added in the management algorithm to identify patients who may be candidates for ALND rather than SLNB (22). However, both AUSG and FNAB are highly operator dependent, and the expertise for assessment of lymph nodes using USG and FNAB may not be widely available in low- and middle-income countries (LMICs). Scaling up facilities and expertise for USG and FNAB in LMICs will improve optimization of patient selection for ALND or SLNB without major financial burden.

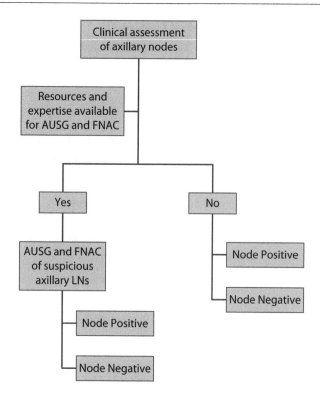

ASSESSMENT OF METASTATIC DISEASE

In EBC, there is a less than 5% chance of distant metastasis. Therefore, routine metastatic workup is not routinely recommended unless there is high tumor burden, aggressive biology, or when symptoms are suggestive of metastases.

- Imaging of chest, abdomen, and bone using CT scan and bone scan or PET scan is recommended for higher-risk patients, who may have one or more risk factors like high tumor burden; aggressive biology; and signs, symptoms, or laboratory values suggesting the presence of metastases.
- In a resource-constrained setup, routine metastatic workup can be initiated with USG of the whole abdomen, chest X-ray, and bone scan. If a CT scan facility is available, then CE CT of the chest, abdomen, and pelvis is preferred. FDG-PET-CT scanning may be useful when conventional methods are inconclusive and may replace traditional imaging for staging in high-risk patients.

Management Principles

The management of EBC includes diagnosis by triple assessment and treatment by a multimodality approach. The multimodality management options include locoregional control using surgery, i.e., breast conservation surgery with radiation therapy (BCT) or mastectomy with or without radiation therapy (RT). The systemic treatment options include chemotherapy, endocrine therapy, and targeted therapy. Chemotherapy may be offered in either the neoadjuvant setting (triple-negative or HER2-enriched molecular subtypes) or in the adjuvant setting based upon the primary tumor characteristics like tumor size, grade, and lymph node involvement. The endocrine therapy and targeted therapy must be added based on the ER/PR-positive status or HER2-positive status, respectively (18, 23).

DCIS

DCIS of the breast is commonly a screen-detected entity and categorized as an EBC. DCIS is usually managed by a multimodality approach incorporating various combinations of surgery, radiation treatment, and hormonal therapy. BCS followed by RT and hormonal therapy reduces the risk of recurrence by 50%. Multiple studies and National Comprehensive Cancer Network (NCCN) guidelines have suggested that radiation treatment after BCS for patients with low-risk DCIS can be avoided, although there are no obvious criteria addressing those with low risk (24, 25). Long-term outcomes after BCS with radiation treatment show high rates of local control and survival (26, 27).

SURGICAL MANAGEMENT

Breast Conservation Surgery versus Mastectomy

The surgical options for EBC are BCS and modified radical mastectomy with or without reconstruction. Axillary nodes need to be addressed as part of the surgical management of EBC. The factors affecting the surgical decisions include:

- *Tumor-related factors*: Tumor size, location, multicentricity, stage, tumor vs breast ratio, and molecular subtypes.
- *Patient-related factors*: Age, family history, mutation status, and desire to conserve the breast.
- The expertise of the treating surgeon.

Several RCTs found that long-term survival rates were not significantly different between breast conservation and mastectomy (28–33). BCS is now the standard surgical option for invasive tumors up to 2 cm in size (T1) or good tumor to breast ratio and luminal subtypes, provided the patient is keen for breast conservation. However, for tumors >2 cm in size and aggressive subtypes (triple-negative or HER2 enriched), neoadjuvant chemotherapy (NACT) followed by reassessment of surgery is increasingly being used (18). The absolute contraindications for BCS include:

- Multicentric disease (tumor involving >1 quadrant).
- Persistent positive margins.
- Diffuse microcalcifications.
- Pregnancy.
- Prior therapeutic chest wall radiation.

Relative contraindications include:

- Poor tumor-to-breast ratio.
- Collagen vascular disease.

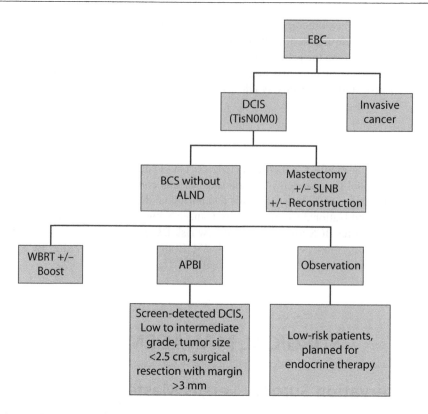

FIGURE 13.1 DCIS treatment algorithm.

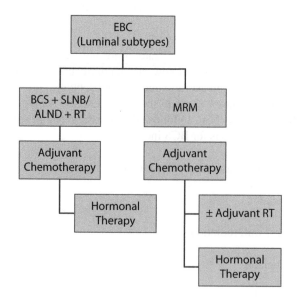

FIGURE 13.2 EBC (luminal subtype) treatment algorithm.

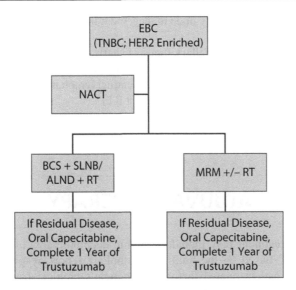

FIGURE 13.3   EBC (TNBC; HER2-enriched) treatment algorithm.

Neoadjuvant Chemotherapy

A complete response or partial response (with adequate downsizing of tumor) after NACT makes breast conservation easier with a good cosmetic outcome. However, an unsatisfactory response or progressive disease after NACT mandates mastectomy. The acceptable margin for invasive cancer is ***no tumor on the inked surface*** (34). After a lumpectomy, the tumor bed should be marked with clips to facilitate treatment planning for the radiation boost. Persistently positive margins even after a reasonable number of attempts at re-excision also warrants mastectomy. For DCIS, BCS with a 2-mm margin followed by whole-breast RT or total mastectomy are acceptable treatment options. Mastectomy is indicated for patients who are not candidates for lumpectomy or for those who are not keen for breast conservation (18, 19, 23). The structures removed in a modified radical mastectomy are breast with pectoral fascia, nipple–areola complex, and part of skin and complete ALND/SLNB.

Management of Axilla

The management of axillary lymph nodes is paramount to improve long-term survival rates. The option for axillary staging includes ALND or SLNB. ALND is considered the standard of care for patients with clinically positive lymph nodes. However, based on results from RCTs (35, 36), SLNB has replaced ALND for clinically node-negative axilla, thereby reducing morbidities of ALND like lymphedema, shoulder stiffness, and paresthesia. For clinically positive lymph nodes, the NCCN panel recommends pathologic confirmation of malignancy using ultrasound-guided fine needle aspiration/core biopsy of suspicious lymph nodes. If positive for malignancy, complete level I and II axillary lymph node dissection is warranted with harvesting of at least 10 lymph nodes. The level III lymph node is also dissected in cases of gross disease in level II or III. SLNB should be done with a combination of techniques (blue dye, radioactive colloid, or indocyanine green dye fluorescence) to increase the accuracy. During SLNB, if sentinel nodes are not identified, low axillary dissection, i.e., removal of fibrofatty tissue overlying the second and third digitation of the serratus anterior below the intercostal nerve should be performed for axillary staging.

Current recommendations for axillary node management include (18):

- SLNB is the standard of care for axillary staging in early, clinically node-negative breast cancer.
- Complete axillary dissection following positive SLNB is not needed in case of low axillary disease burden (micrometastases or one to two sentinel lymph nodes [SLNs] containing metastases, treated with postoperative tangential breast RT).
- Axillary radiation is a valid alternative in patients with positive SLNB, irrespective of the type of breast surgery.

ADJUVANT THERAPY

After surgery, adjuvant treatment may include systemic chemotherapy, hormonal therapy, targeted therapy, and radiotherapy. Based on the final histopathology report, response to NACT, risk stratification tools, and other patient-related factors (the patient's biological age, general health status, comorbidities, and preferences), the patient may receive single therapy or a combination of adjuvant therapies.

Adjuvant Chemotherapy

General recommendations (18):

- Adjuvant systemic therapy should be started without undue delays, as data show an important decrease in efficacy when it is administered >12 weeks after surgery (37).
- Most luminal A–like cancers do not require chemotherapy, except those with high disease burden. Indications for chemotherapy within this subtype depend on the individual's risk of relapse, considering the tumor burden and features suggestive of biological aggressiveness (grade, proliferation, vascular invasion), presumed responsiveness to Endocrine therapy (ET), and patient preferences.
- Data from neoadjuvant studies have demonstrated that chemotherapy sensitivity depends on the intrinsic phenotype, with the highest being for HER2-positive (when combined with anti-HER2 therapy) and triple-negative breast cancer.
- In luminal cancers, ESMO, ASCO, and the NCCN guidelines recommend the use of risk stratification tools for predicting the benefit from adjuvant chemotherapy. The most used is the 21-gene assay (oncotype diagnosis). For patients with a score below 10, adjuvant chemotherapy can be avoided, and the patients receive only hormone therapy. If patients have a score above 31, the risk of recurrence is high and they should receive adjuvant chemotherapy along with adjuvant radiotherapy. For the intermediate group, there is still no guideline. As per the TAILORx study (38), patients below 50 years of age with a score between 16 and 25 appear to benefit from chemotherapy.
- In cases of uncertainty regarding indications for adjuvant chemotherapy (after consideration of all clinical and pathological factors), expression of uPA-PAI1 or gene expression assays, such as MammaPrint, Oncotype DX, Prosigna, Endopredict, or Breast Cancer Index, can be used.
- Luminal A patients with pathologically positive nodes should receive chemotherapy along with hormone therapy. As per the preliminary results of the Rxponder trial (39), postmenopausal women with hormone receptor–positive, HER2-negative (HR+/HER2−) breast cancer, with one to three involved lymph nodes, and a Recurrence Score (RS) ≤25 may avoid adjuvant chemotherapy.

- Patients with TNBC histology receive neoadjuvant chemotherapy before surgery. In case of pathological complete response (CR), the patient is kept for follow-up. In case of residual disease, capecitabine is given for six to eight cycles (create-X trial).
- In patients with HER2-neu–enriched disease, neoadjuvant chemotherapy with trastuzumab +/– pertuzumab is recommended. After surgery, if there is a complete pathological response, then 12–14 months of further trastuzumab +/– pertuzumab is recommended. In the case of residual disease, 12–14 months of adjuvant trastuzumab emtansine is recommended.
- Chemotherapy should not be used concomitantly with ET, with the exception of gonadotropin-releasing hormone (GnRH) analogues used for ovarian protection (40).
- Anti-HER2 therapy may routinely be combined with non-anthracycline-based chemotherapy, ET, and RT.
- Radiation therapy may be delivered safely during anti-HER2 therapy, ET, and non-anthracycline, non-taxane-based chemotherapy. Chemotherapy and RT should be given sequentially, i.e., chemotherapy should be given first.

Systemic treatment recommendations for EBC subtypes (18)

SUBTYPE	RECOMMENDED THERAPY	COMMENT
Luminal A–like	ET alone in most cases	Consider chemotherapy if high tumor burden (≥ 4 LNs, T3 or higher
Luminal B–like (HER2-negative)	Chemotherapy followed by ET for the majority of cases	
Luminal B–like (HER2-positive)	Chemotherapy + anti-HER2 followed by ET for all patients	If contraindications for the use of chemotherapy, one may consider ET + anti-HER2 therapy, although no randomized data exist
HER2-positive (nonluminal)	Chemotherapy + anti-HER2	
Triple-negative (ductal)	Chemotherapy	

HORMONE THERAPY

Hormone-Positive Premenopausal Patients

Tamoxifen for a period of 5–10 years is the standard of care. Annual gynecological assessment is recommended, but transvaginal ultrasound for endometrial thickness is no longer routinely advised.

Numerous studies have demonstrated an advantage of 10 years rather than 5 years of ET, although the optimal duration and regimen of adjuvant ET are currently unknown, and there is a minimal benefit for the use of aromatase inhibitors (AIs) for more than 5 years (41, 42).

Hormone-Positive Postmenopausal Patients

AIs like anastrozole are given for 5 years. After more than 5 years, the benefit is unclear. AIs compared with tamoxifen allow for about 4% absolute benefit in disease-free survival, with no significant impact on overall survival (1%–2%, depending on the choice of an up-front or sequential strategy) (43–45). The patient should be given calcium and vitamin D_3 along with a periodic DEXA scan to assess bone density.

RADIOTHERAPY

All patients undergoing BCS receive radiation to the whole breast along with a boost to the tumor bed.

- **Postoperative whole-breast RT** (WBRT) is strongly recommended after BCS. WBRT alone reduces the 10-year risk of any first recurrence (including locoregional and distant) by 15% and the 15-year risk of breast cancer–related mortality by 4% (46).
- **Boost RT** gives a further 50% relative risk (RR) reduction and is indicated for most patients who have unfavourable risk factors for local control such as age <50 years, grade 3 tumors, presence of vascular invasion or extensive intraductal component, and nonradical tumor excision (focally—otherwise, further surgery should be advocated) (47, 48).
- **Accelerated partial breast irradiation** where only the tumor bed is irradiated is given in cases where the patient is above 50 years of age, hormone positive, unifocal, nonlobular histology, <3 cm in size without extensive intraductal component, and with negative margins (49, 50).
- **Partial mastectomy and radiotherapy** (PMRT) is recommended in patients who have high-risk features, four or more positive axillary nodes, T3/T4 tumor size, and positive margins. It is also recommended in patients with one to three positive nodes; still, an individualized risk assessment can be done (51).
  - PMRT in node-positive patients reduces the 10-year risk of any recurrence (including locoregional and distant) by 10% and the 20-year risk of breast cancer–related mortality by 8% (51).
- **After ALND**, the resected part of the axilla should not be irradiated, except in cases of clear residual disease after surgery. After a positive SLNB without subsequent ALND, regional RT is advised.

Hereditary Breast Cancer

All high-risk breast cancer patients should be offered genetic counseling and testing for germline *BRCA1* and *BRCA2* mutations (52). These groups include patients with a:

- Strong family history of breast, ovarian, pancreatic, and/or high-grade/metastatic prostate cancer.
- Diagnosis of breast cancer before the age of 45 years.
- Diagnosis of TNBC before the age of 60.
- Personal history of ovarian cancer or second breast cancer or male sex.

FERTILITY

For young patients who want to complete their family after treatment, ovarian protection during chemotherapy should be attempted. A GnRH agonist (goserelin) can be started before chemotherapy and continued during chemotherapy (53). Other options include ovum preservation prior to initiation of chemotherapy. Use of oral contraceptive pills for birth control is not recommended. Usually, an intrauterine device (IUD) or barrier methods are advised.

EXTREMES OF AGE

Geriatric breast cancer in the subset of patients means they must be treated according to their biological age rather than their chronological one. Before planning any treatment, these patients must be evaluated comprehensively. There are different geriatric performance status assessment tools like G8 which can provide sufficient information pertaining to tolerability for standard treatment. The general condition of the patient and preexisting comorbidities should be considered when planning chemotherapy (54). In patients suitable for standard chemotherapy, a standard multidrug regimen should be used. Patients in the extremes of age with luminal subtypes can be considered for neoadjuvant hormonal therapy if clinically indicated.

PREGNANCY

Breast cancer is one of the most diagnosed malignancies during pregnancy. Breast cancers occurring during pregnancy are typically aggressive with higher grade, HER2 positive, and hormone receptor negative (55). If breast cancer is diagnosed in the first or second trimester, then termination of the pregnancy is usually advisable. BCS/mastectomy can be performed safely during any trimester of pregnancy and may be appropriate if the multimodality treatment plan is timed such that the woman can receive postsurgical RT after full-term delivery without unduly delaying treatment. For the management of axilla, SLNB is still a bit controversial (56, 57), and therefore ALND is the standard of care.

The risk of congenital malformation from cytotoxic chemotherapy varies. Exposure in the first trimester is associated with risks of 10%–20% and should be avoided. Risks decline to <2% with exposure in the second and third trimesters, enabling chemotherapy administration at that time (58).

The use of trastuzumab in pregnancy is associated with oligohydramnios and is contraindicated. Methotrexate should be avoided during pregnancy because of the risk of abortion and severe fetal malformation. Similarly, tamoxifen and all hormonal approaches should be withheld until after delivery because of concerns for the health of the fetus. When chemotherapy or tamoxifen is given postpartum, breastfeeding should be avoided, as these agents may be excreted in the breast milk. Postsurgical RT can cause fibrosis of the treated breast that precludes successful lactation. Postmalignancy pregnancy should be stratified according to the risk of the index cancer and advised only after completion of multimodality treatment and at least 18 months of hormone therapy.

FOLLOW-UP AND SURVIVAL

Patients are followed up 3 monthly for first 2 years, then 6 monthly for 5 years, and annually thereafter.

- Annual mammography is recommended along with history and physical examination. In patients with genetic disorders, annual MRI is recommended too.
- There is no indication for screening for metastasis in the follow-up period.
- Investigations are ordered according to symptoms that patients may have.
- Patients on tamoxifen who enter menopause should be shifted to aromatase inhibitors. A DEXA scan should be done before the changeover.
- Education about postsurgery lymphedema should be given to every patient who has undergone axillary procedures.
- Patients should have a healthy diet and get regular exercise.

REFERENCES

1. Sung, H, Ferlay, J, Siegel, RL, Laversanne, M, Soerjomataram, I, Jemal, A, Bray, F. Global cancer statistics 2020: GLOBOCAN estimates of incidence and mortality worldwide for 36 cancers in 185 countries. *CA Cancer J Clin.* 2021;71:209–49. doi: 10.3322/caac.21660.
2. Autier P, Boniol M, La Vecchia C, et al. Disparities in breast cancer mortality trends between 30 European countries: Retrospective trend analysis of WHO mortality database. *BMJ.* 2010;341(Aug 11):c3620.
3. Allemani C, Weir HK, Carreira H, et al. Global surveillance of cancer survival 1995–2009: Analysis of individual data for 25,676,887 patients from 279 population-based registries in 67 countries (CONCORD-2). *Lancet.* 2015;385(9972):977–1010.
4. Amin MB, Edge S, Greene F, et al., eds. *AJCC Cancer Staging Manual.* 8th ed. New York: Springer International Publishing; 2017.
5. Giuliano AE, Connolly JL, Edge SB, et al. Breast cancer—Major changes in the American Joint Committee on Cancer Eighth Edition Cancer Staging Manual. *CA Cancer J Clin.* 2017;67(4):290–303.
6. Perry N, Broeders M, de Wolf C et al. European guidelines for quality assurance in breast cancer screening and diagnosis. Fourth edition—Summary document. *Ann Oncol.* 2007;19(4):614–22.
7. Devolli-Disha E, Manxhuka-Kërliu S, Ymeri H, Kutllovci A. Comparative accuracy of mammography and ultrasound in women with breast symptoms according to age and breast density. *Bosn J Basic Med Sci.* 2009;9(2):131–136. doi: 10.17305/bjbms.2009.2832.
8. Menezes GL, Knuttel FM, Stehouwer BL, Pijnappel RM, van den Bosch MA. Magnetic resonance imaging in breast cancer: A literature review and future perspectives. *World J Clin Oncol.* 2014;5(2):61–70. doi: 10.5306/wjco.v5.i2.61.
9. Berg WA, Gutierrez L, NessAiver MS, Carter WB, Bhargavan M, Lewis RS, Ioffe OB. Diagnostic accuracy of mammography, clinical examination, US, and MR imaging in preoperative assessment of breast cancer. *Radiology.* 2004;233:830–49. [PMID: 15486214] doi: 10.1148/radiol.2333031484.
10. Boetes C, Mus RD, Holland R, Barentsz JO, Strijk SP, Wobbes T, Hendriks JH, Ruys SH. Breast tumors: Comparative accuracy of MR imaging relative to mammography and US for demonstrating extent. *Radiology.* 1995;197:743–47. [PMID: 7480749].
11. Boetes C, Strijk SP, Holland R, Barentsz JO, Van Der Sluis RF, Ruijs JH. False-negative MR imaging of malignant breast tumors. *Eur Radiol.* 1997;7:1231–34. [PMID: 9377507].
12. Zhang Y, Ren H. Meta-analysis of diagnostic accuracy of magnetic resonance imaging and mammography for breast cancer. *J Can Res Ther.* 2017;13:862–8.
13. Peters NH, van Esser S, van den Bosch MA, Storm RK, Plaisier PW, van Dalen T, Diepstraten SC, Weits T, Westenend PJ, Stapper G, Fernandez-Gallardo MA, Borel Rinkes IH, van Hillegersberg R, Mali WP, Peeters PH. Preoperative MRI and surgical management in patients with nonpalpable breast cancer: The MONET–randomised controlled trial. *Eur J Cancer.* 2011 Apr;47(6):879–86. doi: 10.1016/j.ejca.2010.11.035. Epub 2010 Dec 30. PMID: 21195605.
14. Turnbull LW, Brown SR, Olivier C, Harvey I, Brown J, Drew P, Hanby A, Manca A, Napp V, Sculpher M, Walker LG, Walker S; COMICE Trial Group. Multicentre randomised controlled trial examining the cost-effectiveness of contrast-enhanced high field magnetic resonance imaging in women with primary breast cancer scheduled for wide local excision (COMICE). *Health Technol Assess.* 2010 Jan;14(1):1–182. doi: 10.3310/hta14010. PMID: 20025837.
15. Houssami N, Ciatto S, Macaskill P, Lord SJ, Warren RM, Dixon JM, Irwig L. Accuracy and surgical impact of magnetic resonance imaging in breast cancer staging: Systematic review and meta-analysis in detection of multifocal and multicentric cancer. *J Clin Oncol.* 2008 Jul 1;26(19):3248–58. doi: 10.1200/JCO.2007.15.2108. Epub 2008 May 12. PMID: 18474876.
16. Bleicher RJ, Ciocca RM, Egleston BL, Sesa L, Evers K, Sigurdson ER, Morrow M. Association of routine pretreatment magnetic resonance imaging with time to surgery, mastectomy rate, and margin status. *J Am Coll Surg.* 2009 Aug;209(2):180–7; quiz 294-5. doi: 10.1016/j.jamcollsurg.2009.04.010. Epub 2009 Jun 18. Erratum in: *J Am Coll Surg.* 2009 Nov;209(5):679. PMID: 19632594; PMCID: PMC2758058.
17. Turnbull L, Brown S, Harvey I, Olivier C, Drew P, Napp V, Hanby A, Brown J. Comparative effectiveness of MRI in breast cancer (COMICE) trial: A randomised controlled trial. *Lancet.* 2010 Feb 13;375(9714):563–71. doi: 10.1016/S0140-6736(09)62070-5. PMID: 20159292.
18. Cardoso, F, Kyriakides, S, Ohno, S, Penault-Llorca, F, Poortmans, P, Rubio, IT, … Senkus, E. Early breast cancer: ESMO Clinical Practice Guidelines for diagnosis, treatment and follow-up. *Ann Oncol.* 2019. doi: 10.1093/annonc/mdz173.

19. Goldhirsch A, Winer EP, Coates AS, et al. Personalizing the treatment of women with early breast cancer: Highlights of the St Gallen International Expert Consensus on the Primary Therapy of Early Breast Cancer 2013. *Ann Oncol*. 2013;24(9):2206–23.
20. Lanng C, Hoffmann J, Galatius H, Engel U. Assessment of clinical palpation of the axilla as a criterion for performing the sentinel node procedure in breast cancer. *Eur J Surg Oncol J Eur Soc Surg Oncol Br Assoc Surg Oncol*. 2007 Apr;33(3):281–4.
21. Bourez RLJH, Rutgers EJT, Van De Velde CJH. Will we need lymph node dissection at all in the future? *Clin Breast Cancer*. 2002 Dec;3(5):315–22; discussion 323-325.
22. van Rijk MC, Deurloo EE, et al. Ultrasonography and fine-needle aspiration cytology can spare breast cancer patients unnecessary sentinel lymph node biopsy. *Ann Surg Oncol*. 2005:13(1):31–35.
23. https://www.nccn.org/guidelines/Breast Cancer, Version 4.2021, NCCN Clinical Practice Guidelines in Oncology (NCCN).
24. Gradishar WJ, Anderson BO, Balassanian R, Blair SL, Burstein HJ, Cyr A, et al. Breast Cancer, Version 4.2017, NCCN Clinical Practice Guidelines in Oncology. *J Natl Compr Cancer Netw*. 2018;16:310–20. doi: 10.6004/jnccn.2018.0012.
25. Moran MS, Bai HX, Harris EER, Arthur DW, Bailey L, Bellon JR, et al. ACR Appropriateness Criteria Ductal Carcinoma In Situ. *Breast J*. 2012;18;8–15. doi: 10.1111/j.1524-4741.2011.01197.x.
26. Moran MS, Zhao Y, Ma S, Kirova Y, Fourquet A, Chen P, et al. Association of radiotherapy boost for ductal carcinoma in situ with local control after whole-breast radiotherapy. *JAMA Oncol*. 2017;3:1060–8. doi: 10.1001/jamaoncol.2016.6948.
27. Lalani N, Paszat L, Sutradhar R, Thiruchelvam D, Nofech-Mozes S, Hanna W, et al. Long-term outcomes of hypofractionation versus conventional radiation therapy after breast-conserving surgery for ductal carcinoma in situ of the breast. *Int J Radiat Oncol Biol Phys*. 2014;90:1017–24. doi: 10.1016/j.ijrobp.2014.07.026.
28. Fisher B, Anderson S, Bryant J, Margolese RG, Deutsch M, Fisher ER, Jeong JH, Wolmark N. Twenty-year follow-up of a randomized trial comparing total mastectomy, lumpectomy, and lumpectomy plus irradiation for the treatment of invasive breast cancer. *N Engl J Med*. 2002 Oct 17;347(16):1233–41.
29. Veronesi U, Cascinelli N, Mariani L, Greco M, Saccozzi R, Luini A, Aguilar M, Marubini E. Twenty-year follow-up of a randomized study comparing breast-conserving surgery with radical mastectomy for early breast cancer. *N Engl J Med*. 2002 Oct 17;347(16):1227–32.
30. Arriagada R, Lê MG, Rochard F, Contesso G. Conservative treatment versus mastectomy in early breast cancer: Patterns of failure with 15 years of follow-up data. Institut Gustave-Roussy Breast Cancer Group. *J Clin Oncol*. 1996 May;14(5):1558–64.
31. Jacobson JA, Danforth DN, Cowan KH, d'Angelo T, Steinberg SM, Pierce L, Lippman ME, Lichter AS, Glatstein E, Okunieff P. Ten-year results of a comparison of conservation with mastectomy in the treatment of stage I and II breast cancer. *N Engl J Med*. 1995 Apr 6;332(14):907–11.
32. van Dongen JA, Voogd AC, Fentiman IS, Legrand C, Sylvester RJ, Tong D, van der Schueren E, Helle PA, van Zijl K, Bartelink H. Long-term results of a randomized trial comparing breast-conserving therapy with mastectomy: European Organization for Research and Treatment of Cancer 10801 trial. *J Natl Cancer Inst*. 2000 Jul 19;92(14):1143–50.
33. Blichert-Toft M, Rose C, Andersen JA, Overgaard M, Axelsson CK, Andersen KW, Mouridsen HT. Danish randomized trial comparing breast conservation therapy with mastectomy: Six years of life-table analysis. Danish Breast Cancer Cooperative Group. *J Natl Cancer Inst Monogr*. 1992;(11):19–25.
34. Moran, MS, Schnitt, SJ, Giuliano, AE, Harris, JR, Khan, SA, Horton, J, … Morrow, M. Society of Surgical Oncology–American Society for Radiation Oncology Consensus Guideline on Margins for Breast-Conserving Surgery with Whole-Breast Irradiation in Stages I and II Invasive Breast Cancer. *Int J Radiat Oncol Biol Phys*. 2014;88(3):553–64. doi: 10.1016/j.ijrobp.2013.11.012.
35. Krag DN, Anderson SJ, Julian TB, Brown AM, Harlow SP, Costantino JP, Ashikaga T, Weaver DL, Mamounas EP, Jalovec LM, Frazier TG, Noyes RD, Robidoux A, Scarth HM, Wolmark N. Sentinel-lymph-node resection compared with conventional axillary-lymph-node dissection in clinically node-negative patients with breast cancer: Overall survival findings from the NSABP B-32 randomised phase 3 trial. *Lancet Oncol*. 2010 Oct;11(10):927–33.
36. Giuliano AE, McCall L, Beitsch P, Whitworth PW, Blumencranz P, Leitch AM, Saha S, Hunt KK, Morrow M, Ballman K. Locoregional recurrence after sentinel lymph node dissection with or without axillary dissection in patients with sentinel lymph node metastases: The American College of Surgeons Oncology Group Z0011 randomized trial. *Ann Surg*. 2010 Sep;252(3):426–32; discussion 432-3.
37. Lohrisch C, Paltiel C, Gelmon K, et al. Impact on survival of time from definitive surgery to initiation of adjuvant chemotherapy for early-stage breast cancer. *J Clin Oncol*. 2006;24(30):4888–94.

38. Sparano, JA, Gray, RJ, Makower, DF, Pritchard, KI, Albain, KS, Hayes, DF, … Sledge, G.W. Adjuvant chemotherapy guided by a 21-gene expression assay in breast cancer. *N Eng J M.* 2018;379(2):111–21. doi: 10.1056/nejmoa1804710.

39. Kalinsky K, Barlow WE, Meric-Bernstam F, et al. First results from a phase III randomized clinical trial of standard adjuvant endocrine therapy +/– chemotherapy in patients with 1-3 positive nodes, hormone receptor-positive and HER2-negative breast cancer with recurrence score <25: SWOG S1007 (RxPonder). *Cancer Res.* 2020;81S:SABCS #GS3-00.

40. Albain KS, Barlow WE, Ravdin PM, et al. Adjuvant chemotherapy and timing of tamoxifen in postmenopausal patients with endocrineresponsive, node-positive breast cancer: A phase 3, open-label, randomised controlled trial. *Lancet.* 2009;374(9707):2055–63.

41. Goss PE, Ingle JN, Pater JL, et al. Late extended adjuvant treatment with letrozole improves outcome in women with early-stage breast cancer who complete 5 years of tamoxifen. *J Clin Oncol.* 2008;26(12):1948–55.

42. Davies C, Pan H, Godwin J, et al. Long-term effects of continuing adjuvant tamoxifen to 10 years versus stopping at 5 years after diagnosis of oestrogen receptor-positive breast cancer: ATLAS, a randomised trial. *Lancet.* 2013;381(9869):805–16.

43. Bliss JM, Kilburn LS, Coleman RE, et al. Disease-related outcomes with long-term follow-up: An updated analysis of the intergroup exemestane study. *J Clin Oncol.* 2012;30(7):709–17.

44. Regan MM, Neven P, Giobbie-Hurder A, et al. Assessment of letrozole and tamoxifen alone and in sequence for postmenopausal women with steroid hormone receptor-positive breast cancer: The BIG 1-98 randomised clinical trial at 8.1 years median follow-up. *Lancet Oncol.* 2011;12(12):1101–08.

45. Cuzick J, Sestak I, Baum M, et al. Effect of anastrozole and tamoxifen as adjuvant treatment for early-stage breast cancer: 10-year analysis of the ATAC trial. *Lancet Oncol.* 2010;11(12):1135–41.

46. Darby S, McGale P, Correa C, et al. Effect of radiotherapy after breast conserving surgery on 10-year recurrence and 15-year breast cancer death: Meta-analysis of individual patient data for 10, 801 women in 17 randomised trials. *Lancet.* 2011;378(9804):1707–16.

47. van Werkhoven E, Hart G, van Tinteren H, et al. Nomogram to predict ipsilateral breast relapse based on pathology review from the EORTC 22881-10882 boost versus no boost trial. *Radiother Oncol.* 2011;100(1):101–7.

48. Bartelink H, Maingon P, Poortmans P, et al. Whole-breast irradiation with or without a boost for patients treated with breast-conserving surgery for early breast cancer: 20-year follow-up of a randomised phase 3 trial. *Lancet Oncol.* 2015;16(1):47–56.

49. Coles CE, Griffin CL, Kirby AM, et al. Partial-breast radiotherapy after breast conservation surgery for patients with early breast cancer (UK IMPORT LOW trial): 5-year results from a multicentre, randomised, controlled, phase 3, non-inferiority trial. *Lancet.* 2017;390(10099):1048–60.

50. Livi L, Meattini I, Marrazzo L, et al. Accelerated partial breast irradiation using intensity-modulated radiotherapy versus whole breast irradiation: 5-year survival analysis of a phase 3 randomised controlled trial. *Eur J Cancer.* 2015;51(4):451–63.

51. McGale P, Taylor C, Correa C, et al. Effect of radiotherapy after mastectomy and axillary surgery on 10-year recurrence and 20-year breast cancer mortality: Meta-analysis of individual patient data for 8135 women in 22 randomised trials. *Lancet.* 2014;383(9935):2127–35.

52. Paluch-Shimon S, Cardoso F, Sessa C et al. Prevention and screening in BRCA mutation carriers and other breast/ovarian hereditary cancer syndromes: ESMO Clinical Practice Guidelines for cancer prevention and screening. *Ann Oncol.* 2016;27(Suppl 5):v103–v10.

53. Moore HC, Unger JM, Phillips KA, et al. Goserelin for ovarian protection during breast-cancer adjuvant chemotherapy. *N Engl J Med.* 2015;372(10):923–32.

54. Biganzoli L, Wildiers H, Oakman C, et al. Management of elderly patients with breast cancer: Updated recommendations of the International Society of Geriatric Oncology (SIOG) and European Society of Breast Cancer Specialists (EUSOMA). *Lancet Oncol.* 2012;13(4):e148–e60.

55. Amant F, von Minckwitz G, Han SN, et al. Prognosis of women with primary breast cancer diagnosed during pregnancy: Results from an international collaborative study. *J Clin Oncol.* 2013;31(20):2532–39.

56. Gentilini O, Cremonesi M, Trifirò G, et al. Safety of sentinel node biopsy in pregnant patients with breast cancer. *Ann Oncol.* 2004;15(9):1348–51.

57. Han SN, Amant F, Cardonick EH, et al. Axillary staging for breast cancer during pregnancy: Feasibility and safety of sentinel lymph node biopsy. *Breast Cancer Res Treat.* 2018;168(2):551–57.

58. Ebert U, Löffler H, Kirch W. Cytotoxic therapy and pregnancy. *Pharmacol Ther.* 1997;74(2):207–20.

Controversies and Consensus in the Management of Axilla

14

Soumen Das

IMPORTANCE OF THE AXILLA

Axillary nodal status is the single most important prognostic factor of breast cancer. The Halstedian philosophy was to treat breast cancer as a local disease. The spectrum theory of breast cancer states that systemic spread without axillary involvement is very rare, and the axilla is the site of host-tumor interaction. Early breast cancer (EBC) without any axillary nodal involvement is considered a local disease, whereas EBC with axillary nodal involvement is considered a systemic disease.

STAGING OF AXILLA

Breast cancer is staged both on the basis of clinically detected findings (known as cTNM) and postoperative pathological observations (known as pTNM). Clinically detected is defined as detected by imaging studies (excluding lymphoscintigraphy) or by clinical examination having characteristics highly suspicious for malignancy or a presumed pathologic macrometastasis based on fine needle aspiration.

Evaluation of Axillary Lymph Node Status

The axilla is initially evaluated by clinical examination. If clinically significant nodes are palpable, then fine needle aspiration cytology (FNAC) from the node helps to confirm the staging. Clinically impalpable axilla is then evaluated with ultrasonography. The ultrasonographic features of a malignant node are loss of fat hilum, increased cortical thickness >3 mm, irregular shape, markedly hypoechoic cortex, round shape, and increased peripheral blood flow.

DOI: 10.1201/9780367821982-14

Regional Lymph Nodes (N)

Clinical

NX	Regional lymph nodes cannot be assessed (e.g., previously removed)
N0	No regional lymph node metastasis
N1	Metastases to movable ipsilateral level I, II axillary lymph node(s)
N2	Metastases in ipsilateral level I, II axillary lymph nodes that are clinically fixed or matted; or in clinically detected* ipsilateral internal mammary nodes in the *absence* of clinically evident axillary lymph node metastases
N2a	Metastases in ipsilateral level I, II axillary lymph nodes fixed to one another (matted) or to other structures
N2b	Metastases only in clinically detected* ipsilateral internal mammary nodes and in the *absence* of clinically evident level I, II axillary lymph node metastases
N3	Metastases in ipsilateral infraclavicular (level III axillary) lymph node(s) with or without level I, II axillary lymph node involvement; or in clinically detected* ipsilateral internal mammary lymph node(s) with clinically evident level I, II axillary lymph node metastases; or metastases in ipsilateral supraclavicular lymph node(s) with or without axillary or internal mammary lymph node involvement
N3a	Metastasis in ipsilateral infraclavicular lymph node(s)
N3b	Metastasis in ipsilateral internal mammary lymph node(s) and axillary lymph node(s)
N3c	Metastasis in ipsilateral supraclavicular lymph node(s)

Note: Clinically detected is defined as detected by imaging studies (excluding lymphoscintigraphy) or by clinical examination and having characteristics highly suspicious for malignancy or a presumed pathologic macrometastasis based on fine needle aspiration.

Pathologic (pN)*

pNX	Regional lymph nodes cannot be assessed (e.g., previously removed, or not removed for pathologic study)
pN0	No regional lymph node metastasis histologically

Note: Isolated tumor cell clusters (ITC) are defined as small clusters of cells not greater than 0.2 mm, or single tumor cells, or a cluster of fewer than 200 cells in a single histologic cross-section. ITCs may be detected by routine histology or by immunohistochemical (IHC) methods. Nodes containing only ITCs are excluded from the total positive node count for purposes of N classification but should be included in the total number of nodes evaluated.

pN0(i–)	No regional lymph node metastasis histologically, negative IHC
pN0(I+)	Malignant cells in regional lymph node(s) no greater than 0.2 mm (detected by H&E or IHC including ITC)
pN0(mol–)	No regional lymph node metastases histologically, negative molecular findings (RT-PCR)
pN0(mol+)	Positive molecular findings (RT-PCR),** but no regional lymph node metastases detected by histology or IHC

*Classification is based on axillary lymph node dissection with or without sentinel lymph node biopsy. Classification based solely on sentinel lymph node biopsy without subsequent axillary lymph node dissection is designated (sn) for "sentinel node," for example, pN0(sn).

**RT-PCR: reverse transcriptase/polymerase chain reaction.

FIGURE 14.1   Clinical axillary staging (1).

Axillary lymph node dissection (ALND) is the standard of care for node-positive axilla. Clinicoradiologically negative axilla is further evaluated by sentinel lymph node biopsy (SLNB).

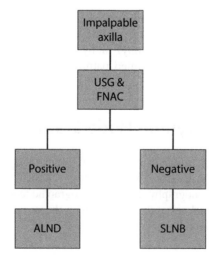

Regional Lymph Node (N)
Pathologic (pN)

pN1 Micrometastases; or metastases in 1–3 axillary lymph nodes; and/or in internal mammary nodes with metastases detected by sentinel lymph node biopsy but not clinically detected***

pN1mi Micrometastases (greater than 0.2 mm and/or more than 200 cells, but none greater than 2.0 mm)

pN1a Metastases in 1–3 axillary lymph nodes, at least one metastasis greater than 2.0 mm

pN1b Metastases in internal mammary nodes with micrometastases or macrometastases detected by sentinel lymph node biopsy but not clinically detected***

pN1c Metastases in 1–3 axillary lymph nodes and in internal mammary lymph nodes with micrometastases or macrometastases detected by sentinel lymph node biopsy but not clinically detected

pN2 Metastases in 4–9 axillary lymph nodes; or in clinically detected**** internal mammary lymph nodes in the *absence* of axillary lymph node metastases

pN2a Metastases in 4–9 axillary lymph nodes (at least one tumor deposit greater than 2.0 mm)

pN2b Metastases in clinically detected**** internal mammary lymph nodes in the *absence* of axillary lymph node metastases

pN3 Metastases in ten or more axillary lymph nodes; or in infraclavicular (level III axillary) lymph nodes; or in clinically detected**** ipsilateral internal mammary lymph nodes in the *presence* of one or more positive level I, II axillary lymph nodes; or in more than three axillary lymph nodes and in internal mammary lymph nodes with micrometastases or macrometastases detected by sentinel lymph node biopsy but not clinically detected***; or in ipsilateral supraclavicular lymph nodes

pN3a Metastases in ten or more axillary lymph nodes (at least one tumor deposit greater than 2.0 mm); or metastases to the infraclavicular (level III axillary lymph) nodes

pN3b Metastases in clinically detected**** ipsilateral internal mammary lymph nodes in the *presence* of one or more positive axillary lymph nodes; or in more than three axillary lymph nodes and in internal mammary lymph nodes with micrometastases or macrometastases detected by sentinel lymph node biopsy but not clinically detected***

pN3c Metastasis in ipsilateral supraclavicular lymph nodes

*** "Not clinically detected" is defined as not detected by imaging studies (excluding lymphoscintigraphy) or not detected by clinical examination.

*** "Clinically detected" is defined as detected by imaging studies (excluding lymphoscintigraphy) or by clinical examination and having characteristics highly suspicious for malignancy or a presumed pathologic macrometastasis based on fine needle aspiration biopsy with cytologic examination.

Distant Metastasis (M)

M0 No clinical or radiographic evidence of distant metastases

cM0(I+) No clinical or radiographic evidence of distant metastases, but deposits of molecularly or microscopically detected tumor cells in circulating blood, bone marrow, or other nonregional nodal tissue that are no larger than 0.2 mm in a patient without symptoms or signs of metastases

M1 Distant detectable metastases as determined by classic clinical and radiographic means and/or histologically proven larger than 0.2 mm

FIGURE 14.2 Pathological axillary staging (2).

AXILLARY LYMPH NODE DISSECTION

ALND involves the removal of axillary lymph nodes routinely up to level II, it can be extended up to level III depending upon involvement, as the incidence of skip metastasis is not high. A minimum of 10 lymph nodes must be removed to be regarded as adequate axillary dissection. ALND is associated with significant morbidity like lymphedema, arm movement restriction, etc.

SENTINEL LYMPH NODE DISSECTION

SLNB is the recommended method of axillary staging in node-negative disease. The sentinel node is the first node that lymph from the breast drains into. In SLNB, the node/nodes are identified by various methods (blue dye/radioactive colloid/indigo cyanine green) and surgically removed and sent for biopsy. If this node is found to be involved by a tumor, then a standard ALND is carried out.

Methods of Sentinel Node Detection

- Blue dye
- Radioactive colloid
- SentiMag
- ICG
- OSNA

SLNB with SentiMag

- Nonradioactive detection system
- Handheld magnetometer, the SentiMag
- *Magnetic tracer*: Sienna+, superparamagnetic iron oxide (SPIO)

SLNB with OSNA

- One-step nucleic acid amplification
- Isothermal technology to amplify nucleic acid (RT-LAMP)
- CK19 mRNA

The reaction procedure is based on specific isothermal technology to amplify nucleic acid (RT-LAMP) and allows the detection of cytokeratin 19 (CK19) mRNA expression. CK19 is an epithelial cell marker and is not normally present in lymph node tissue. The expression rate of CK19 mRNA correlates with the size of the metastatic foci. The benefits of using OSNA include prompt availability of results, automated and standardized test procedure, high levels of sensitivity and specificity, and the entire lymph node can be analyzed. This is a simple test to perform even without molecular biological expertise.

Sentinel Lymph Node Biopsy after Neoadjuvant Chemotherapy—Axillary De-Escalation Surgery: Targeted Axillary Dissection

Locally advanced breast cancers and some early breast cancers (HER-positive/triple-negative breast cancer [TNBC]) are treated with neoadjuvant chemotherapy (NACT) first. In the post-NACT setting, the use of SLNB is not yet well established.

Node-Negative Disease at Presentation (cN0)

Up-front SLNB can prior to NACT is feasible. This can identify unexpected lymph node metastasis and facilitate planning for axillary treatment/reconstruction. If macrometastases are seen, then treatment options are ALND or radiation as per the AMAROS trial. If micrometastases/negative SLNB is seen, no further treatment is required in selected cases. But the disadvantage is the patient will require two surgeries: SLNB prior to NACT and definitive surgery after NACT.

Patients who are node negative at the time of diagnosis and received NACT and remained node negative are candidates for SLNB as per the NSABP B-27 study. SLNB with a dual method in these patients had a sensitivity of 85%–96%, and the false-negative rate (FNR) was 6%–11%. There is emerging evidence that the prognostic value of SLNB performed after NACT is higher than SLNB performed prior to NACT. Information on the nodal metastasis response and residual cancer burden can be obtained if SLNB is done after NACT. These are prognostic factors independent of breast response.

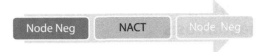

In patients who become node negative after NACT, SLNB becomes challenging. Patients with extensive axillary disease may always proceed to ALND.

The German SENTINA trial looked into patients with limited axillary disease who became node negative after NACT and reported a high FNR. Removal of four sentinel lymph nodes (SLNs), use of a dual method, and removal of the marked node is associated with lower FNR.

If SLNB shows a complete pathological response within the nodes, axillary radiotherapy is recommended. If SLNB shows Isolated Tumour Cell (ITC), micrometastases or macrometastatses, ALND is offered.

Targeted Axillary Dissection

This is an axillary staging technique whereby the lymph node positive for metastatic disease at diagnosis is marked using different methods (like carbon tattooing, radioiodine, metallic clips, ferromagnetic seeds) prior to NACT so that this marked lymph node can be removed during breast cancer surgery.

Targeted axillary dissection (TAD) is associated with 5% FNR.

Can we avoid ALND in SLNB-positive cases?
Can radiotherapy be an alternative to surgery?

AMAROS (After Mapping of Axilla: Radiotherapy or Surgery)
This study compared outcomes of ALND vs radiation therapy (RT) in SLNB-positive breast cancer patients. The 10-year follow-up data did not show any significant difference between two modalities. They concluded that ALND and axillary radiotherapy after a positive sentinel node provide excellent and comparable axillary control for patients with T1–2 primary breast cancer and no palpable lymphadenopathy. Axillary radiotherapy results in significantly less morbidity.

Can we avoid axillary treatment (surgery and RT)?
ACOSOG Z0011 Trial

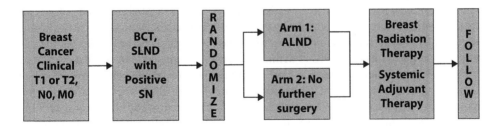

ASBS Statement
The results from ACOSOG Z0011 are potentially practice-changing, and ALND may no longer be routinely required for patients who meet all of the following criteria:

• T1–2 tumors
• One to two positive SLNs without extracapsular extension
• Patient acceptance and completion of whole-breast RT
• Patient acceptance and completion of adjuvant therapy (hormonal, cytotoxic, or both)

Axillary Reverse Mapping and Primary Lymphovenous Anastomosis

Lymphedema is a common and troublesome complication of ALND. SLNB and TAD are the major advancements to avoid ALND and subsequent lymphedema. Still, the majority of node-positive patients will require ALND.

The axilla receives lymphatics both from the arm and breast. Damage of arm lymphatics during ALND results in lymphedema. Axillary reverse mapping (ARM) is a method of delineating arm lymphatics and differentiating them from that of the breast during ALND. Once demonstrated, arm lymphatics are preserved during surgery. A total of 6%–15% of patients undergoing ALND will have a significant node on the arm lymphatics. In these cases, ALND with adequate lymph node dissection is done, and the cut end of the arm lymphatic channel is anastomosed with any of the available tributaries of the axillary vein (known as primary lymphovenous anastomosis). This allows the flow of lymph from the arm into the axillary vein thereby preventing arm edema.

NCCN RECOMMENDATIONS FOR SURGICAL AXILLARY STAGING (3)

In patients with clinically positive nodes, to determine whether ALND is needed, the panel recommends pathologic confirmation of malignancy using ultrasound-guided fine needle aspiration (FNA) or core biopsy of suspicious nodes. According to the National Comprehensive Cancer Network (NCCN) panel, the recommendation for axillary dissection of level I and II nodes is limited to patients with biopsy-proven axillary metastases. Traditional level I and level II axillary lymph nodes require that at least 10 lymph nodes be provided for pathological evaluation to accurately stage the axilla. ALND should be extended to include level III nodes only if gross disease is apparent in the level II and III nodes. In the absence of gross disease in level II nodes, lymph node dissection should include tissue inferior to the axillary vein from the latissimus dorsi muscle laterally to the medial border of the pectoralis minor muscle (level I and II).

If axillary lymph nodes are clinically negative at the time of diagnosis or if FNA/core biopsy results of suspicious nodes are negative, the panel recommends sentinel lymph node (SLN) mapping and excision. SLNs can be assessed for the presence of metastases by both hematoxylin and eosin (H&E) staining and cytokeratin immuno Histo Chemistry (IHC). The clinical significance of a lymph node that is negative by H&E staining but positive by cytokeratin IHC is not clear. Because the historical and clinical trial data on which treatment decisions are based have relied on H&E staining, the panel does not recommend routine cytokeratin IHC to define node involvement and believes that current treatment decisions should be made based solely on H&E staining. This recommendation is further supported by a randomized clinical trial (ACOSOG Z0010) for patients with H&E-negative nodes where further examination by cytokeratin IHC was not associated with improved overall survival over a median of 6.3 years. In the uncommon situation in which H&E staining is equivocal, reliance on the results of cytokeratin IHC is appropriate.

Based on the ACOSOG Z0011 trial results, for patients with T1 or T2 tumors, one to two positive SLNs, treated with lumpectomy but no preoperative systemic therapy, and where whole-breast RT (WBRT) has been received, the NCCN panel recommends no further axillary surgery. If any of the previous criteria are not met, the panel recommends level I and II axillary dissection. In the 2017 version of the NCCN guidelines, based on the results of the IBCSG 23-01 trial, the NCCN panel recommends no ALND for patients with positive SLN when that disease is only micrometastatic. According to the American Joint Committee on Cancer (AJCC) staging, micrometastatic nodal involvement is defined as a metastatic deposit >0.2 mm but ≤2.0 mm.

When sentinel nodes are not successfully identified, the panel recommends level I and II axillary dissection be performed for axillary staging.

For patients undergoing mastectomy with clinically negative axillae but with positive SLNs, the panel notes that for regional control of disease, axillary radiation may replace ALND.

REFERENCES

1. https://www.nccn.org/professionals/physician_gls/pdf/breast_blocks.pdf, page ST-1
2. https://www.nccn.org/professionals/physician_gls/pdf/breast_blocks.pdf, page ST-2
3. https://www.nccn.org/professionals/physician_gls/pdf/breast_blocks.pdf, page MS-16

Locally Advanced Breast Cancer

15

Diptendra Kumar Sarkar

DEFINITION

Locally advanced breast cancer (LABC) comprises a subset of patients who present with a large (>5 cm) mass with or without skin involvement (peau d'orange, ulceration, skin nodules) and/or involvement of the chest wall (intercostal muscles, serratus anterior, and ribs) and/or fixed axillary lymph nodes without any demonstrable systemic metastasis. Clinically, the lesions can be subclassified into large operable lesions (mostly T3 lesions in a moderate- to large-volume breast) or inoperable lesions (T4a, T4b, T4c, T4d, and/ or N2, N3 lesions).

EVALUATION OF LOCALLY ADVANCED BREAST CANCER

- *Clinical breast examination*: The hallmark of skin involvement includes peau d'orange, skin ulceration, and the presence of satellite nodules. The exact size of the lesion also needs to be assessed clinically. The surgeon needs to assess the operability of the mass if primary surgery is planned (mastectomy or breast conservation, as the case may be). Clinical evaluation of axillary node should be done to note the fixity to the surrounding structure.
- *Radiology*: Mammogram and high-resolution ultrasonography (HRUSG) of both breasts is the standard of care in most centers. Many centers prefer to use MRI (1) and PET-CT (2) to assess the mass. Apart from diagnosis, radiological evaluation of the size (helps in assessing the response to systemic therapy) of the mass, multicentricity and multifocality of the lesion, and screening the opposite breast play a major role in planning treatment.
- *Core biopsy*: Core biopsy is the gold standard for diagnosis. A marker should be placed at the center of the lesion during core biopsy. The marker helps in localizing the residual footprints of the lesions after systemic therapy. Cytology from the axillary node is done to confirm the diagnosis. Markers can also be placed in the metastatic node. The role the marking the axilla is

DOI: 10.1201/9780367821982-15

to plan for targeted axillary dissection after neoadjuvant systemic therapy (NST). While HPE remains the gold standard diagnostic tool, immunohistochemistry (IHC) (estrogen receptor [ER], progesterone receptor [PR], HER2-neu, and Ki67) plays a crucial role in planning the type and duration of NST.

- *Systemic staging*: All LABCs should have a pretreatment systemic evaluation. This includes CT of the thorax, abdomen, and pelvis and a bone scan. The PET-CT scan is being used in some centers. The sensitivity of PET in picking up liver and brain lesions and the cost involved are hindrances to its liberal use.

PRINCIPLES OF TREATMENT

- NST followed by surgery is the standard of care. The advantages of NST are as follows:
  - It takes care of systemic micrometastasis.
  - Downsizes the lump and increases incidence of breast conservation surgery.
- *In vivo* assessment of the effectivity of particular systemic therapy.
- In triple-negative and HER2-neu–enriched tumors, a complete pathological response is associated with improved survival (3). However, in luminal cancers such benefits are not observed (4).
- Radiotherapy following systemic therapy and surgery is associated with reduced locoregional failure by 20% and 5.4%–10% improved overall survival (randomized controlled trial [RCT] Danish 82b and 82c) (5, 6).
- Appropriate endocrine therapy in hormone receptor–positive cancers is indicated.

TREATMENT OPTIONS IN LABC

NST in LABC

- *Pattern of response*: NST is associated with a high complete clinical response rate ranging between 50% and 80%. A complete pathological response rate is observed between 0% and 30% (7), while a partial response is observed in most. In 60%–90% of cases, the response is concentric in nature while in the rest a patchy response is observed.
- *Evaluation of response*: The response pattern is best observed using MRI. However, MRI suffers from overdiagnosis bias in some cases. Clinicoradiological assessment using mammogram and/or HRUSG is commonly used in most centers. A pathological complete response may occur in a significant number of triple-negative breast cancer (TNBC)/HER2-neu–enriched tumors; thus, it is important to place a marker at the core of the tumor.
- *Number of cycles*: Luminal cancers are less sensitive to systemic therapy. In patients with luminal cancers, three to four cycles of systemic therapy are instituted. If the lesion is operable (mastectable or able to perform breast-conserving surgery), surgery is proceeded with. In TNBC, all the cycles are given up-front with the idea of cPR. In HER2-neu–enriched tumors, a combination of chemotherapy with trastuzumab is preferred. Pertuzumab may be added along with trastuzumab. The idea of NST is to achieve cPR. In cases where response is inadequate, TDM1 may be used.

Neoadjuvant endocrine therapy

- Neoadjuvant endocrine therapy is associated with a significant response in luminal cancers. In postmenopausal hormone receptor breast cancers, use of an aromatase inhibitor (AI) or tamoxifen is associated with an increase in the incidence of breast conservation surgery. It takes 3–4 months to achieve an appreciable response. The cPR and cCR rates are very low. These two factors are responsible for its restrictive use. In the real world, neoadjuvant endocrine therapy use is reserved for patients not considered fit for chemotherapy (typically more than 70 years of age).

Surgery in LABC

- *Surgery of the breast*: There is strong evidence (8) to recommend an increase in the incidence of breast conservation surgery after NST. In patients with cCR, marker-guided excision is preferred. In inflammatory cancers and in cancers with extensive involvement, mastectomy remains the standard of care. In patients with a patchy response and multicentric disease, breast conservation may not be feasible. Use of oncoplasty is necessary to expand the spectrum of breast conservation surgery. In gross extensive disease after NST, chest wall coverage may be achieved using latissimus dorsi myocutaneous flaps, transverse rectus abdominis myocutaneous (TRAM), and thoracoabdominal flaps. In patients with limited chest wall involvement (fewer than three ribs) without systemic disease, resection of the chest wall followed by composite reconstruction using absorbable mesh and flaps may be used.
- *Surgery of the axilla*: The standard of care in LABC is axillary lymph node dissection. The results of sentinel lymph node biopsy (SLNB) in LABC is inconclusive. Though it has shown acceptable results in a T3N0 subset, the INR and false-negative rate (FNR) are unacceptably low in T4 lesions. With the advent of NST as the standard of care, targeted axillary dissection (TAD) is fast becoming the standard. TAD involves the placement of markers (iodine seeds, marker clips, or carbon tattooing) in the metastatic node before initiation of NST. After NST, surgery is planned. The axillary surgery involves SLNB (dual technique) and dissection of pre-NST marked nodes.

Adjuvant therapy in LABC

- *Adjuvant systemic therapy*: The remaining chemotherapy and molecular targeted therapy are completed after surgery. In hormone receptor–positive cancer, appropriate endocrine therapy is given (depending on the menstrual status of the patient).
- *Adjuvant radiation therapy*: All patients with breast conservation surgery undergo standard radiation. In patients undergoing mastectomy, radiation becomes mandatory. The indications of chest wall irradiation are large tumors (>5 cm), tumors with involvement of the skin and underlying structures, close negative (<1 mm), and focal R1 status. The indications for radiotherapy to the regional nodal basin after axillary lymph node dissection (ALND) are extensive axillary nodal metastasis (>4 nodal metastasis), perinodal/extranodal disease, and inadequate axillary dissection (<10 node yield).

The indications for axillary radiation after SLNB is the presence of nodal metastasis in one to three nodes.

Inflammatory Carcinoma of the Breast

- Inflammatory carcinoma of the breast is an aggressive subtype of LABC and is characterized by:
  - *Signs of inflammation*: Rapid onset of erythema, edema.
  - *Short duration and rapid progression*: Presence of these lesions for less than 6 months.
  - Lack of a well-defined palpable lump.

- Peau d'orange that involves more than one-third of the surface area of the breast. Genetically, these cancers are different from noninflammatory invasive cancers. According to TNM staging, they are classified as T4 lesions.

Diagnosis

Triple assessment:

- Clinical characteristics.
- Radiology shows dermal thickening with metastatic nodes. Frequently a lump is not picked up, as the parenchymal involvement is diffuse and is nondescript in dense breasts.
- Radiology-guided core biopsy is the procedure of choice. In patients without well-defined parenchymal lesions, full-thickness dermal biopsy may demonstrate blockade of dermal lymphatics by cancer cells.
- Axillary nodal metastasis is a common finding, and guided fine needle aspiration cytology (FNAC) may be helpful. HPE is followed by IHC. Most patients have TNBC, and the scope of wider NST is limited.

Systemic involvement: All patients with inflammatory breast cancer (IBC) are mandatorily investigated for systemic metastasis.

Treatment

Up-front systemic therapy is the treatment of choice. In TNBC resistant to chemotherapy, immunotherapy is advocated. If local control is inadequate after systemic therapy, neoadjuvant radiation is attempted. Surgery in most circumstances is used for palliation and salvage.

PROGNOSIS IN LABC

- LABCs have a poorer prognosis with an estimated 5-year survival of only 50%–60%.
- Inflammatory breast cancer has an even lower survival rate at 35% (9).

REFERENCES

1. Radhakrishna S, Agarwal S, Parikh PM, Kaur K, Panwar S, Sharma S, et al. Role of magnetic resonance imaging in breast cancer management. *South Asian J Cancer [Internet]*. 2018 [cited 2022 Apr 14];7(2):69–71. Available from: https://www.ncbi.nlm.nih.gov/pmc/articles/PMC5909298/
2. Groheux D, Espié M, Giacchetti S, Hindié E. Performance of FDG PET/CT in the clinical management of breast cancer. *Radiology [Internet]*. 2013 Feb [cited 2022 Apr 14];266(2):388–405. Available from: https://pubs.rsna.org/doi/full/10.1148/radiol.12110853
3. Spring LM, Fell G, Arfe A, Sharma C, Greenup R, Reynolds KL, et al. Pathological complete response after neoadjuvant chemotherapy and impact on breast cancer recurrence and survival: A comprehensive meta-analysis. *Clin Cancer Res [Internet]*. 2020 Jun 15 [cited 2022 Jan 30];26(12):2838–48. Available from: https://www.ncbi.nlm.nih.gov/pmc/articles/PMC7299787/
4. Pennisi A, Kieber-Emmons T, Makhoul I, Hutchins L. Relevance of pathological complete response after neoadjuvant therapy for breast cancer. *Breast Cancer (Auckl) [Internet]*. 2016 Jul 25 [cited 2022 Jan 30]; 10:103–6. Available from: https://www.ncbi.nlm.nih.gov/pmc/articles/PMC4961053/

5. Overgaard M, Jensen MB, Overgaard J, Hansen PS, Rose C, Andersson M, et al. Postoperative radiotherapy in high-risk postmenopausal breast-cancer patients given adjuvant tamoxifen: Danish Breast Cancer Cooperative Group DBCG 82c randomised trial. *Lancet.* 1999 May 15;353(9165):1641–8.

6. Overgaard M, Hansen PS, Overgaard J, Rose C, Andersson M, Bach F, et al. Postoperative radiotherapy in high-risk premenopausal women with breast cancer who receive adjuvant chemotherapy. *N Engl J Med [Internet].* 1997 Oct 2 [cited 2022 Jan 30];337(14):949–55. Available from: https://doi.org/10.1056/NEJM199710023371401

7. Romeo V, Accardo G, Perillo T, Basso L, Garbino N, Nicolai E, et al. Assessment and prediction of response to neoadjuvant chemotherapy in breast cancer: A comparison of imaging modalities and future perspectives. *Cancers (Basel) [Internet].* 2021 Jul 14 [cited 2022 Apr 16];13(14):3521. Available from: https://www.ncbi.nlm.nih.gov/pmc/articles/PMC8303777/

8. Sun Y, Liao M, He L, Zhu C. Comparison of breast-conserving surgery with mastectomy in locally advanced breast cancer after good response to neoadjuvant chemotherapy: A PRISMA-compliant systematic review and meta-analysis. *Medicine (Baltimore).* 2017 Oct;96(43):e8367.

9. Genomic Biomarkers of Locally Advanced Breast Cancer (LABC) and Inflammatory Breast Cancer (IBC) – Duke OTC [Internet]. [cited 2022 Apr 14]. Available from: https://otc.duke.edu/technologies/genomic-biomakers-of-locally-advanced-breast-cancer-labc-and-imflammatory-breast-cancer-ibc/

Special Considerations in Breast Cancer Management

16

16A Breast Cancer and Fertility

Diptendra Kumar Sarkar, Ronit Roy, and Srija Basu

INTRODUCTION

There is an increased incidence of breast cancer in the younger population in India as compared to the West. The median age of presentation of breast cancer is 49 years in India versus 62 in the Western population (1). According to GLOBOCAN 2020 data, the estimated number of new cases of breast cancer in 2020 in India in those less than age 49 years was 1,084,868 cases (out of 3,417,166 female cancers under the age of 49 years) (2). With a later age at marriage and delayed childbearing, many premenopausal women might not have started a family or completed their family when they get diagnosed with breast cancer. Thus, fertility preservation is extremely important and a vital part in their cancer treatment.

EFFECTS OF BREAST CANCER TREATMENT ON FERTILITY

The Effects of Adjuvant Chemotherapy on Fertility

There is ovarian dysfunction following chemotherapy, which may be transient or permanent. Alkylating agents like cyclophosphamide and ifosfamide have a high risk for ovarian failure (3). The rate of chemotherapy-related amenorrhea is 30%–40% in women less than 40 years and 76%–95% in women of age 40 or more following cyclophosphamide, methotrexate, and 5-fluorouracil for at least 3 months (4) A

DOI: 10.1201/9780367821982-16

prospective study of women with breast cancer undergoing multiagent chemotherapy found an incidence of amenorrhea of 10% in women less than 35 years and 50% for women between 35 and 40 years (5). A survey revealed the prevalence of infertility in survivors of breast cancer was 15%–30% in women age less than 25 years and 25%–50% among women diagnosed by age 35 years (6).

The Effects of Adjuvant Endocrine Therapy on Fertility

Although endocrine therapies like tamoxifen don't usually cause permanent infertility, they require years of treatment (5–10 years) during which pregnancy is contraindicated. The POSITIVE trial has evaluated the temporary interruption of adjuvant endocrine therapy to attempt pregnancy in young women with previous breast cancer.It has concluded that among select group of women with hormone receptor-positive early breast cancer, temporary cessation of endocrine therapy to attempt pregnancy did not confer a higher short-term risk of breast cancer events (7).

Effect of Pregnancy on Breast Cancer Recurrence

As breast cancer is responsive to various endocrine changes, there have been concerns that pregnancy after breast cancer may worsen the prognosis. The concern is that of dormant micrometastases stimulated by gestational hormones. However, recent studies have found that subsequent pregnancy does not alter overall survival for women (8). Some believe that recurrence rates of breast carcinoma are highest during the first 2 years after treatment; thus, it may be advisable to defer pregnancy until 2 years after the end of therapy.

TABLE 16A.1   Fertility preservation methods

TECHNIQUE	ADVANTAGES	DISADVANTAGES
Surgical method of preservation of fertility		
Embryo banking	• Established technique • Predictable success rates	• Requires male gamete • Time required for ovarian stimulation • Potential for ethical issues with embryo disposition
Oocyte banking	• No male gamete required	• Time required for ovarian stimulation
In vitro maturation of oocytes	• Greater reproductive flexibility • Avoids ovarian stimulation	• Inferior oocyte yield compared to embryo/oocyte banking • Similar time required for procedure as for embryo/oocyte banking
Nonsurgical method of preservation of fertility		
Ovarian tissue cryopreservation	• Restoration of hormonal function • Potential for future pregnancy without need for artificial reproduction technology (ART) • Option for prepubertal girls	• Experimental procedure • Unproven success rates

FERTILITY PRESERVATION METHODS (3)

Nonsurgical Methods of Preserving Fertility Post–Breast Cancer Treatment

Gonadotropin-releasing hormone (GnRH) agonists: In the POEMS study, premenopausal women with operable hormone receptor–negative breast cancer were randomized to receive both standard chemotherapy and the GnRH agonist goserelin versus standard chemotherapy alone. Women randomized to receive the GnRH agonist were found less likely to experience ovarian failure. Pregnancy was more common among women in the goserelin group than in the control group. Women in the GnRH agonist group experienced longer disease-free survival as well as overall survival compared to controls (9). Another meta-analysis of five randomized controlled trials (RCTs) found ovarian sufficiency and conception rates were preserved post-chemotherapy in both hormone receptor (HR)-positive and -negative breast cancer (10). Thus, GnRH agonists may be quite useful for fertility preservation post-adjuvant therapy in both HR-positive and -negative breast cancer.

CHALLENGES AHEAD

Although with scientific advancement conceiving post–breast cancer treatment is no longer impossible, there are still quite a few hurdles. Often at the time of diagnosis the patient is overwhelmed with the disease itself and the treatment plan and is unable to take the decision for fertility preservation. Hence, it is of utmost importance that a reproductive counselor be part of her multidisciplinary team. The different methods of fertility preservation are quite expensive and may not be affordable to many. With the rise of breast cancer in younger women, fertility preservation needs to be a part of comprehensive cancer care for every premenopausal woman.

REFERENCES

1. Parmar V. Rising incidence of breast cancer in the young fertile Indian population—A reality check. *Indian J Surg Oncol [Internet]*. 2018 Sep [cited 2022 Mar 20];9(3):296–9. Available from: http://link.springer.com/10.1007/s13193-018-0800-4
2. Cancer Today [Internet]. [cited 2022 Mar 20]. Available from: http://gco.iarc.fr/today/home
3. McLaren JF, Bates GW. Fertility preservation in women of reproductive age with cancer. *Am J Obstet Gynecol [Internet]*. 2012 Dec [cited 2022 Mar 20];207(6):455–62. Available from: https://linkinghub.elsevier.com/retrieve/pii/S0002937812008617
4. Kim H, Kim SK, Lee JR, Hwang KJ, Suh CS, Kim SH. Fertility preservation for patients with breast cancer: The Korean Society for Fertility Preservation clinical guidelines. *Clin Exp Reprod Med [Internet]*. 2017 Dec [cited 2022 Mar 20];44(4):181–6. Available from: https://www.ncbi.nlm.nih.gov/pmc/articles/PMC5783914/
5. ResearchGate Link [Internet]. [cited 2022 Mar 20]. Available from: https://www.researchgate.net/publication/246806741_The_Incidence_of_Chemotherapy-induced_Amenorrhea_and_Recovery_in_Young_45-year-old_Breast_Cancer_Patients

6. Letourneau JM, Ebbel EE, Katz PP, Oktay KH, McCulloch CE, Ai WZ, et al. Acute ovarian failure underestimates age-specific reproductive impairment for young women undergoing chemotherapy for cancer. *Cancer [Internet]*. 2012 Apr 1 [cited 2022 Mar 20];118(7):1933–9. Available from: https://europepmc.org/articles/PMC3220922

7. International Breast Cancer Study Group. A Study Evaluating the Pregnancy Outcomes and Safety of Interrupting Endocrine Therapy for Young Women With Endocrine Responsive Breast Cancer Who Desire Pregnancy [Internet]. clinicaltrials.gov; 2021 Feb [cited 2022 Mar 17]. Report No.: NCT02308085. Available from: https://clinicaltrials.gov/ct2/show/NCT02308085

8. Averette HE, Mirhashemi R, Moffat FL. Pregnancy after breast carcinoma: The ultimate medical challenge. *Cancer [Internet]*. 1999 Jun 1 [cited 2022 Mar 20];85(11):2301–4. Available from: https://onlinelibrary.wiley.com/doi/10.1002/(SICI)1097-0142(19990601)85:11<2301::AID-CNCR1>3.0.CO;2-A

9. Gerber B, Ortmann O. Prevention of Early Menopause Study (POEMS): Is it possible to preserve ovarian function by gonadotropin releasing hormone analogs (GnRHa)? *Arch Gynecol Obstet*. 2014 Dec;290(6):1051–3.

10. Lambertini M, Cinquini M, Moschetti I, Peccatori F, Anserini P, Menada M, et al. Temporary ovarian suppression during chemotherapy to preserve ovarian function and fertility in breast cancer patients: A GRADE approach for evidence evaluation and recommendations by the Italian Association of Medical Oncology. *Eur J Cancer*. 2017 Jan 31;71:25–33.

Special Considerations in Breast Cancer Management

16

16B Pregnancy-Associated Breast Cancer

Diptendra Kumar Sarkar, Ronit Roy, and Srija Basu

Breast cancer is the most common form of cancer diagnosed during pregnancy, and the incidence has varied among different studies from 1:10,000 to 1:3,000 of all pregnancies (1) with a median age at diagnosis of 33 years (2). This incidence is expected to rise due to a delay in childbearing combined with the increased incidence of breast cancer in the younger population.

Pregnancy-associated breast cancer is defined as breast cancer diagnosed during pregnancy or within a year after delivery. These breast cancers are often identified in women at an earlier age, often estrogen receptor (ER)-negative, and with an advanced stage, suggesting they have some distinct characteristics (3).

RISK FACTORS

No specific risk factors for breast cancer in pregnancy are known yet. Genetic or environmental risk factors are similar to those for age-adjusted breast cancer in the general population. BRCA1- or BRCA2-positive patients may be at increased risk, but they do not have an increased incidence of pregnancy-associated breast cancer (4).

HISTORY AND CLINICAL EXAMINATION

Breast cancer in pregnancy typically presents as a painless lump palpated by the woman (5).

DOI: 10.1201/9780367821982-17

131

Physiological breast changes associated with pregnancy, including hypertrophy, mastalgia, breast engorgement, and nipple discharge, make the detection of breast cancer difficult. Therefore, a delay in diagnosis is common, leading to more advanced stages at diagnosis than in the general population. As a consequence, breast cancer in pregnancy is associated with more metastases, and subsequently poorer outcomes, than breast cancer in nonpregnant women (6).

Although about 80% of breast lesions during pregnancy are benign, any clinically suspicious or persisting breast mass during pregnancy should be investigated further (7).

DIAGNOSIS

The diagnosis of pregnancy-associated breast cancer is more difficult due to a low level of suspicion.

- A diagnostic strategy should be established in a multidisciplinary setting to reduce fetal radiation exposure. Most of the time it is indifferent from other scenarios where triple assessment plays the most crucial role.
- Breast ultrasound is highly sensitive and specific in diagnosing during pregnancy and lactation, and is considered a standard method for the evaluation of a breast lump. It is the first diagnostic instrument used by clinicians when a breast mass and the axillary area need to be assessed in a pregnant woman, since it is nonionizing and has high sensitivity and specificity (8).
- The safety and efficacy of mammography during pregnancy have been supported, with sensitivity rates from 78% to 90% in detecting suspicious features of malignancy (3). When the fetus is shielded adequately, it has been established that the estimated dose of radiation from a standard two-view mammogram is not associated with any fetal harm (3).
- Noncontrast MRI can be used when ultrasonography is inadequate. MRI of the spine can be used to asses bone metastasis (9).
- All suspicious breast masses must undergo evaluation by core needle biopsy for a tissue diagnosis.
- Fine needle aspiration cytology is not recommended as it has high false-positive as well as false-negative results in pregnancy (10).
- CT scan and nuclear imaging are contraindicated during pregnancy (11).
- Chest X-ray with abdominal shielding and abdominal ultrasonography can be used if indicated to look for metastasis (11).

TREATMENT

Once a diagnosis of malignancy is established, the treatment approach to each patient must be individualized, taking into account gestational age at presentation, stage of disease, and patient preference (Figures 16B.1 and B.2). The goal should be curative treatment of the breast cancer and preservation of pregnancy without injury to the fetus. Termination of pregnancy in the hope of minimizing hormonal stimulation of the tumor does not alter maternal survival and is not recommended (3).

Genetic counseling is also recommended for all women with breast cancer during pregnancy (3).

A multidisciplinary team with all involved specialties should assess the medical, ethical, and psychological issues.

Surgical treatment of gestational breast cancer is generally identical to that of nongestational breast cancer. There is no evidence that extraabdominal surgical procedures are associated with premature labor or that the typically used anesthetic agents are teratogenic (3).

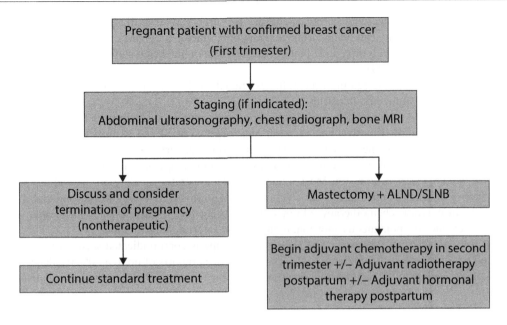

FIGURE 16B.1   Depicting the management of pregnancy-associated breast cancer in the first trimester.

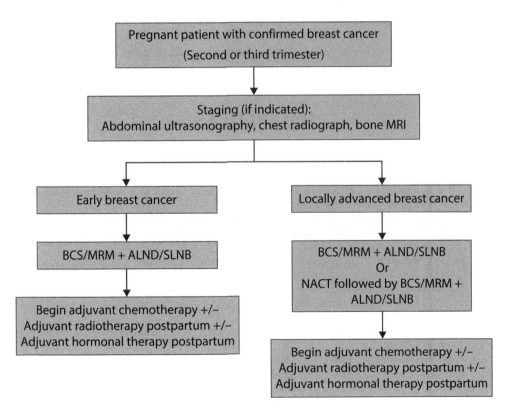

FIGURE 16B.2   Depicting the management of pregnancy-associated breast cancer in the second and third trimesters.

Modified radical mastectomy or breast-conserving surgery with axillary lymph node dissection (ALND) as primary therapy can be undertaken at any point during pregnancy. Although study numbers are relatively small, sentinel lymph node biopsy (SLNB) with radiolabeled sulfur colloid is safe in pregnant breast cancer patients (11).

The surgery may be deferred until the 12th gestational week to avoid the risk of spontaneous abortion, which is highest in the first trimester.

Radiation therapy is contraindicated during pregnancy during all trimesters (3, 11). For cancers detected during the third trimester, breast-conserving surgery (BCS) and axillary surgery can be performed safely, and radiation therapy can be delayed until after delivery.

The decision to administer neoadjuvant or adjuvant chemotherapy is difficult, as fears of congenital malformations are a serious concern. Most studies have demonstrated a safety profile and no increased risk of fetal malformation associated with chemotherapy administered during the second and third trimesters (3). In contrast, chemotherapy administration during the first trimester is associated with an increased incidence of spontaneous abortion, teratogenesis, or fetal malformations.

The role of endocrine therapy or anti-HER2-neu therapy is contraindicated secondary to teratogenicity and possible fetal malformation (3, 11). There have been reports of up to a 20% incidence of fetal abnormalities, leading to the recommendation that endocrine therapy be delayed until after delivery.

CONCLUSION

Pregnant women are more likely to be diagnosed with advanced disease than nonpregnant women. But published studies have found that patients with pregnancy-associated breast cancer have similar survivals compared to those with nonpregnancy-associated breast cancer. These findings emphasize that definitive treatment and local control of breast cancer during pregnancy are feasible and effective.

REFERENCES

1. Ruiz R, Herrero C, Strasser-Weippl K, et al. Epidemiology and pathophysiology of pregnancy-associated breast cancer: a review. *Breast* 2017; 35:136–41.
2. Beadle BM, Woodward WA, Middleton LP, et al. The impact of pregnancy on breast cancer outcomes in women < or ¼ 35 years. *Cancer* 2009; 115: 1174–84.
3. *MD Anderson Surgical Oncology Handbook*, Sixth ed., Copyright © 2019 Wolters Kluwer.
4. Wohlfahrt J, Olsen JH, Melby M. Breast cancer risk after childbirth in young women with family history (Denmark). *Cancer Causes Control* 2002; 13: 169–74.
5. Molckovsky A, Madarnas Y. Breast cancer in pregnancy: a literature review. *Breast Cancer Res Treat* 2008; 108: 333–38.
6. Ulery M, Carter L, McFarlin BL, Giurgescu C. Pregnancy-associated breast cancer: significance of early detection. *J Midwifery Womens Health* 2009; 54: 357–63.
7. Breast cancer in pregnancy. *Lancet Oncol*.
8. Navrozoglou I, Vrekoussis T, Kontostolis E, et al. Breast cancer during pregnancy: a mini-review. *Eur J Surg Oncol* 2008; 34: 837–43.
9. Oto A, Ernst R, Jesse MK, Chaljub G, Saade G. Magnetic resonance imaging of the chest, abdomen, and pelvis in the evaluation of pregnant patients with neoplasms. *Am J Perinatol* 2007; 24: 243–50.
10. Amant F, Deckers S, Van Calsteren K, et al. Breast cancer in pregnancy: recommendations of an international consensus meeting. *Eur J Cancer* 2010; 46: 3158–68.
11. NCCN Guidelines Version 5.2021: Breast Cancer during Pregnancy. https://www.nccn.org/professionals/physician_gls/pdf/breast.pdf

Male Breast Cancer

17

Raghavan Vidya, Matt Green, and Sharat Chopra

INTRODUCTION

Breast cancer in men is rare and usually accounts for nearly 1% of cases of the disease. About 350 men are diagnosed each year in the UK (1). There are a few similarities between male breast cancer and female breast cancer, but the two are different at a molecular level. Nearly 95% of male breast cancers are either luminal A or B as opposed to 73% of cases of female breast cancer (2, 3). The worldwide female-to-male incidence rate ratio of breast cancer is 122:1 (4). The lifetime risk of breast cancer in a man is about 1:1,000, whereas it is 1:8 for a woman. Breast cancer incidence rates steadily rise with age in men as in women. However, the average age for a new breast cancer diagnosis is 5 years older in men (67 years) than for women (62 years). Given the rarity of this disease, male breast cancer treatment follows similar principles as that of female breast cancer.

RISK FACTORS

Several risk factors are associated with the development of male breast cancer, including genetic, endocrine, and environmental factors. These are highlighted in Table 17.1.

The most potent risk factor for male breast cancer noted is Klinefelter syndrome. A rare condition results from the inheritance of an additional X chromosome (XXY). With increased estrogen-testosterone ratio, it is hypothesized that this leads to abnormal hormonal stimulation of cell proliferation in the mammary ductal epithelium (5).

Various testicular conditions associated with an increased risk of male breast cancer include undescended testis (cryptorchidism), orchitis, and testicular injury.

Nearly 5%–10% of female breast cancers are hereditary, with most of these mutations occurring in two genes, namely breast cancer type 1 and 2 susceptibility genes (*BRCA1* and *BRCA2*). The breast cancer risk also appears to be higher with *BRCA2* mutations as opposed to *BRCA1*. Deleterious *BRCA2* mutations are found in 4%–14% of men with breast cancer in the United Kingdom and the United States (6, 7). Approximately 15%–20% of male breast cancers are associated with a positive family history as opposed to 7% of the general male population. Other genetic mutations like Cowden syndrome, an autosomal dominant syndrome, are associated with germline mutations in the tumor suppressor gene *PTEN*, located on chromosome 10, which may also predispose to males developing

DOI: 10.1201/9780367821982-18

TABLE 17.1   Risk factors for male breast cancer

Klinefelter syndrome

Testicular conditions

Gynecomastia

Liver disease

Diabetes mellitus

Nutritional/Lifestyle

Low physical activity

Alcohol use

Obesity

Family history

BRCA carrier (*BRCA2* > *BRCA1*)

Cowden syndrome

Li–Fraumeni syndrome

Hereditary nonpolyposis colorectal cancer (Lynch) syndrome

breast cancer. Similarly, mutations in DNA repair genes such as *CHEK2* and *PALB2* are also associated with male breast cancer risk.

CLINICAL PRESENTATION AND DIAGNOSIS

Unfortunately, due to the absence of a screening program and decreased awareness, male breast cancer has been typically diagnosed later in males than in females. It often exhibits advanced disease features, such as larger tumor size, lymph node involvement, or distant metastases at the time of diagnosis. Like women, male breast cancer typically presents as a subareolar painless mass/lump (40%–50%) associated with skin/nipple retraction (9%), tethering, or rash around the nipple–areolar complex (8). Other symptoms include blood-stained nipple discharge (6%) or an enlarged axillary lymph node. Other rare presentations include association with gynecomastia. Typically, men in the clinic present with concentric enlargement often referred to as gynecomastia, a benign condition that occurs due to tissue growth behind the nipple–areolar complex. It is tender and usually bilateral but can sometimes be unilateral, as opposed to male breast cancers, which present as an eccentric hard lump sometimes fixed to the chest wall.

Initial assessment of the male patient referred to the rapid access breast clinic should follow very similar processes as a female patient. A thorough triple assessment is mandated with a high index of suspicion in a breast clinic. Ultrasound-guided core/fine needle biopsy of the breast lump and axilla assessment are usually the first modality of choice, followed by mammography (sensitivity of 92% and specificity of 90%) (9). Further assessment is generally done with a CT scan or an MRI scan to stage the disease appropriately in advanced cases.

Following confirmation of the diagnosis in the multidisciplinary setting, tumor biomarkers such as estrogen receptor, progesterone receptor, and HER2-neu receptors are also evaluated. Pathologically, nearly 10% of male breast cancers diagnosed are ductal carcinoma *in situ* (DCIS), while the remaining 90% are attributed to infiltrating ductal carcinoma (10). Very rarely, medullary, lobular, or tubular cancers are found on pathology.

Standardized TNM staging is the same as for female breast cancers and is used to classify tumors into either early breast cancers, locally advanced, or metastatic cancers.

MANAGEMENT FOR EARLY-STAGE BREAST CANCER

Surgical

The standard approach traditionally has been modified radical mastectomy with axillary lymph node clearance or sentinel lymph node biopsy (SNLB) for male breast cancers. This is due to the small size of breast tissue and its usually aggressive presentation. The role of breast-conserving treatment (BCT) is still controversial as there have been no randomized controlled trials (RCTs) to compare the safety of mastectomy vs. BCT in men. Various case series published have established the feasibility of sentinel lymph node biopsy (SNLB) (11–13) in male breast cancer patients. The American Surgical and Oncological Society has endorsed SNLB as an acceptable method of assessing the axilla in men (14). Rarely, oncoplastic techniques can be used in men because of the significant psychological and emotional impact of the physical consequences of treatment in male breast cancer management.

Endocrine Treatment

Nearly 90% of male breast cancers express the estrogen receptor (ER), and approximately 81% express the progesterone receptor (PR). In contrast, in females, 60%–70% of breast cancers are ER or PR positive (3).

The androgen receptor (AR) expression has been reported recently in some series ranging from 34% to 95% with no apparent association with other clinicopathologic features or measures of outcome (15).

Tamoxifen, a selective estrogen regulator modulator, is commonly used to treat ER+ male breast cancers for 5 years. The role of the aromatase inhibitor (AI) is extremely limited. It may cause a partial decrease in estrogens but also cause an increase in androgens, presumably from a lack of estradiol negative feedback on gonadotropin release (16). If an AI is used, it is recommended that it be coadministered with chemical or surgical castration.

Although tamoxifen is the standard treatment for ER+ tumors, it may be tolerated worse by men than by women. A series reported that men had serious side effects, such as deep vein thrombosis, decreased libido (29%), weight gain (25%), mood alterations (21%), hot flashes (21%), and depression (17%). Nearly 20%–25% of men had poor compliance because of side effects (17). This percentage is greater than the 4%–7% rate reported in women receiving adjuvant tamoxifen.

Adjuvant Radiotherapy

There are limited data on the role of radiotherapy (RT) use in male breast cancer. Men tend to get more RT than women due to their aggressive presentation. In some retrospective series, adjuvant RT appears to prevent local recurrences but without any survival benefit. It is recommended that all patients who undergo BCS have adjuvant RT. Adjuvant postmastectomy RT is often recommended for men with involved lymph nodes or tumors > 5 cm or with positive resection margins (18).

Role of Neoadjuvant or Adjuvant Chemotherapy

The data for using systemic treatment in male breast cancers are limited and are derived mainly from female breast cancer treatments. Adjuvant chemotherapy should be considered for men with intermediate- or high-risk primary breast cancer and is mandatory in ER-negative or triple-negative tumors. Although there are no long-term data regarding the benefit of trastuzumab in male breast cancers (19), its use in

Her-2+ patients is recommended based on female breast cancers. Use of neoadjuvant systemic treatment in male breast cancer has been reported in a study from Chennai, India, showing a pathological complete response rate of 45% (20).

MANAGEMENT OF METASTATIC MALE BREAST CANCER

Male breast cancers are almost always ER+; the preferred first-line therapy of metastatic disease is endocrine therapy with tamoxifen unless relapse occurs while on treatment with this agent. The other therapeutic options are an AI (preferably associated with a luteinizing hormone–releasing agonist) or fulvestrant (21). Chemotherapy may be reserved for use in highly symptomatic patients or in visceral crisis. Combinations of endocrine with targeted agents, such as mTOR and CDK inhibitors can be used in metastatic patients. Recently, the Food and Drug Administration (FDA) approved the use of palbociclib, a selective cyclin-dependent kinase 4/6 inhibitor with proven efficacy for HR-positive/HER2-negative cancer in combination with an AI or fulvestrant for advanced male breast cancers.

GENE EXPRESSION ASSAY STUDIES

Of all the available gene assays, only Oncotype DX has been tested on male breast cancer. This assay examines the expression of 16 cancer-associated genes and 5 reference genes to estimate a recurrence risk score (RS): (low < 18, intermediate 18 to < 31, and high score > 31). Various studies have demonstrated the use of the Oncotype DX scoring in providing adjuvant chemotherapy in selected male breast cancer patients with a higher recurrence score (22–25). A study involving nearly 668 node-negative ER+ cancers randomized to tamoxifen or placebo followed by Oncotype DX assay showed the 10-year distant recurrence rate in the low RS group to be 7% compared with 14% in the intermediate group and 31% in the high-risk group (26). The study showed that the Oncotype DX test had predictive power independent of tumor grade or size. This study validates the 21-gene reverse transcriptase polymerase chain reaction (RT-PCR) assay and recurrence score algorithm's ability to quantify the likelihood of distant recurrence in breast cancer patients who are node-negative and ER-positive and have been treated with tamoxifen.

FOLLOW-UP

- Regular clinical follow-ups to check for recurrences, bone pain, and new lumps should be offered along with mammography.
- Genetic referral should be done to look for any germline mutations.
- Psychological and other forms of counseling should be offered.
- Avoid the use of testosterone/androgen supplementation in male breast cancer patients.

KEY POINTS

- Male breast cancer accounts for 1% of breast cancers.
- Male breast cancer is similar to female breast cancer but has a more aggressive presentation.

- It is treated mainly with modified radical mastectomy and SLNB or axillary lymph node clearance.
- More than 90% of male breast cancers are ER+ tumors, so endocrine treatment plays a crucial role in adjuvant management.
- There is a role of the gene expression assay in managing male breast cancers similar to female breast cancers.

REFERENCES

1. https://www.cancerresearchuk.org/about-cancer/breast-cancer/stages-types-grades/types/male-breast-cancer.
2. Shaaban AM, Ball GR, Brannan RA, Cserni G, Di Benedetto A, Dent J, Fulford L, Honarpisheh H, Jordan L, Jones JL, et al. A comparative biomarker study of 514 matched cases of male and female breast cancer reveals gender-specific biological differences. *Breast Cancer Res Treat.* 2012;133:949–958. DOI: 10.1007/s10549-011-1856-9.
3. Ge Y, Sneige N, Eltorky MA, Wang Z, Lin E, Gong Y, Guo M. Immunohistochemical characterisation of subtypes of male breast carcinoma. *Breast Cancer Res.* 2009;11:R28. DOI: 10.1186/bcr2258.
4. Ly D, Forman D, Ferlay J, et al. An international comparison of male and female breast cancer incidence rates. *Int J Cancer.* 2013;132:1918–1926.
5. Louise A Brinton. Breast cancer risk among patients with Klinefelter syndrome. *Acta Paediatr.* 2011;100:814–818.
6. Friedman LS, Gayther SA, Kurosaki T, et al. Mutation analysis of BRCA1 and BRCA2 in a male breast cancer population. *Am J Hum Genet.* 1997;60(2):313–319.
7. Basham VM, Lipscombe JM, Ward JM, et al. BRCA1 and BRCA2 mutations in a population-based study of male breast cancer. *Breast Cancer Res.* 2002;4(1):R2.
8. Fentiman IS, Fourquet A, Hortobagyi GN. Male breast cancer. *Lancet.* 2006;367:595–604.
9. Evans GF, Anthony T, Turnage RH, et al. The diagnostic accuracy of mammography in the evaluation of male breast disease. *Am J Surg.* 2001;181:96–100.
10. Giordano SH, Schröder CP, Poncet C, van Leeuwen-Stok E, Linderholm B, Abreu MH, et al. Clinical and biological characterisation of male breast cancer (BC) EORTC 10085/TBCRC 029/BOOG 2013–02/BIG 2–07: baseline results from the prospective registry. *Cancer Res.* 2018;78(4 Supplement):P5-23-01.
11. Albo D, Ames FC, Hunt KK, et al. Evaluation of lymph node status in male breast cancer patients: a role for sentinel lymph node biopsy. *Breast Cancer Res Treat.* 2003;77:9–14.
12. Goyal A, Horgan K, Kissin M, et al. Sentinel lymph node biopsy in male breast cancer patients. *Eur J Surg Oncol.* 2004;30:480–483.
13. Gentilini O, Chagas E, Zurida S, et al. Sentinel lymph node biopsy in male patients with early breast cancer. *Oncologist.* 2007;12:512.
14. Lyman GH, Giuliano AE, Smerfield MR, et al. American Society of Clinical Oncology guideline recommendations for sentinel lymph node biopsy in early stage breast cancer. *J Clin Oncol.* 2005;23:7703.
15. Kidwai N, Gong Y, Sun X, et al. Expression of androgen receptor and prostate-specific antigen in male breast carcinoma. *Breast Cancer Res.* 2004;6:R18–R23.
16. Mauras N, O'Brien KO, Klein KO, Hayes V. Estrogen suppression in males: metabolic effects. *J Clin Endocrinol Metab.* 2000;85(7):2370–2377.
17. Anelli TF, Anelli A, Tran KN, et al. Tamoxifen administration is associated with a high rate of treatment-limiting symptoms in male breast cancer patients. *Cancer.* 1994;74:74–77.
18. Schuchart U, Seegenschmiedt MH, Kirschner MJ, et al. Adjuvant radiotherapy for breast carcinoma in men: a 20-year clinical experience. *Am J Clin Oncol.* 1996;19:330.
19. Giordano SH, Perkins GH, Broglio K, et al. Adjuvant systemic therapy for male breast carcinoma. *Cancer.* 2005;104(11):2359–2364.
20. Shanta V, Swaminathan R, Rama R, Radhika R. Retrospective analysis of locally advanced noninflammatory breast cancer from Chennai, South India, 1990–1999. *Int J Radiat Oncol Biol Phys.* 2008;70:51–58.
21. Masci G, Gandini C, Zuradelli M, Pedrazzoli P, Torrisi R, Lutman FR, et al. Fulvestrant for advanced male breast cancer patients: a case series. *Ann Oncol.* 2011;22(4):985.
22. Henry LR, Stojadinovic A, Swain SM, Prindiville S, Cordes R, Soballe PW. The influence of a gene expression profile on breast cancer decisions. *J Surg Oncol.* 2009;99:319e23.

23. Kiluk JV, Lee MC, Park CK, Meade T, Minton S, et al. Male breast cancer: management and follow-up recommendations. *Breast J.* 2011;17:503e9.
24. Grenader T, Yerushalmi R, Tokar M, Fried G, Kaufman B, et al. The 21-gene recurrence score assay (Oncotype DX™) in estrogen receptor-positive male breast cancer: experience in an Israeli cohort. *Oncology.* 2014;87:1e6.
25. Turashvili G, Gonzalez-Loperena M, Brogi E, Dickler M, Norton L, Morrow M, Wen HY. The 21-gene recurrence score in male breast cancer. *Ann Surg Oncol.* 2018 Jun;25(6):1530–1535. DOI: 10.1245/s10434-018-6411-z.
26. Paik S, Shak S, Tang G, Kim C, Baker J, Cronin M, Baehner FL, Walker MG, Watson D, Park T, Hiller W, Fisher ER, Wickerham DL, Bryant J, Wolmark N. A multigene assay to predict recurrence of tamoxifen-treated, node-negative breast cancer. *N Engl J Med.* 2004 Dec 30;351(27):2817–2826. DOI: 10.1056/NEJMoa041588.

Prognostication in Breast Cancer

18

Srija Basu and Diptendra Kumar Sarkar

Breast cancer is considered a heterogenous disease.

- A prognostic factor is defined as the likely outcome (disease-free or overall survival) of a cancer at the time of diagnosis or surgery in the absence of any systemic treatment.
- A predictive factor of a cancer is defined as factors which measure the likely response to a particular form of treatment.

The outcome of a cancer depends on tumor characteristics and host factors.

Demographic factors

- Age
- Sex
- Menopausal status
- Ethnicity

Tumor characteristics

- Tumor size
- Nodal status
- Grade
- Metastasis
- Histological subtypes

Tumor growth factors or biomarkers

- Estrogen and progesterone receptor status
- HER2-neu receptor expression
- Ki67 status
- Androgen receptor status
- *Others*: Mitotic index, thymidine labeling index, and S phase fraction
- Molecular subtypes
- Proliferative genes (gene expression)
- Host immune status

DOI: 10.1201/9780367821982-19

IMPLICATIONS OF PROGNOSTICATION AND PREDICTION

- To identify a subset of patients in whom systemic therapy and its side effects can be avoided.
- To identify poor prognostic cancers where aggressive treatment is needed.
- To predict appropriate treatment according to the biological character.

The Key Prognostic Factors and Their Impact on Treatment

TABLE 18.1 Demographic factors

FACTOR	STATUS	IMPACT
Age	• Young cancers are associated with poorer outcome	• Aggressive systemic treatment is recommended
Sex	• The prognosis of breast cancer is the same in both sexes according to T status but there is faster stage migration	• In males breast cancer is likely to become inoperable earlier
Menopausal status	• Premenopausal cancers are more likely to be TNBC • Postmenopausal cancers are more likely to be luminal (1, 2)	• Premenopausal cancers require aggressive treatment
Ethnicity	• The survival in Asian, African, and African American and Hispanic patients is relatively poorer compared to Whites (3, 4)	• This may be related to later detection and higher incidence of TNBC

TABLE 18.2 Tumor characteristics

FACTOR	STATUS	IMPACT
Tumor size	• The risk of recurrence increases in a linear fashion for patients with fewer than four lymph nodes. • Thereafter, nodal status plays a larger role.	• In lesions less than 1–2 cm, adjuvant systemic therapy is based on risk stratification. • In lesions more than 5 cm, the chance of occult metastasis is high, and feasibility of breast conservation reduces. • In these patients, NST is standard of care.
Nodal status	• It can be stratified into N0, N1–3, N3–9, and N > 9 nodes. • The larger the number of nodes involved, the poorer the outcome.	• N0 axilla: SLNB N1–3 nodes: Axillar RT N > 3 nodes: ALND • Or NST followed by TAD
Grade	• Higher grade associated with poor prognosis.	• Aggressive adjuvant therapy recommended.
Metastasis	• M1 disease has poor prognosis.	• Palliative treatment.
Histopathological subtypes	• Invasive carcinoma of no special type (NOS) refers to infiltrating duct carcinoma. • It shows a higher incidence of lymph node metastasis and carries a poorer outcome compared to special subtypes. • Infiltrating lobular carcinoma shows a higher chance of contralateral spread (5%–19%). • Other special types (mucinous, papillary, medullary, tubular) carry a better outcome. • Metaplastic carcinoma carries a poor outcome.	• Attempts have been made to correlate with HP subtype and biological subtype. • Presence of LVI, PNI in HPE indicates need for aggressive treatment. • Presence of E-cadherin expression in ILC signifies loss of adhesion.

TABLE 18.3   Biomarkers and growth factors

FACTOR	STATUS	IMPACT
Hormone receptor status (ER/PR)	• ER/PR-negative cancers carry poorer prognosis compared to dual positive lesions • At least 1% positive nuclear staining	• Selection of hormone therapy depends on menopausal and hormone receptor status
Androgen receptor status		
HER2-neu–enriched cancer	• Associated with high cell survival, proliferation, and metastasis • IHC staining of 3+ is considered positive • In 2+ (equivocal cases) cases, FISH confirmation is necessary • These cancers are likely to be of higher grade, lack hormone receptors, and have a higher nodal burden and poorer prognosis	• Selection of targeted therapy (trastuzumab, pertuzumab, TDM1, and lapatinib) depends on overexpression
Ki67	• It is associated with cell proliferation • Ki67 is present in G1, G2, S, and mitotic phase but is absent in resting cells (G0) • A cutoff of 20% is considered positive	• Grade is considered a surrogate marker • It helps in differentiating between luminal A and B cancers
OTHERS: Mitotic index, thymidine labelling index and S phase fraction	• Thought of as promising tools • Except for mitotic index, the rest are usually nonspecific markers	• Not useful in clinical practice

Molecular Subtypes

The understanding of the microscopic anatomy of the breast has revolutionized the prognostication. Each lining duct has inner luminal cells and outer myoepithelial cells. Cancer arising from different layers tends to behave differently. Broadly, they are classified into luminal A, luminal B, HER2-neu–enriched, and basal-like (triple-negative breast cancer [TNBC]).

The TNBC, HER2-neu–enriched, and luminal B cancers have a higher propensity for earlier recurrence compared to luminal A cancers. Typically, TNBCs show higher recurrence rates in the first 5 years after detection and treatment. By the end of 7 years, both the TNBC and non-TNBC recurrence curves meet (5).

The predictive value of molecular subtypes is very high. Luminal cancers are likely to be less chemosensitive. Luminal cancers with early breast cancers are best treated with surgery followed by systemic therapy. In locally advanced luminal subtype cancers, three cycles of neoadjuvant systemic therapy (NST) are preferred followed by surgery (the number of cycles can be increased depending on operability). In HER2-neu–enriched cancers, NST is used in most tumors more than 2 cm in size. In TNBC, the same principle is followed. This is based on the fact that complete pathological response is associated with improved survival in these two subtypes (6, 7). In luminal lesions, cPR is not associated with improved survival.

Thus, molecular subtypes have both prognostic and predictive importance. They also lay the foundation for personalized therapy in breast cancer treatment.

Gene Expression and Prognostication

Complete gene sequencing has opened up a new understanding in breast cancer. Gene expression profiling can stratify breast cancer into high-, intermediate-, or low-risk cancers. Treatment can also be tailor-made according to the expression scores. The genes involved in assessing risk stratification of breast cancers are proliferating, antiapoptotic, and angiogenesis-promoting ones. Various gene expressions are evaluated and validated based on clinical trials.

MOLECULAR TEST	ELIGIBILITY	IMPLICATIONS
Oncotype DX	• ER-positive, HER2-neu–negative EBC, node negative or positive (1 to 3 nodes) • RTPCR is used to measure expression of 16 tumor-related and 5 reference genes	• TAILORx trial established it as the standard of care. Patients with recurrence score (RS) • *0 to 25*: Endocrine therapy alone • *26 to 100*: Significant benefit with chemotherapy
MammaPrint	• ER-positive/ER-negative EBC with fewer than 3 nodes • 70-gene assay using microarray technique	• The MINDACT (EORTC 10041/BIG3-04) study, a multicenter, randomized phase 3 clinical trial confirmed the clinical utility of MammaPrint to identify patients with early breast cancer who may safely avoid postsurgery chemotherapy
Prosigna Breast Cancer Prognostic Gene Signature Assay	• ER-positive/ER-negative EBC with fewer than 3 nodes	• The Prosigna Assay measures tumor expression levels of 50 genes used in the PAM50 classification algorithm, weighted together with clinical variables, to predict the risk of distant breast cancer recurrence within 10 years
EndoPredict Test	• ER-positive/ER-negative EBC with fewer than 3 nodes • The test combines a 12-gene molecular score with tumor size and node to give a risk score	• EXET trial is an ongoing trial The purpose of this study is to evaluate the impact of using EndoPredict clinically to inform treatment decisions for extended endocrine therapy and the subsequent impact on patient outcomes
CanAssist Breast	• ER-positive/ER-negative EBC with fewer than 3 nodes	• CanAssist Breast (CAB) is an immunohistochemistry (IHC)–based test • This test uses a machine learning algorithm • It assesses the expression of five biomarkers (CD44, ABCC4, ABCC11, N-cadherin, pan-cadherin) and arrives at a score predictive of distant recurrence, along with three clinical parameters (tumor size, grade, and node status)

Host Immunity

Breast cancer outcome traditionally has been viewed from the point of view of the tumor characteristic. Cancer outcome depends on host-tumor interactions. Thus, host immunity plays an important role in disease outcome.

- *Tumor infiltrating lymphocyte (TIL)*: Infiltration of lymphocytes is thought of as a good prognostic marker (8). However, recent studies show contradictory data (9).
- *T-regulatory and T-cytotoxic cells*: Presence of cytotoxic-effector cells is likely to lead to tumor destruction, whereas T-regulatory cells inhibit cell destruction.
- *Immune checkpoint inhibitors*: Tumor cells evade the host immunity and remain unaffected. This is because the cancer cells have a protein, PD L-1, which is expressed on its surface. Upregulation of PD L-1 makes the cancer cell evade the host immune system. High expression

of PD L-1 is associated with aggressive behavior and poorer outcome. The PD L-1 interacts with the PD-1, which is situated on the surface of the T lymphocytes. There is higher expression of PD L-1 in TNBC and HER2-neu–enriched cancers. Overexpression of PD L-1 and PD-1 is associated with a poor prognosis. Overexpression is predictive of therapeutic immunotherapy.

REFERENCES

1. vanBarele M, Heemskerk-Gerritsen BAM, Louwers YV, Vastbinder MB, Martens JWM, Hooning MJ, Jager A . Estrogens and progestogens in triple negative breast cancer: Do they harm? *Cancers* 2021;13:2506. [Internet]. [cited 2022 Jan 14]. Available from: https://www.ncbi.nlm.nih.gov/pmc/articles/PMC8196589/pdf/cancers-13-02506.pdf
2. Mills M, Liveringhouse C, Lee F, Nanda RH, Ahmed KA, Washington IR, et al. The prevalence of luminal B subtype is higher in older postmenopausal women with ER+/HER2− breast cancer and is associated with inferior outcomes. J Geriatr Oncol. 2021 Mar;12(2):219–26.
3. Yedjou CG, Sims JN, Miele L, Noubissi F, Lowe L, Fonseca DD, et al. Health and racial disparity in breast cancer. Adv Exp Med Biol [Internet]. 2019 [cited 2022 Jan 14];1152:31–49. Available from: https://www.ncbi.nlm.nih.gov/pmc/articles/PMC6941147/
4. Özdemir BC, Dotto G-P. Racial differences in cancer susceptibility and survival: More than the color of the skin? Trends Cancer [Internet]. 2017 Mar [cited 2022 Jan 14];3(3):181–97. Available from: https://www.ncbi.nlm.nih.gov/pmc/articles/PMC5518637/
5. Jatoi I, Anderson WF, Jeong J-H, Redmond CK. Breast cancer adjuvant therapy: Time to consider its time-dependent effects. J Clin Oncol [Internet]. 2011 Jun 10 [cited 2022 Mar 21];29(17):2301–4. Available from: http://ascopubs.org/doi/10.1200/JCO.2010.32.3550
6. Spring LM, Fell G, Arfe A, Sharma C, Greenup R, Reynolds KL, et al. Pathological complete response after neoadjuvant chemotherapy and impact on breast cancer recurrence and survival: A comprehensive meta-analysis. Clin Cancer Res [Internet]. 2020 Jun 15 [cited 2022 Jan 30];26(12):2838–48. Available from: https://www.ncbi.nlm.nih.gov/pmc/articles/PMC7299787/
7. Pennisi A, Kieber-Emmons T, Makhoul I, Hutchins L. Relevance of pathological complete response after neoadjuvant therapy for breast cancer. Breast Cancer Basic Clin Res [Internet]. 2016 Jul 25 [cited 2022 Jan 30];10:103–6. Available from: https://www.ncbi.nlm.nih.gov/pmc/articles/PMC4961053/
8. Chen T-H, Zhang Y-C, Tan Y-T, An X, Xue C, Deng Y-F, et al. Tumor-infiltrating lymphocytes predict prognosis of breast cancer patients treated with anti-HER-2 therapy. Oncotarget. 2017 Jan 17;8(3):5219–32.
9. Tumor-infiltrating lymphocytes are associated with poor prognosis in invasive lobular breast carcinoma. Mod Pathol [Internet]. [cited 2022 Jan 14]. Available from: https://www.nature.com/articles/s41379-020-0561-9

Management of Metastatic Breast Cancer

19

Kakali Choudhury

INTRODUCTION

Metastatic breast cancer (MBC) is defined as the breast cancer spreading beyond the breast, chest wall, and ipsilateral regional lymph nodes. The most common sites for metastasis are bone, lung, liver, lymph nodes, chest wall, and brain. Although MBC is not curable, it is always treatable. As the treatments are continually improving, there is an increasing chance of higher survival with better quality of life for MBC patients.

EPIDEMIOLOGY

MBC comprises 6%–10% of the newly diagnosed breast cancer cases in the United States and is higher in developing countries (1). Breast cancer is the second most common cause of cancer death worldwide (1). MBC is mostly the cause of this death. The 5-year survival of MBC is 28% and 22% in females and males, respectively.

PATHOPHYSIOLOGY

Every breast cancer patient has the potential to metastasize, and this is difficult to predict beforehand. There is an increased chance of metastasis with higher tumor staging and grading, skin infiltration, and higher nodal involvement. Tumor size and nodal involvement are the strongest prognostic factors. Among histological subtypes metaplastic, undifferentiated, and other rare subtypes have poorer outcomes; tubular, mutinous, and medullary are better in terms of outcome than the invasive ductal or lobular variety.

DOI: 10.1201/9780367821982-20

Other factors like younger age, premenopausal status, obesity, smoking, and pregnancy are also associated with a higher risk of metastasis. Hormonal receptor status and gene signatures are also important. HER2-neu overexpression is an independent risk factor for metastasis. A higher Oncotype DX score is associated with a higher risk of recurrence. Hormone receptor–positive disease mostly metastasizes to bones, whereas hormone receptor–negative/HER2-neu–positive patients have visceral spread initially. Lobular carcinoma has a tendency for a serosal spread like to the pleura or peritoneum.

CLASSIFICATION

Most commonly, metastasis occurs in a person previously treated for breast cancer at the early stage and locally advanced stage. If a patient presents with metastasis, it is called *de novo* MBC. MBC can be divided according to the tumor burden, e.g., bone-only metastasis, oligometastasis (one to five lesions), and visceral metastasis with or without organ crisis. It can be divided also by hormonal receptor status, HER2-neu overexpression, and Ki67 (proliferative index). These classifications are useful in management decisions for MBC patients.

CLINICAL FEATURES

The clinical presentation of MBC depends on the site of metastasis. Symptoms are nonspecific and need further investigation for confirmation. Bone metastasis presents with bone, back, neck or joint pain, bone fracture (pathological), swelling, paraplegia, or paresis (spinal cord compression). Headache, nausea, seizures, dizziness, confusion, vision changes, personality changes, and loss of balance are common symptoms for brain metastasis. Lung metastasis may cause shortness of breath, chest pain, persistent dry cough, etc. Nausea, loss of appetite, pain in the abdomen, and jaundice may be the presentation of liver metastasis. Weight loss, loss of appetite, fatigue, and nausea are the nonspecific symptoms for spread of the disease.

Metastasis can also present without any symptoms and be detected by routine staging workup in a newly diagnosed case or during follow-up investigations in a previously treated patient. When a patient is diagnosed with MBC, a thorough investigation should be performed to confirm the histology and to know the extent of metastasis. FDG PET-CT scan is helpful to know the extent of disease and also response evaluation after treatment. Biopsy is needed to confirm the histology and also hormone receptor status and HER2-neu overexpression.

MANAGEMENT

MBC is not considered a curative disease, and the goals of the treatment are to increase survival, relieve symptoms and complications, decrease tumor burden, and improve quality of life. A small group of MBC patients with oligometastasis or bone-only metastasis may have a longer survival (in years) with a good quality of life.

Management of MBC requires a multidisciplinary team consisting of a medical oncologist, surgical oncologist, radiation oncologist, radiologist, and pathologist along with physician support, oncology nurses, counselors, dietitian, genetic counselors, etc.

Treatment options for MBC depend on the site of metastasis, hormone receptor status, and Her 2 neu overexpression of tumor cells; genetic mutations of tumor cells; and also symptoms of metastasis, previous cancer treatment received, and performance status of the patient. Hence, a detailed medical history and thorough physical examination, along with appropriate investigations, are needed to assess the symptoms, disease extent and tumor biology, functional status, and any residual toxicity of previous treatments. The outcome of treatment mostly depends on the extent of previous treatment received and disease-free interval with bone or soft tissue metastasis and good performance status; hormone-positive and HER2-neu–positive patients also show longer survival compared to heavily treated patients with a shorter treatment-free period and visceral metastasis with more symptoms and comorbidities.

Clinical guidelines for the management of MBC are quite open ended, and patient preference and illness experience are equally important along with clinical decision for treatment selection. The options for treatment are hormone therapy, chemotherapy, targeted therapy, and immunotherapy along with some role for radiotherapy and surgery.

Hormone Therapy

Hormone therapy, also known as endocrine therapy (ET), is a major treatment option in hormone-positive tumors. The patients with hormone-sensitive tumors with minimal symptoms and without visceral crisis are suitable candidates for ET. Single-agent therapy is the standard of care. A combination of ET has not shown any benefit. Chemoendocrine therapy has not shown any improvement in survival (2). Sequential treatment with a single agent is recommended until the third line, although the duration of response gradually decreases. Table 19.1 contains the list of available ETs for MBC.

In premenopausal MBC, ovarian suppression or ablation improves survival along with tamoxifen or an aromatase inhibitor (AI) (3). For postmenopausal patients, ET options are tamoxifen, AIs, fulvestrant, or progestin agents. AIs are the ET of choice in a patient treated with tamoxifen in adjuvant setting (3, 4) and have a moderate clinical advantage as initial therapy in MBC (5, 6). In treatment-naive patients, the SWOG 0226 trial has shown a combination of AI with fulvestrant improved progression-free survival (PFS) and overall survival (OS), but this advantage is not present in patients previously treated with tamoxifen or AI. The FALCON trial compared fulvestrant and anastrozole in hormone therapy–naive advanced breast cancer, and there is a comparable outcome in its use as first-line therapy for ER-positive MBC (7). Hence, first-line ET for MBC includes AI, fulvestrant, or a combination, especially for hormone-naive patients.

Resistance to AI therapy is mostly due to acquired mutation in the ER gene (*ESR1*) and develops in approximately 40% of patients with recurrent or progressive disease with AI therapy. Fulvestrant is still active in this condition (8).

Cyclin-dependent kinases (CDKs) are important cell cycle regulators. CDK4/6 inhibitors are studied with AIs in first-line ET and with fulvestrant in a second-line setting, and in both conditions shows improved PFS compared to ET alone, but not OS. Table 19.2 shows the list of trials (9–13).

TABLE 19.1   Endocrine therapies for metastatic breast cancer

- Ovarian suppression/Ablation (premenopausal women)
- Selective estrogen receptor modulators (tamoxifen, toremifene)
- Aromatase inhibitors (anastrozole, letrozole, exemestane; postmenopausal women)
- Antiestrogens (fulvestrant, postmenopausal women)
- Progestins (megestrol and medroxyprogesterone)
- Other steroid hormones (high-dose estrogens, androgens, principally of historical interest)

TABLE 19.2   Trials of CDK4/6 inhibitors in ER-positive, HER2-negative metastatic breast cancer

LINE OF THERAPY	STUDY NAME	SCHEMA	MEDIAN PFS (mo)	HAZARD RATIO
First	PALOMA-2 427	Letrozole +/– palbociclib	14.5 vs. 24.8	0.58
First	MONALEESA-2 428	Letrozole +/– ribociclib	14.7 vs. <26	0.56
First	MONARCH-3 429	AI +/– Abemaciclib	14.7 vs. <25	0.54
Second	PALOMA-3 430	Fulvestrant +/– Palbociclib	3.8 vs. 9.2	0.42
Second	MONARCH-2 431	Fulvestrant +/– Abemaciclib	9.3 vs. 16.4	0.55

AI: Sromatase inhibitor, CDK: Cyclin-dependent kinase, ER: Estrogen receptor, HER2: Human epidermal growth factor receptor, MONALEESA: Mammary Oncology Assessment of LEE011's Efficacy and Safety, MONARCH: Nonsteroidal Aromatase Inhibitors plus Abemaciclib in Postmenopausal Women with Breast Cancer, PALOMA: Palbociclib: Ongoing Trials in the Management of Breast Cancer, PFS: Progression-free survival.

Palbociclib and ribociclib have a greater risk of neutropenia, and abemaciclib causes diarrhea.

Everolimus, an mTOR inhibitor, shows enhanced activity of ET in a resistant setting (14). A combination of exemestane and everolimus shows increased PFS in AI-resistant patients but with significant toxicities like stomatitis, hyperglycemia, and pneumonitis.

Chemotherapy

Cytotoxic chemotherapy is the standard of care in MBC irrespective of hormone receptor status and also along with other targeted therapies. As chemotherapy has several toxicities like nausea, vomiting, alopecia, fatigue, diarrhea, myelosuppression, neuropathy, and cardiac toxicities, the benefit of palliation and toxicities should be compared carefully. Tumor response to chemotherapy is a surrogate for increased disease control and survival (15).

Single-agent chemotherapy is the preferred choice for MBC, as there is better understanding of benefit from the drug and usually lesser toxicity. Combination chemotherapy can be preferred in extensive visceral disease or impending visceral crisis, but benefit is not proven in prospective trials. Duration of response gradually decreases with the subsequent line of chemotherapy. Chemotherapy can be withheld with adequate response and symptom relief and can be restarted after disease progression or symptom recurrence. Table 19.3

TABLE 19.3   Approved chemotherapy agents and combinations for advanced breast cancer

SINGLE AGENTS	COMBINATION REGIMENS
Anthracyclines (doxorubicin, epirubicin, pegylated liposomal doxorubicin)	Cyclophosphamide/Anthracycline ± 5 fluorouracil regimens (such as AC, EC, CEF, CAF, FEC, FAC)
Taxanes (paclitaxel, docetaxel, nanoparticle albumin-bound paclitaxel)	CMF
5-Fluorouracil (5-fluorouracil by IV infusion or oral capecitabine)	Anthracyclines/Taxanes (such as Doxorubicin/Paclitaxel or doxorubicin/Docetaxel)
Vinca alkaloids (vinorelbine, vinblastine)	Docetaxel/Capecitabine
Gemcitabine	Gemcitabine/Paclitaxel
Platinum salts (cisplatin, carboplatin)	Taxane/Platinum regimens (such as paclitaxel/Carboplatin or docetaxel/Carboplatin)
Ixabepilone	Ixabepilone/Capecitabine
Cyclophosphamide	
Eribulin	

A: Doxorubicin, C: Cyclophosphamide, E: epirubicin, F: 5-Fluorouracil, M: Methotrexate, IV: Intravenous.

shows chemotherapeutic agents approved for treatment of MBC (16). Anthracyclines and taxanes are the most effective drugs for breast cancer. The regimen or drug selection is guided by previous chemotherapeutic agent received, residual toxicities of previous treatments (like neuropathy and cardiac morbidity), performance status of patient, and patient's preference.

Dose escalation and bone marrow or stem cell transplant have not shown any benefit in MBC.

Anti-HER2 Therapy

HER2 targeted therapy has revolutionized the treatment outcome in HER2-positive breast cancer which had short disease-free survival (DFS) and OS when treated with conventional therapy. Signal transduction by the HER2 family promotes proliferation, survival, and invasiveness of cancer cells. Table 19.4 shows the list of anti-HER2 agents.

Trastuzumab, a humanized monoclonal anti-HER2 antibody, is the first one in clinical practice and shows improvement in response rate, TTP, and OS in MBC (17, 18). Trastuzumab should not be used along with anthracyclines as its main toxicity is cardiomyopathy. Regular monitoring of left ventricular ejection fraction is mandatory during trastuzumab treatment.

Pertuzumab is another anti-HER2 antibody with different binding sites in both HER2 and HER3 receptors, and it inhibits dimerization of receptors and thus inhibits their activation. The CLEOPETRA study showed improvement in PFS and OS when pertuzumab is added with trastuzumab and docetaxel in HER2-positive breast cancer in first-line treatment (19).

Hence, first-line treatment in HER2-positive MBC is a combination of trastuzumab, pertuzumab, and chemotherapy. Although single-agent trastuzumab or trastuzumab and pertuzumab have shown responses (20) in MBC, the major benefits are with a chemotherapy combination (21). After the induction phase, chemotherapy is withheld and anti-HER2 therapy is continued with or without hormone therapy.

Lapatinib, the first-in-class oral small molecule inhibitor of HER2 tyrosine kinase, blocks singling though HER2 and epidermal growth factor receptor (EGFR) homodimers and heterodimers. In trastuzumab-refractory HER2-positive MBC, lapatinib is used along with capecitabine and showed improvement in response rate and tumor control but not OS (22).

Aldo-trastuzumab emtansine (T-DM1) is a novel antibody drug conjugate consisting of the monoclonal antibody trastuzumab and the cytotoxic drug DM1, a highly potent tubulin destabilizer linked by tether systemically stable linker. In trastuzumab-refractory MBC, T-DM1 showed improved PFS and OS with better tolerability compared to the lapatinib and capecitabine combination (23).

Multiple lines of anti-HER2 therapies are clinically beneficial even after progression with T-DM1.

Immunotherapy

The discovery of immune checkpoint inhibitors and their success in cancer treatment led to an exploration of the role of immunotherapy in breast cancer especially in triple-negative breast cancer (TNBC). These newer agents are studied mostly in advanced-stage breast cancer alone or with chemotherapy. In TNBC, due to a lack of targeted therapy and higher rate of mutations and presence of tumor-infiltrating lymphocytes, immunotherapy has shown to have a clinical promising outcome. Pembrolizumab,

TABLE 19.4 Anti-HER2 agents

MONOCLONAL ANTIBODY	TKI
TRASTUZUMAB	LAPATINIB
PERTUZUMAB	NERATINIB
ADO – TRASTUZUMAB	TUCATINIB

a programmed cell death protein 1(PD-1) inhibitor, has shown a response rate of 10%–20% as single agent in previously treated TNBC (24). Avelumab, a programmed cell death protein ligand 1 (PDL1) inhibitor alone also showed lower response rates in previously treated HER2-positive and TNBC patients (25). In a few studies anti-PDL1 and chemotherapy improve outcomes in first-line treatment of metastatic TNBC.

BRCA-ASSOCIATED BREAST CANCER

BRCA1- and *BRCA2*-associated breast cancer (mostly hereditary) are deficient in *BRCA*-dependent DNA repair and depend on the poly-adenosine diphosphate-ribose (PARP) enzyme complex for repair. Hence, the PARP inhibitors, a novel class of drugs, are particularly active in this group of breast cancer. Olaparib, a PARP inhibitor, shows better response, DFS, and lesser toxicities compared to different chemotherapy regimens in refractory *BRCA*-associated MBC in a randomized trial (26). Talazoparib also shows good response in these groups of patients.

Platinum-based chemotherapy is also another option for *BRCA*-associated MBC. In the TNT trial carboplatin showed a better response and PFS compared to docetaxel in *BRCA*-associated MBC in first-line treatment.

SURGERY

Radiotherapy

The role of radiation is mainly for symptom palliation in MBC patients. External beam radiation is helpful with focal pain at skeletal metastasis, impending fracture, and pathological fracture in MBC.

As there is improvement in the survival of MBC patients due to newer systemic therapies, the incidence of central nervous system (CNS) metastases is also increased, particularly in HER2-positive and TNBC (27). Whole-brain radiation is the standard treatment for brain metastasis and leptomeningeal disease. Stereotactic radiotherapy or stereotactic radio surgery may be a good option for single or oligometastases. Isolated pulmonary nodules, isolated contralateral lymph node, or bone lesions may be aggressively treated with curative intent (28). The role of local therapy (like radiation) in oligometastatic MBC is an area of active ongoing investigation (29).

Miscellaneous

Bisphosphonates (pamidronate or zoledronic acid) and the RANK ligand inhibitor denosumab are useful in skeletal metastases and alleviate pain and prevent pathological fracture and hypercalcemia (30, 31).

In CNS metastasis, there are systemic therapies like endocrine treatments; chemotherapy like alkylations, anthracyclines, and capecitabine; and anti-HER2 therapies like lapatinib, TDM-1, and neratinib. But the data are limited and can't replace local therapy of the brain (32).

The standard of care for MBC is still systemic therapy like hormone or chemotherapy and other targeted agents, and local therapy is mostly for symptom relief. For oligometastasis, local approaches are under trial. There are many more newer approaches and new molecules under investigation to improve the outcome of treatment of MBC.

REFERENCES

1. Cancer.Net Editorial Board, 01/2021.
2. Rugo HS, Rumble RB, Macare E, et al. Endocrine therapy for hormone receptor positive metastatic breast cancer: American Society of Clinical Oncology guideline. *J Clin Oncol* 2016:34(25):3069–3103.
3. Buzdar AU, Jonat W, Howell A, et al. Anastrozole versus megestrol acetateinthe treatment of postmenopausal women with advanced breast carcinoma: results of survival update based on a combined analysis of data from two mature phase III trials, Arimidix Study Group. *Cancer* 1998;83(6):1142–1152.
4. Budzar A, Douma J, Davidson N, et al. Phase III, multicentered, double-blinded, randomised studios letrozole, an aromatase inhibitor, for advanced breast cancer versus megestrol acetate. *J Clin Oncol* 2001;19(14):3357–3366.
5. Bonneterre J, Thurlimann B, Robertson JF, et al. Anastrazole versus tamoxifen as first line therapy for advanced breast cancer in 668 postmenopausal women: results of the Tamoxifen or Arimidix Randomized Group Efficacy and Tolerability Study. *J Clin Oncol* 2000;18(22):3748–3757.
6. Mouridsen H, Gershanovich M, Sun Y, et al. Superior efficacy of letrozole versus tamoxifen as first line therapy for post menopausal women with advanced breast cancer: results of a phase III study the International Letrozole Breast Cancer Group. *J Clin Oncol* 2001;19(10):2596–2606.
7. Robertson JFR, Bondarenko IM, Trishkina E, et al. Fulvestrant 500 mg versus anastrazole 1 mg for hormone receptor positive advanced breast cancer (FALCON): an international, randomised, double blind, phase 3 trial. *Lancet* 2016;388(10063):2997–3005.
8. Fribbens C, O'Leary B, Kilburn L, et al. Plasma ERS1 mutations and the treatment of oestrogen receptor positive advanced breast cancer. *J Clin Oncol* 2016;34(25):2961–2968.
9. Finn RS, Martin M, Rugo HS, et al. Palbociclib and letrozole in advanced breast cancer. *N Engl J Med* 2016;375(20):1925–1936.
10. Hortobagyi GN, Stemmer SM, Burris HA, et al. Ribociclib as first-line therapy for HR-positive, advanced breast cancer. *N Engl J Med* 2016;375(18):1738–1748.
11. Goetz MP, Toi M, Campone M, et al. MONARCH 3: abemaciclib as initial therapy for advanced breast cancer. *J Clin Oncol* 2017;35(32):3638–3646.
12. Turner NC, Ro J, André F, et al. Palbociclib in hormone-receptor-positive advanced breast cancer. *N Engl J Med* 2015;373(3):209–219.
13. Sledge GW Jr, Toi M, Neven P, et al. MONARCH 2: abemaciclib in combination with fulvestrant in women with HR+/HER2-advanced breast cancer who had progressed while receiving endocrine therapy. *J Clin Oncol* 2017;35(25):2875–2884.
14. Baselga J, Campone M, Piccart M, et al. Everolimus in postmenopausal hormone-receptor-positive advanced breast cancer. *N Engl J Med* 2012;366(6):520–529.
15. Geels P, Eisenhauer E, Bezjak A, et al. Palliative effect of chemotherapy: objective tumor response is associated with symptom improvement in patients with metastatic breast cancer. *J Clin Oncol* 2000;18(12):2395–2405.
16. Cardoso F, Costa A, Senkus E, et al. 3rd ESO-ESMO International Consensus Guidelines for Advanced Breast Cancer (ABC 3). *Ann Oncol* 2017;28(1):16–33.
17. Marty M, Cognetti F, Maraninchi D, et al. Randomized phase II trial of the efficacy and safety of trastuzumab combined with docetaxel in patients with human epidermal growth factor receptor 2-positive metastatic breast cancer administered as first-line treatment: the M77001 study group. *J Clin Oncol* 2005;23(19):4265–4274.
18. Slamon DJ, Leyland-Jones B, Shak S, et al. Use of chemotherapy plus a monoclonal antibody against HER2 for metastatic breast cancer that overexpresses HER2. *N Engl J Med* 2001;344(11):783–792.
19. Baselga J, Cortés J, Kim SB, et al. Pertuzumab plus trastuzumab plus docetaxel for metastatic breast cancer. *N Engl J Med* 2012;366(2):109–119.
20. Vogel CL, Cobleigh MA, Tripathy D, et al. Efficacy and safety of trastuzumab as a single agent in first-line treatment of HER2-overexpressing metastatic breast cancer. *J Clin Oncol* 2002;20(3):719–726.
21. von Minckwitz G, du Bois A, Schmidt M, et al. Trastuzumab beyond progression in human epidermal growth factor receptor 2-positive advanced breast cancer: a German Breast Group 26/Breast International Group 03-05 study. *J Clin Oncol* 2009;27(12):1999–2006.
22. Geyer CE, Forster J, Lindquist D, et al. Lapatinib plus capecitabine for HER2-positive advanced breast cancer. *N Engl J Med* 2006;355(26):2733–2743.
23. Verma S, Miles D, Gianni L, et al. Trastuzumab emtansine for HER2-positive advanced breast cancer. *N Engl J Med* 2012;367(19):1783–1791.

24. Nanda R, Chow LQ, Dees EC, et al. Pembrolizumab in patients with advanced triple-negative breast cancer: phase Ib KEYNOTE-012 Study. *J Clin Oncol* 2016;34(21):2460–2467.
25. Dirix LY, Takacs I, Jerusalem G, et al. Avelumab, an anti-PD-L1 antibody, in patients with locally advanced or metastatic breast cancer: a phase 1b JAVELIN Solid Tumor Study. *Breast Cancer Res Treat* 2018;167(3):671–686.
26. Robson M, Im SA, Senkus E, et al. Olaparib for metastatic breast cancer in patients with a germline BRCA mutation. *N Engl J Med* 2017;377(6):523–533.
27. Lin NU, Bellon JR, Winer EP. CNS metastases in breast cancer. *J Clin Oncol* 2004;22(17):3608–3617.
28. Rivera E, Holmes FA, Buzdar AU, et al. Fluorouracil, doxorubicin, and cyclophosphamide followed by tamoxifen as adjuvant treatment for patients with stage IV breast cancer with no evidence of disease. *Breast J* 2002;8(1):2–9.
29. Chmura SJ, Winter KA, Salama JK, et al. NRG BR002: a phase IIR/III trial of standard of care therapy with or without stereotactic body radiotherapy (SBRT) and/or surgical ablation for newly oligometastatic breast cancer. *J Clin Oncol* 2016;34(15 Suppl):TPS1098.
30. Van Poznak C, Somerfield MR, Barlow WE, et al. Role of bone-modifying agents in metastatic breast cancer: an American Society of Clinical Oncology–Cancer Care Ontario focused guideline update. *J Clin Oncol* 2017;35(35):3978–3986.
31. Stopeck AT, Lipton A, Body JJ, et al. Denosumab compared with zoledronic acid for the treatment of bone metastases in patients with advanced breast cancer: a randomized, double-blind study. *J Clin Oncol* 2010;28(35):5132–5139.
32. Lin NU, Carey LA, Liu MC, et al. Phase II trial of lapatinib for brain metastases in patients with human epidermal growth factor receptor 2-positive breast cancer. *J Clin Oncol* 2008;26(12):1993–1999.

CORE AREA VI: OPERATIVE SURGERY IN BREAST CANCER

Breast Conservation Therapy

20

Rudradeep Banerjee and Diptendra Kumar Sarkar

Breast conservation therapy (BCT) includes breast conservation surgery (BCS) followed by radiation therapy (RT) in all cases and adjuvant chemotherapy (CT) if indicated. Over the last three decades, BCT is the treatment of choice for early breast cancers, but there are still a significant proportion of patients who choose to undergo mastectomies for early breast cancer in day-to-day clinical practice.

There have been a significant number of trials that have proven that BCT is not at all inferior to mastectomy or modified radical mastectomy; rather, BCT is superior to mastectomies in terms of overall survival, disease-free survival, and cancer recurrence (1–5).

In this chapter, the following will be discussed:

- Components of BCT
- Contraindications to BCT
- Advantages of BCT

COMPONENTS OF BCT

Usually, BCT is performed for early breast cancers. But in today's era, with the improvements of neo-adjuvant chemotherapy (NACT), BCT is possible for locally advanced breast cancers (LABCs) as well.

For early breast cancer, after confirmation of the diagnosis, hormonal status evaluation, and metastatic workups, depending on the patient's choice, BCS is performed. There are multiple techniques for OPS which provide excellent postoperative outcomes. Different OPS techniques have been discussed in the relevant chapters of this book.

During surgery, wide local excision of the tumor is done with a rim of healthy tissue. Following resection either the cavity is obliterated in layers or drain is placed with the idea to reduce seroma. For invasive ductal cancers, an ink-free margin is adequate, and for ductal carcinoma *in situ*, at least a 2-mm tumor-free margin is considered adequate. The axillary nodal management is the same for BCS or mastectomy. If there are clinicoradiologically negative axilla, during BCS, sentinel lymph node biopsy is performed

DOI: 10.1201/9780367821982-21

and is treated accordingly. For patients with clinicoradiologically positive axilla, either targeted axillary dissection is planned or conventional axillary lymph nodal clearance is performed.

During BCS, the specimen is properly marked for orientation and the tumor cavity and the tumor base are marked with radiopaque markers for future irradiation.

Intraoperatively, the negative margin can be confirmed by various methods like frozen section from the margin, specimen mammography, etc.

Postoperatively once the wound is healed properly, the patient is sent for adjuvant chemotherapy if indicated followed by RT with or without hormonal therapy. After completion of therapy, the patient is followed up as per the standard guidelines. Local tumor bed boost irradiation is needed in a few selected cases with a high risk of recurrence.

Recently, accelerated partial bed irradiation has become more relevant, where the tumor bed and surrounding 1–2 cm of healthy breast tissues are irradiated. Patients who are considered ideal for partial breast irradiation fulfill the following criteria (6):

- *BRCA*-negative patient
- Older than 50 years of age
- Having invasive ductal carcinoma, size than 2 cm with 2-mm free resection margin
- No lymphovascular invasion
- Estrogen receptor (ER)-positive
- Low/Intermediate nuclear grade
- Screening-detected ductal carcinoma *in situ* (DCIS) measuring ≤ 2.5 cm with negative margin widths of ≥3 mm

For patients with LABC, after tissue diagnosis, a radiopaque marker is placed at the center of the tumor and the patient is given NACT. The response is evaluated clinicoradiologically after every three cycles of NACT. If there is acceptable response after the first three cycles, breast conservation is possible without any major morbid reconstruction procedure; then after this the patient is taken up for surgery. Otherwise, the patient is given the full course of NACT. However, in triple-negative and HER2-positive breast cancer, regardless of the response, the full course NACT is completed before surgery ().

CONTRAINDICATIONS TO BCT (6)

Absolute contraindications

- If radiotherapy is needed during pregnancy
- Multifocal or diffuse disease, which needs extensive excision to achieve tumor-free margins, resulting in poor cosmetic outcome
- Homozygous for ATM mutation

Relative contraindications

- Prior RT to the chest wall or breast
- Active connective tissue disease
- Repeatedly positive pathologic margin
- Patients with a known or suspected genetic predisposition to breast cancer

ADVANTAGES OF BCT

The major advantage of BCT is that the breast need not be sacrificed. With the development of different oncoplastic techniques, the cosmetic outcomes are acceptable in most of the cases. The improvement of psychosocial impact after BCS compared to mastectomy still remains a matter of debate. Some of the literature suggests that BCS is associated with more anxiety and fear and less compliance, whereas others have shown that BCS leads to an overall better psychosocial impact (7–11). But most of these studies have shown that BCS gives better body image perception and improved sexual function (8–10, 12). Considering all these issues, the patient should be properly counseled regarding the available and suitable treatment options for breast cancer and treated with the best possible option.

REFERENCES

1. Veronesi U, Zucali R, Luini A. Local control and survival in early breast cancer: the Milan trial. *Int J Radiat Oncol Biol Phys.* 1986 May;12(5):717–20.
2. Blichert-Toft M, Nielsen M, Düring M, Møller S, Rank F, Overgaard M, et al. Long-term results of breast conserving surgery vs. mastectomy for early stage invasive breast cancer: 20-year follow-up of the Danish randomized DBCG-82TM protocol. *Acta Oncol Stockh Swed.* 2008;47(4):672–81.
3. Corradini S, Reitz D, Pazos M, Schönecker S, Braun M, Harbeck N, et al. Mastectomy or breast-conserving therapy for early breast cancer in real-life clinical practice: outcome comparison of 7565 cases. *Cancers.* 2019 Jan 31;11(2):160.
4. Veronesi U, Cascinelli N, Mariani L, Greco M, Saccozzi R, Luini A, et al. Twenty-year follow-up of a randomized study comparing breast-conserving surgery with radical mastectomy for early breast cancer. *N Engl J Med.* 2002 Oct 17;347(16):1227–32.
5. Fisher B, Anderson S, Bryant J, Margolese RG, Deutsch M, Fisher ER, et al. Twenty-year follow-up of a randomized trial comparing total mastectomy, lumpectomy, and lumpectomy plus irradiation for the treatment of invasive breast cancer. *N Engl J Med.* 2002 Oct 17;347(16):1233–41.
6. Breast.pdf [Internet]. [cited 2022 Nov 16]. Available from: https://www.nccn.org/professionals/physician_gls/pdf/breast.pdf
7. Ng ET, Ang RZ, Tran BX, Ho CS, Zhang Z, Tan W, et al. Comparing quality of life in breast cancer patients who underwent mastectomy versus breast-conserving surgery: a meta-analysis. *Int J Environ Res Public Health [Internet].* 2019 Dec [cited 2022 Nov 16];16(24):4970. Available from: https://www.ncbi.nlm.nih.gov/pmc/articles/PMC6950729/
8. Arndt V, Stegmaier C, Ziegler H, Brenner H. Quality of life over 5 years in women with breast cancer after breast-conserving therapy versus mastectomy: a population-based study. *J Cancer Res Clin Oncol.* 2008 Dec;134(12):1311–8.
9. Ahn S kyung, Oh S, Kim J, Choi JS, Hwang KT. Psychological impact of type of breast cancer surgery: a National Cohort Study. *World J Surg [Internet].* 2022 Sep 1 [cited 2022 Nov 16];46(9):2224–33. Available from: https://doi.org/10.1007/s00268-022-06585-y
10. Quality of life and sexual functioning of women after breast cancer surgery | *Open Access Maced J Med Sci.* 2021 Oct 13 [cited 2022 Nov 16]; Available from: https://oamjms.eu/index.php/mjms/article/view/6015
11. Sun MQ, Meng AF, Huang XE, Wang MX. Comparison of psychological influence on breast cancer patients between breast-conserving surgery and modified radical mastectomy. *Asian Pac J Cancer Prev [Internet].* 2013 [cited 2022 Nov 16];14(1):149–52. Available from: http://www.koreascience.or.kr/article/JAKO201312855329444.page
12. Aerts L, Christiaens MR, Enzlin P, Neven P, Amant F. Sexual functioning in women after mastectomy versus breast conserving therapy for early-stage breast cancer: a prospective controlled study. *Breast Edinb Scotl.* 2014 Oct;23(5):629–36.

Principles in Oncoplastic Breast Surgery

21

Heba Khanfar, Saima Taj, and Debashis Ghosh

ONCOPLASTIC BREAST SURGERY

Oncoplastic breast surgery (OPS) represents a major advance in breast cancer surgery. The term was first introduced in the 1980s by Werner Audretsch. OPS is not a technique; it's a way of thinking. It's a comprehensive approach to surgical planning that combines the principles of surgical oncology with plastic surgery and reconstructive surgery (1–4).

AIMS OF ONCOPLASTIC SURGERY

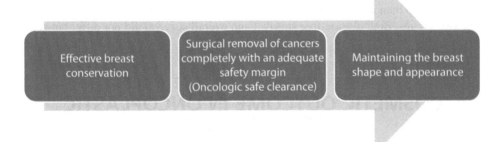

Effective breast conservation

Surgical removal of cancers completely with an adequate safety margin (Oncologic safe clearance)

Maintaining the breast shape and appearance

Development of Oncoplastic Breast-Conserving Surgery

Breast-conserving surgery allowed the resection of the tumor with adequate margins and preservation of the breast, which reduced the psychological morbidities. However, a considerable proportion of patients had bad cosmetic outcomes. This could be attributed to poorly planned incisions, leaving the lumpectomy

DOI: 10.1201/9780367821982-22

157

cavity open to fill with seroma, which would give a false satisfactory appearance directly after surgery, but upon finishing radiotherapy, fibrosis would result in retraction and poor cosmetic outcome. In response, breast surgeons across the globe joined forces to improve their techniques. This resulted in the emergence of a new concept: OPS (5).

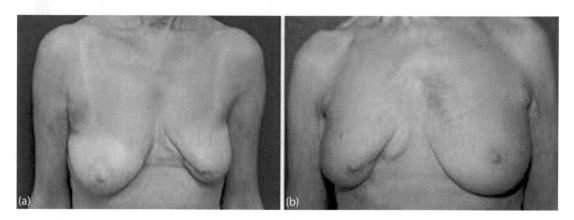

CASE EXAMPLE 21.1   Breast deformity after breast conservation surgery.

Advantages of Oncoplastic Breast Surgery

Oncologic safety of oncoplastic breast surgery

Breast conservation surgery (BCS) is oncologically and surgically safe, with long-term survival comparable to total mastectomy. Previous studies reported positive margins were found in 10%–40% and the re-excision rate was up to 60% (6–10). OPS allows wider excision; this leads to reduces positive margins and results in fewer re-excision rates as compared with standard BCS (11, 12). A systematic review assessed over 5,000 patients treated with OPS in 49 studies and reported an average positive margin rate of 10.8%, re-excision rate of 6.0%, and conversion to mastectomy rate of 6.2% (13). In addition, a recent meta-analysis that included 3,789 patients from 11 studies with 2,691 in the BCS-alone group and 1,098 in BCS plus OPS compared the short-term and long-term oncological outcomes between two groups. Re-excision was less common, and the positive margin rate was lower, but not significantly, in the BCS-plus oncoplastic group than in the BCS-alone group. The local and distal recurrence rates were similar between the two groups. Both disease-free survival and overall survival did not differ between the two groups (14).

COSMETIC OUTCOME IN ONCOPLASTIC BREAST SURGERY

Breast aesthetics is an important aspect of the female body, which is valuable for women's self-confidence and physical attractiveness (15). The aesthetic outcome of BCS is unsatisfactory in 30% of patients, while the cosmetic rate of OPS is 0%–18%. Furthermore, when breast conservation is employed with OPS techniques, the failure rate decreases to < 7% at 2 years (2, 14, 16). A systemic review included 25 studies that assessed the cosmetic outcome of OPS patients (n = 1962). About 55.2% patients had excellent outcomes, while 31.0% had good, 9.4% had fair, and 4.4% had a poor cosmetic outcome. Further, the studies reported a good cosmetic outcome after OPS in approximately 90% of patients (17).

PATIENTS SELECTION

Indications and Contraindications for OPS

There are some established indications for OPS. Therefore, the main indication is for breast cancer patients who require more than 20% resection of the breast volume, which significantly leads to breast deformity (1, 2, 18). The OPS techniques are more often used for tumors located in the central, medial, or inferior quadrants due to aesthetic problems (1, 15, 19).

TABLE 21.1 Indications and relative contraindications for oncoplastic surgery in breast-conserving surgery

INDICATIONS	CONTRAINDICATIONS
• More than 20% resection of breast volume	• Diffuse microcalcification
• Multifocal	• Inflammatory breast cancer
• Central, medial, and inferior tumors	• Previous radiotherapy
• Severe ptosis	• Multicentric tumors
• Macromastia	• Small-volume breast without ptosis
• *In situ* cancer presence	• Uncontrolled diabetes, smoking, collagen disease
• Patient and surgeon preference	• Patient and surgeon preference

Source: From References (1, 15).

PREOPERATIVE PLANNING

Preoperative planning is vital for optimizing surgical resection and achieving an acceptable breast appearance without compromising oncological effectiveness.

Several factors need to be considered when planning OPS. These include breast size, tumor location, breast density, ptosis, and patient and surgeon preference (1, 2).

Breast Size

The most important factor that affects the cosmetic results are tumor size to the breast size. Some oncoplastic techniques are indicated for large breasts such as reduction mammoplasties. Alternatively, round block mammoplasty or rotation patterns are more appropriate for small and medium breasts.

Tumor Location

Some zones are at high risk of deformity during breast cancer surgery. The upper outer quadrant is a favorable location for large-volume excision. Conversely, the lower pole or upper inner quadrants of the breast often produce a major risk for deformity; for instance, "bird's beak deformity" is typically seen on excision of tumors from the lower pole of the breast.

Glandular Density

The breast density predicts the fatty composition of the breast and determines the ability to perform extensive breast undermining and reshaping without complications. It is evaluated clinically and radiologically. However, mammographic evaluation is a more reproducible method to determine breast density (20, 21).

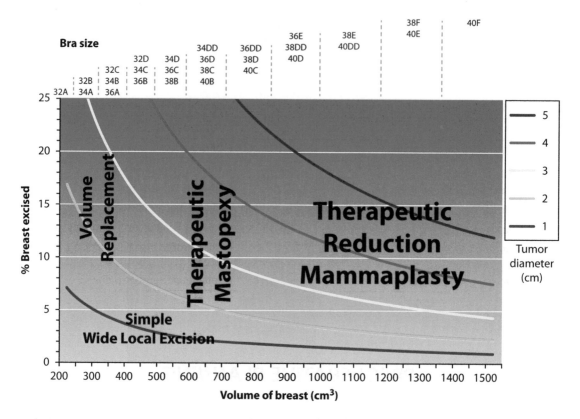

FIGURE 21.1   The graph illustrates the role of the main techniques of oncoplastic breast conservation surgery according to breast size, size of the cancer, and estimated percentage of breast volume that would be removed (4).

ONCOPLASTIC TECHNIQUE CLASSIFICATION

Level I Oncoplastic Technique

When less than 20% of breast volume is excised with a simple parenchymal advancement flap to fill the defect and the nipple–areolar complex (NAC) is repositioned if required.

Level II Oncoplastic Technique

The resection of 20%–50% of breast volume requires level II techniques. This involves extensive skin resection with a variety of volume displacement or replacement methods (20, 22).

TECHNIQUES TO RECONSTRUCT A BREAST PARENCHYMAL DEFECT

Volume Displacement

In this technique, the local breast parenchyma is repositioned to fill the defect with either simple breast parenchymal advancement or more complex mammoplasties.

Volume Replacement

In this technique, autologous tissue is used to replace volume loss. The volume replacement technique is used for reconstruction of a small breast with a large resection volume (15).

STEPS OF LEVEL I ONCOPLASTIC TECHNIQUES

Clough defined six steps for level I oncoplastic surgery:

1. Skin incision.
2. Undermining of the skin.
3. NAC.
4. A full-thickness glandular excision is performed from subcutaneous fat to the pectoralis fascia.
5. Closure of glandular defect with tissue approximation followed by specimen X-ray to determine the complete radiological response.
6. If required, an area in the shape of a crescent bordering the areola is de-epithelized to reposition the NAC to avoid its displacement (20).

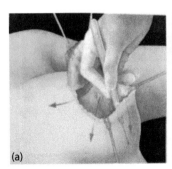 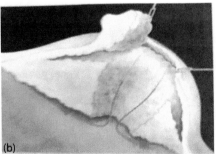 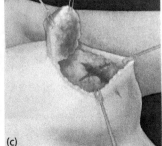

(a)   (b)   (c)

FIGURE 21.2   Level I OPS: (a) Skin undermining. (b) Excision of tumor. (c) Reapproximation and suturing of gland (20).

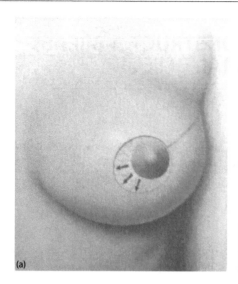
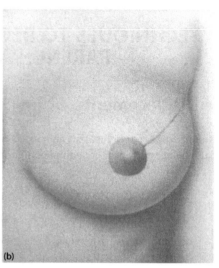

FIGURE 21.3   Level I OPS nipple recentralization: (a) Skin crescent de-epithelized opposite to lumpectomy in upper outer quadrant. (b) NAC recentralized to avoid NAC deviation (20).

VOLUME DISPLACEMENT TECHNIQUES

Round Block Mammoplasty

Round block mammoplasty is also known as doughnut mammoplasty or peri-areolar mammoplasty. It was originally described by Benelli. It is an appropriate technique for small- to-medium-sized breasts without ptosis and upper pole tumor, but it can easily be adapted for tumors in any location of the breast (23–25).

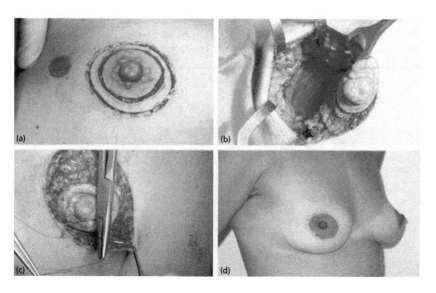

CASE EXAMPLE 21.2   Round block mammoplasty: (a) Two peri-areolar incisions followed by de-epithelialization. (b) Tumor removal and excision cavity. (c) Closure. (d) Final result.

TENNIS RACKET MAMMOPLASTY

The tennis racket method is used for upper outer quadrant tumors. In this technique, a large portion of the upper outer quadrant can be excised by a direct incision over the tumor, from the NAC toward the axilla (20, 26).

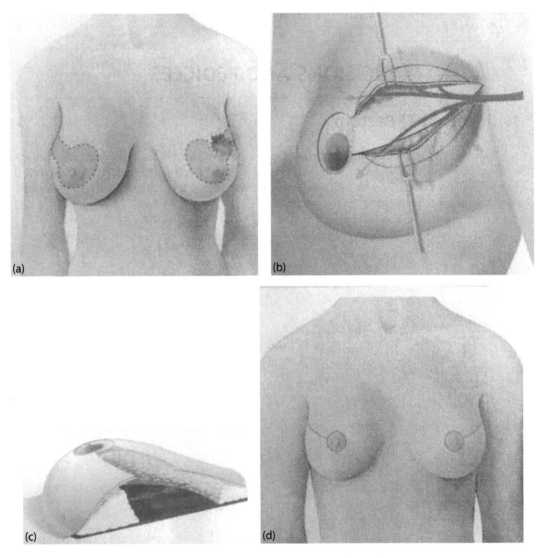

FIGURE 21.4   Level II OPS: Tennis racquet mammoplasty. (a) Preoperative marking. (b) Skin excision and quadrant undermining. (c) Reapproximation and NAC recentralization. (d) Peri-areolar and lateral scar (20).

THERAPEUTIC MAMMOPLASTY

Therapeutic mammoplasty is a well-established oncoplastic technique that combines the principles of reduction mammoplasty and mastopexy with excision of the tumor to reshape the breast. It is particularly useful for large tumor resection in medium- to large-sized breasts, providing an alternative to mastectomy with or without reconstruction in a ptotic breast.

The skin pattern selected is indicated by breast size, degree of ptosis, need to remove skin over a tumor, and tumor site. The pedicle positioning will be dictated by location of the tumor (27, 28).

INCISIONS AND PEDICLES

Wise (Inverted T) Pattern

It is most widely used technique and can be used with most pedicles but is most commonly associated with inferior pedicles. It allows larger skin excision and is good for very large reduction. Therefore, it is suitable for medium to large breasts with moderate to severe ptosis. It is indicated for tumors located in the lower pole or upper pole.

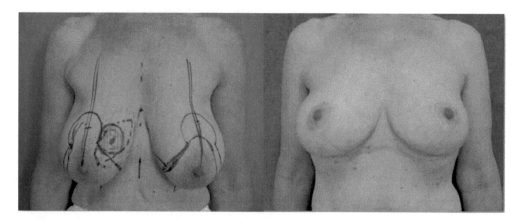

CASE EXAMPLE 21.3 Wise pattern mammoplasty for excision of upper pole tumor.

Vertical Pattern

The vertical mammoplasty is indicated in small- or medium-sized breasts with mild to moderate ptosis for tumors in the center of the lower pole. This pattern is usually used with superior, superomedial, or medial pedicles.

Pedicles

The most important factor when choosing a pedicle is the location of the tumor. An inferior-based pedicle is used for tumors located in the upper breast, and a superiorly based pedicle is used if the tumor is located in the lower breast (21, 29, 30).

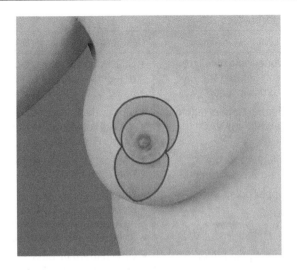

FIGURE 21.5 Vertical pattern incision marking (29).

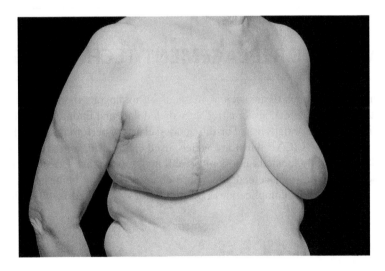

CASE EXAMPLE 21.4 Vertical mammoplasty excision of central tumor.

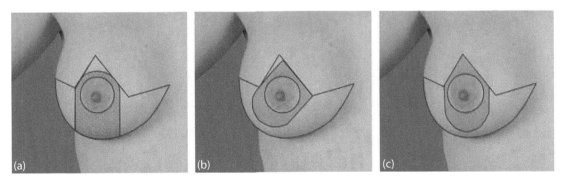

FIGURE 21.6 Wise pattern (inverted T) with (a) inferior pedicle, (b) superomedial pedicle, and (c) superior pedicle (29).

TABLE 21.2   Mammoplasty techniques

PROCEDURE	TUMOR LOCATION	DESCRIPTION/COMMENTS
Round block benelli	Upper pole mainly, but can be used for any tumor location	• Utilizes two concentric peri-areolar incisions with de-epithelialization of intervening skin • Blood supply to NAC maintained by posterior
Grisotti flap	Central tumors requiring excision of NAC	• Aids in the immediate reconstruction of NAC through preservation of skin island on advancement flap
Vertical scar/Lejour type	Inferior pole or retroareolar tumors	• The scar should avoid reaching the inframammary fold
Inferior pedicle mammoplasty	Upper pole tumor	• Wise pattern incision • Blood supply to NAC based on inferior and posterior glandular attachment • Inverted T and peri-areolar scar
Superior pedicle mammoplasty	Lower pole tumor	• Wise pattern incision • Blood supply to NAC based on superior dermoglandular attachment • Inverted T and peri-areolar scar

VOLUME REPLACEMENT TECHNIQUES

This involves using nonautologous tissue such as implants or autologous tissue that is harvested from a remote site to fill the resection defect, either a free or pedicled flap, and lipomodeling techniques.

Recently, pedicled perforator flaps based on thoracodorsal artery perforators (TDAP flaps) and lateral intercostal artery perforators (LICAP flaps) are widely used. They offer an excellent option for reconstruction after BCS for laterally located tumors in a small nonptotic breast. Perforator flaps provide skin and subcutaneous fat for tissue replacement. They are characterized by being quick to perform, with a faster recovery, and with fewer complications and morbidities compared to other flap reconstruction techniques (31).

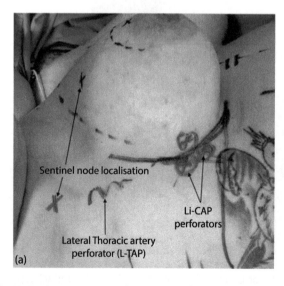

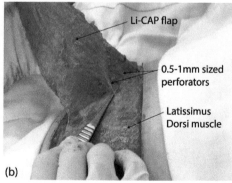

CASE EXAMPLE 21.5   Chest wall perforator flap.

DISADVANTAGES ONCOPLASTIC BREAST SURGERY

OBS procedures, depending on the technique, can be complex, lengthy, and potentially associated with relatively high postoperative complication rates. The experience of the surgeon is paramount in patient and technique selection, as complications after oncoplastic reduction may cause a delay in adjuvant treatment (16, 17).

A recent systemic review of postoperative complications in OPS patients reported problems in 14.3% of patients; these include fat necrosis (3.3%), hematoma (2.5%), delayed wound healing (2.2%), infection (1.9%), seroma (1%), skin necrosis (0.5%), and nipple necrosis (0.4%) (13).

Tenofsky et al. compared OPS with BCS and reported a higher rate of nonhealing wounds in the OPS group, although this did not prolong the time to radiation therapy in OPS (32).

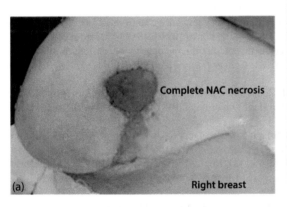
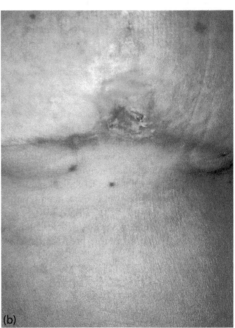

CASE EXAMPLE 21.6   Complications of OPS: (a) Complete NAC necrosis and (b) delayed wound healing in T junction.

REFERENCES

1. Urban C, Lima R, Schunemann E, Spautz C, Rabinovich I, Anselmi K. Oncoplastic principles in breast conserving surgery. *Breast.* 2011;20(Suppl 3):S92–S95. doi:10.1016/S0960-9776(11)70302-2
2. Bertozzi N, Pesce M, Santi PL, Raposio E. Oncoplastic breast surgery: comprehensive review. *Eur Rev Med Pharmacol Sci.* 2017;21(11):2572–2585.
3. Munhoz AM, Montag E, Gemperli R. Oncoplastic breast surgery: indications, techniques and perspectives. *Gland Surg.* 2013;2(3):143–157. doi:10.3978/j.issn.2227-684X.2013.08.02
4. Macmillan RD, McCulley SJ. Oncoplastic breast surgery: what, when and for whom?. *Curr Breast Cancer Rep.* 2016;8:112–117. doi:10.1007/s12609-016-0212-9.

5. Kaufman CS. Increasing role of oncoplastic surgery for breast cancer. *Curr Oncol Rep.* 2019;21(12):111. Published 2019 Dec 14. doi:10.1007/s11912-019-0860-9

6. Fisher B, Anderson S, Bryant J, et al. Twenty-year follow-up of a randomized trial comparing total mastectomy, lumpectomy, and lumpectomy plus irradiation for the treatment of invasive breast cancer. *N Engl J Med.* 2002;347(16):1233–1241. doi:10.1056/NEJMoa022152

7. Veronesi U, Cascinelli N, Mariani L, et al. Twenty-year follow-up of a randomized study comparing breast-conserving surgery with radical mastectomy for early breast cancer. *N Engl J Med.* 2002;347(16):1227–1232. doi:10.1056/NEJMoa020989

8. Clough KB, Cuminet J, Fitoussi A, Nos C, Mosseri V. Cosmetic sequelae after conservative treatment for breast cancer: classification and results of surgical correction. *Ann Plast Surg.* 1998;41(5):471–481. doi:10.1097/00000637-199811000-00004

9. Wanis ML, Wong JA, Rodriguez S, Wong JM, Jabo B, Ashok A, et al. Rate of re-excision after breast-conserving surgery for invasive lobular carcinoma. *Am Surg.* 2013;79:1119–1122

10. Biglia N, Ponzone R, Bounous VE, et al. Role of re-excision for positive and close resection margins in patients treated with breast-conserving surgery. *Breast.* 2014;23(6):870–875. doi:10.1016/j.breast.2014.09.009

11. Houssami N, Macaskill P, Marinovich ML, et al. Meta-analysis of the impact of surgical margins on local recurrence in women with early-stage invasive breast cancer treated with breast-conserving therapy. *Eur J Cancer.* 2010;46(18):3219–232.doi:10.1016/j.ejca.2010.07.043

12. Singletary SE. Surgical margins in patients with early-stage breast cancer treated with breast conservation therapy. *Am J Surg.* 2002;184(5):383–393. doi:10.1016/s0002-9610(02)01012-7

13. De La Cruz L, Blankenship SA, Chatterjee A, et al. Outcomes after oncoplastic breast-conservings in breast cancer patients: a systematic literature review. *Ann Surg Oncol.* 2016;23(10):3247–3258. doi:10.1245/s10434-016-5313-1

14. Chen JY, Huang YJ, Zhang LL, Yang CQ, Wang K. Comparison of oncoplastic breast-conserving surgery and breast-conserving surgery alone: a meta-analysis. *J Breast Cancer.* 2018;21(3):321–329. doi:10.4048/jbc.2018.21.e36

15. Emiroğlu M, Sert İ, İnal A. The role of oncoplastic breast surgery in breast cancer treatment. *J Breast Health.* 2015;11(1):1–9. Published 2015 Jan 1. doi:10.5152/tjbh.2014.2215

16. Fitoussi AD, Berry MG, Famà F, et al. Oncoplastic breast surgery for cancer: analysis of 540 consecutive cases [outcomes article]. *Plast Reconstr Surg.* 2010;125(2):454–462. doi:10.1097/PRS.0b013e3181c82d3e

17. Campbell EJ, Romics L. Oncological safety and cosmetic outcomes in oncoplastic breast conservation surgery, a review of the best level of evidence literature. *Breast Cancer (Dove Med Press).* 2017;9:521–530. Published 2017 Aug 4. doi:10.2147/BCTT.S113742

18. Hernanz F, Regaño S, Vega A, Gómez Fleitas M. Reduction mammaplasty: an advantageous option for breast conserving surgery in large-breasted patients. *Surgical Oncology.* 2010 Dec;19(4):e95–e102. doi: 10.1016/j.suronc.2009.08.001.

19. Kollias J, Davies G, Bochner MA, Gill PG. Clinical impact of oncoplastic surgery in a specialist breast practice. *ANZ J Surg.* 2008;78(4):269–272. doi:10.1111/j.1445-2197.2008.04435.x

20. Clough KB, Kaufman GJ, Nos C, Buccimazza I, Sarfati IM. Improving breast cancer surgery: a classification and quadrant per quadrant atlas for oncoplastic surgery. *Ann Surg Oncol.* 2010;17(5):1375–1391. doi:10.1245/s10434-009-0792-y

21. Rose M, Manjer J, Ringberg A, Svensson H. Surgical strategy, methods of reconstruction, surgical margins and postoperative complications in oncoplastic breast surgery. *Eur J Plast Surg.* 2014;37(4):205–214. doi:10.1007/s00238-013-0922-4

22. Kaviani A, Zand S, Ashraf-Ganjouei A, Younan R, Jacques Salmon R. A novel level I oncoplastic surgery technique for tumors located in UIQ of the breast far from the nipple: the "Cross" technique. *Plast Reconstr Surg Glob Open.* 2019;7(7):e2269. Published 2019 Jul 26. doi:10.1097/GOX.0000000000002269

23. Bramhall RJ, Lee J, Concepcion M, et al. Central round block repair of large breast resection defects: oncologic and aesthetic outcomes. *Gland Surg.* 2017;6(6):689–697. doi:10.21037/gs.2017.06.11

24. Ogawa T. Usefulness of breast-conserving surgery using the round block technique or modified round block technique in Japanese females. *Asian J Surg.* 2014;37(1):8–14. doi:10.1016/j.asjsur.2013.07.007

25. Zaha H, Onomura M, Unesoko M. A new scarless oncoplastic breast-conserving surgery: modified round block technique. *Breast.* 2013;22(6):1184–1188. doi:10.1016/j.breast.2013.07.056

26. Yang JD, Lee JW, Cho YK, et al. Surgical techniques for personalized oncoplastic surgery in breast cancer patients with small- to moderate-sized breasts (part 1): volume displacement. *J Breast Cancer.* 2012;15(1):1–6. doi:10.4048/jbc.2012.15.1.1

27. Aggarwal S, Marla S, Nyanhongo D, Kotecha S, Basu NN. Current practice of therapeutic mammaplasty: a survey of oncoplastic breast surgeons in England. *Int J Surg Oncol.* 2016;2016:1947876. doi:10.1155/2016/1947876er. 2012;15(1):1-6. doi:10.4048/jbc.2012.15.1.1

28. Baker E, Kim B, Rattay T, et al. The team (*Therapeutic Mammaplasty*) study: protocol for a prospective multi-centre cohort study to evaluate the practice and outcomes of therapeutic mammaplasty. *Int J Surg Protoc.* 2016;1:3–10. Published 2016 Sep 14. doi:10.1016/j.isjp.2016.08.001

29. Wong C, Vucovich M, Rohrich R. Mastopexy and reduction mammoplasty pedicles and skin resection patterns. *Plast Reconstr Surg Glob Open.* 2014;2(8):e202. Published 2014 Sep 8. doi:10.1097/GOX.0000000000000125

30. McCulley SJ, Macmillan RD. Planning and use of therapeutic mammoplasty – Nottingham approach. *Br J Plast Surg.* 2005;58(7):889–901. doi:10.1016/j.bjps.2005.03.008

31. Roy PG, Tenovici AA. Staged approach to partial breast reconstruction to avoid mastectomy in women with breast cancer. *Gland Surg.* 2017;6(4):336–342. doi:10.21037/gs.2017.03.08

32. Tenofsky PL, Dowell P, Topalovski T, Helmer SD. Surgical, oncologic, and cosmetic differences between onco-plastic and nononcoplastic breast conserving surgery in breast cancer patients. *Am J Surg.* 2014;207(3):398–402. doi:10.1016/j.amjsurg.2013.09.017

Principles of Breast Reconstruction

22

Jajini Susan Varghese and Afshin Mosahebi

INTRODUCTION

The goal of breast reconstruction is to restore the appearance of the breast and to improve a woman's psychological health after cancer treatment. Rates of breast reconstruction continue to rise through a combination of an increased range of reconstructive techniques, wider availability of appropriate surgical skills, and higher patient expectations (1). The psychosocial benefits of breast reconstruction through restoration of body image, improvement in self-esteem, and improved quality of life have been well-documented (2).

However, even the most sophisticated reconstruction will not fully replicate the native breast in its movement, feel, and sensation, and it is important that the patient understands this at the outset, or they will be disappointed with the outcome. Mastectomy involves removal of breast tissue and varying amounts of skin, with or without nipple removal. The aim of breast reconstruction is to produce a breast mound that matches the contralateral breast. Improvement on preoperative breast aesthetics is sometimes possible.

Breast reconstruction after mastectomy can be performed using autologous tissue, implants, or a combination of both, with the use of symmetrizing mastopexy, reduction, or augmentation surgery if necessary. Women must be fully informed of all options and the possible need for multiple surgeries at the time of initial planning so they can make informed choices, be that delayed reconstruction or none at all. The timing and technique of reconstruction should be decided by the patient guided by a multidisciplinary breast cancer team, which should involve reconstructive surgeons who are able to provide a full range of reconstructive procedures.

ONCOLOGICAL CONSIDERATIONS AND SAFETY

The principal aim of breast surgery is to provide safe and successful oncological treatment. With increasing use of neoadjuvant systemic treatments, more women than ever are able to conserve their breasts through downsizing of tumors (3). They are able to undergo breast-conserving surgery where the tumor and margins are excised, and the rest of the breast tissue is refashioned through application of oncoplastic techniques. This is followed by treatment with adjuvant radiotherapy (4).

DOI: 10.1201/9780367821982-23

However, two-thirds of affected women still undergo mastectomy due to residual tumor extent, location, and cancer stage. These factors also dictate the need for adjuvant chemoradiotherapy. The extent of disease should not, however, be a contraindication to reconstruction. Even women with advanced disease (stages IIb and III) have been shown to benefit from reconstruction through an improvement in quality of life (5). However, patients with early breast cancer (stages 0, I, and IIa) stand to benefit most from reconstruction as they not only have longer life expectancy, but they are also less likely to need adjuvant radiotherapy. Radiotherapy can affect the cosmetic outcome of any reconstruction (6). Conversely, reconstruction can also affect the timing and delivery of adjuvant radiotherapy (7). Patients with diffuse metastatic disease are usually not offered reconstruction.

Most studies to date confirm the oncological adequacy of skin-sparing mastectomy and confirm that local recurrence rates are comparable to those of simple mastectomy (8). Nipple-sparing mastectomy can be offered to patients with peripherally placed small tumors. Most centers, however, undertake an additional retro-areolar biopsy and warn patients that the nipple – areolar complex will need excision if found to be involved. Patients often also need reassurance that immediate reconstruction with implants or autologous flap tissue does not lead to significant masking, as most cases of local recurrence present as a skin-flap mass, lying anterior to the reconstruction (9).

TIMING

Immediate Breast Reconstruction

The main advantage of immediate breast reconstruction, where the reconstruction is performed at the same time as the mastectomy, is that the patient does not spend any time without a breast mound, minimizing the psychological trauma. This technique allows the preservation of the native breast skin envelope and landmarks such as the inframammary fold (IMF) and the breast footprint, allowing a natural shape when volume is restored. When nipple preservation is possible, it's associated with higher patient satisfaction (10). The need for contralateral symmetrizing surgery may also be reduced.

However, there is concern that patients may struggle to fully appreciate all aspects of reconstructive options, as they also have to come to terms with their oncological diagnosis in a relatively short frame of time. As the oncological procedure and the reconstruction are all done in one sitting, there is concern that a longer operating time may lead to higher complication rates. If higher complication rates generate delays in the administration of adjuvant chemoradiotherapy, disease-free and overall survival may be affected. However, a systematic review of 14 studies showed that in clinical practice, immediate breast reconstruction did not significantly delay the start of adjuvant treatment (11).

These concerns are now further reduced with the increasing use of neoadjuvant chemotherapy in that systemic therapy is completed before the surgical procedure, and the 6 months taken for neoadjuvant chemotherapy allows women ample time to make a better-informed decision while the tumor response to the chemotherapy informs the need for adjuvant therapy. The current guidelines therefore recommend that immediate breast reconstruction be offered to many women undergoing mastectomy with the exception of inflammatory breast cancer and those in whom severe comorbidities would increase risks associated with longer operating times.

Delayed Breast Reconstruction

Some patients choose to undergo delayed breast reconstruction, allowing time for decision making and psychological adjustment following the diagnosis of breast cancer. Clinicians may support this approach in advanced stages of disease where the risk of recurrence is higher (>20% chance of locoregional relapse at 10 years), where adjuvant therapy is indicated, and if the patient is unfit to undergo a long operation.

Technically, delayed breast reconstruction is challenging. Patient expectations need to be managed carefully, as loss of mastectomy skin envelope, effect of scarring, and adjuvant therapy will all lead to an inferior cosmetic outcome when compared to immediate reconstruction. Interestingly, patient satisfaction scores were higher among women who underwent reconstruction under a delayed setting compared to immediate, as their starting point was a flat chest, and they appreciated the symmetry achieved through delayed reconstruction.

Autologous options are preferred in a delayed reconstruction setting, as the skin paddle on the flap can be used to create ptosis. The use of expanders in the delayed setting to re-create a pocket into which a definitive implant is placed in a second stage can also be done. This may be associated with increased complications, especially in a post-radiotherapy setting (12).

Delayed Immediate Breast Reconstruction

This staged approach can be useful when there is uncertainty regarding the need for postoperative radiotherapy (13). This technique attempts to combine the aesthetic benefits of skin preservation and effective radiotherapy delivery. Here, a skin-sparing mastectomy is performed at the time of cancer surgery and a temporary tissue expander is placed to preserve the skin envelope. If the final histology indicates a need for radiotherapy, the expander is deflated to allow for effective radiotherapy. The expander is subsequently reinflated to maintain the three-dimensional skin envelope prior to definite breast reconstruction.

TECHNIQUES

Autologous Reconstruction

Gillies principles of reconstruction guide replacing "like with like," and autologous breast reconstruction allows the creation of a breast with a texture and appearance reasonably matched with what is removed. In addition, the aesthetics and patient satisfaction improve with time (2). Autologous flaps can be used in the immediate setting or delayed or when implant reconstruction has failed. In addition, autologous tissue can withstand radiotherapy better than implant-based reconstructions (12).

The deep inferior epigastric flap (DIEP) remains the first choice for breast reconstruction because of the relative abundance of tissue and favorable donor site scar profile, essentially providing an abdominoplasty. Despite the initial increased costs associated with long operation times, the reduction in revisional operations means that autologous reconstructions are more cost-effective in the long run (14). Patients, however, need to be relatively fit to undergo this long procedure. The only absolute contraindications to DIEP are actual ligation of the flap pedicle or previous abdominoplasty. Abdominal surgical scars and liposuction are the only relative contraindications, and imaging to assess vascularity can help. When increased volume is required in relatively thinner women, bipedicled flap technique or stacking of DIEP flaps are all preferred to autologous tissue from other donor sites.

Other commonly used autologous flap options include gluteal flaps, superior and inferior gluteal artery perforator flaps (SGAPs/IGAPs), thigh-based flaps, and transverse upper gracilis (TUG)/profunda artery perforator (PAP) flaps (15). The latissimus dorsi (LD) pedicled flap offers a robust, relatively quick autologous option for higher-risk women. The volume can be augmented with immediate or delayed lipofilling, although it is commonly combined with an implant when extra volume is required (16). The flap can also provide a relatively large skin paddle for reconstruction. The donor site scar can be designed to be hidden under a bra, but associated complications such as seromas can be troublesome. Although the function of the LD muscle is compensated by the teres major muscle, women who place a high demand on upper limbs through activities such as climbing and swimming may experience a function deficit.

Implant-Based Reconstruction

Despite strong evidence showing the superiority of autologous reconstructions, there has been a world-wide trend toward increased implant-based reconstructions. This is partially driven by socioeconomic and health care system–related reasons (17, 18).

Implant-based reconstructions are most suitable for patients with small- to moderate-sized breasts with minimal ptosis. Excellent reconstructive outcomes are possible with careful patient and implant selection. The patient group that benefits the most from this procedure are women undergoing bilateral reconstructions without the need for adjuvant therapy, such as women undergoing risk-reducing mastectomies for high-risk gene carrier status.

Women undergoing unilateral reconstruction with implants must be counseled clearly in terms of long-term results. In larger breasts, use of skin-reducing patterns with contralateral symmetrizing surgery can produce good results. With time, however, the results deteriorate, revealing asymmetry between reconstructed and nonreconstructed breast, implant failure, or capsular contractures. However, implant reconstructions provide the shortest operating time and inpatient stay and fastest recovery. In slimmer or younger women, this option may work well while they complete their family or put on weight to allow for replacement with an autologous flap.

Advancements in prosthetic device designs and the advent of acellular dermal matrices (ADMs) have led to evolution of this technique (19). Traditionally, implant-based reconstruction involved placement of the implant in a fully submuscular position. This often led to the implant being placed too high on the chest. Increasingly, ADM is being used to cover the lower pole of the device while a pectoralis major muscle flap covers the upper pole. This allows for some degree of a natural-appearing ptosis and, along with definition of the IMF, improving the overall cosmesis. While a submuscular placement gives a smooth take-off of the reconstructed breasts and somewhat reduced capsular contracture rates, patients can suffer from serious animation deformities associated with the muscle pulling up on the implant when it is engaged. Women with ptotic breasts can benefit from the use of a dermal sling instead of ADM, which is essentially vascularized, de-epithelized inferior pole skin that is secured to the caudal edge of the pectoralis muscle (20).

Recently, there has been increased interest in prepectoral or subcutaneous placement of implants (21). Here the implant is wrapped in a mesh pocket and anchoring sutures are placed to the pectoralis muscle. Careful patient selection is key, as women with decent subcutaneous coverage get better cosmetic results. The main advantage is avoidance of animation deformity, as the muscle is not detached, and patients also have reduced postoperative pain. Visible rippling or palpable implant edges can be addressed with lipofilling in a separate sitting. Although initial outcome data are promising, it is currently too limited to make a definitive conclusion as to whether prepectoral placement is better than the subpectoral lower pole sling technique.

Growing concerns regarding the risk of breast implant–related anaplastic large-cell lymphoma (BIA-ALCL), thought to be related to implant texturing and breast implant illness (BII), may see a trend reverse to women requesting more autologous-based reconstructions (22, 23).

Role of Autologous Fat Grafting in Breast Reconstruction

Fat grafting plays a major role in both the immediate and delayed breast reconstruction settings (24). It has been shown to be an oncologically safe procedure following both mastectomy and breast-conserving surgery (25). The procedure can be used to not only correct contour defects and improve mastectomy flap thickness, improving cosmesis, but also mitigate some of the effects of radiotherapy in the delayed setting. All autologous flaps can be volume augmented using fat grafting in the delayed setting using the vascularized matrix principle, while musculocutaneous flaps such as the LD muscle can be volume augmented in the immediate setting to avoid implant usage.

CONCLUSION

- Breast reconstruction plays a significant role in the woman's physical, emotional, and psychological recovery from breast cancer.
- Surgical options include the use of tissue expanders or implants and the use of pedicled or free autologous flaps.
- Decisions regarding the type and timing of reconstruction need to be made with the patient guided by a multidisciplinary breast cancer team, which should involve reconstructive surgeons who are able to provide a full range of reconstructive procedures.

REFERENCES

1. Doherty C, Pearce S, Baxter N, *et al.* Trends in immediate breast reconstruction and radiation after mastectomy: a population study. *Breast J* 2020. DOI:10.1111/tbj.13500.
2. Hu ES, Pusic AL, Waljee JF, *et al.* Patient-reported aesthetic satisfaction with breast reconstruction during the long-term survivorship period. *Plast Reconstr Surg* 2009. DOI:10.1097/PRS.0b013e3181ab10b2.
3. Asselain B, Barlow W, Bartlett J, *et al.* Long-term outcomes for neoadjuvant versus adjuvant chemotherapy in early breast cancer: meta-analysis of individual patient data from ten randomised trials. *Lancet Oncol* 2018. DOI:10.1016/S1470-2045(17)30777-5.
4. van Maaren MC, de Munck L, de Bock GH, *et al.* 10 year survival after breast-conserving surgery plus radiotherapy compared with mastectomy in early breast cancer in the Netherlands: a population-based study. *Lancet Oncol* 2016. DOI:10.1016/S1470-2045(16)30067-5.
5. Crisera CA, Chang EI, Da Lio AL, Festekjian JH, Mehrara BJ. Immediate free flap reconstruction for advanced-stage breast cancer: Is it safe? *Plast Reconstr Surg* 2011. DOI:10.1097/PRS.0b013e3182174119.
6. Ho AY, Hu ZI, Mehrara BJ, Wilkins EG. Radiotherapy in the setting of breast reconstruction: types, techniques, and timing. *Lancet Oncol* 2017. DOI:10.1016/S1470-2045(17)30617-4.
7. Yun JH, Diaz R, Orman AG. Breast reconstruction and radiation therapy. *Cancer Control* 2018. DOI:10.1177/1073274818795489.
8. Tokin C, Weiss A, Wang-Rodriguez J, Blair SL. Oncologic safety of skin-sparing and nipple-sparing mastectomy: a discussion and review of the literature. *Int J Surg Oncol* 2012. DOI:10.1155/2012/921821.
9. Lim W, Ko BS, Kim HJ, *et al.* Oncological safety of skin sparing mastectomy followed by immediate reconstruction for locally advanced breast cancer. *J Surg Oncol* 2010. DOI:10.1002/jso.21573.
10. Howard MA, Sisco M, Yao K, *et al.* Patient satisfaction with nipple-sparing mastectomy: a prospective study of patient reported outcomes using the BREAST-Q. *J Surg Oncol* 2016. DOI:10.1002/jso.24364.
11. Xavier Harmeling J, Kouwenberg CAE, Bijlard E, Burger KNJ, Jager A, Mureau MAM. The effect of immediate breast reconstruction on the timing of adjuvant chemotherapy: a systematic review. *Breast Cancer Res Treat* 2015. DOI:10.1007/s10549-015-3539-4.
12. Jagsi R, Momoh AO, Qi J, *et al.* Impact of radiotherapy on complications and patient-reported outcomes after breast reconstruction. *J Natl Cancer Inst* 2017. DOI:10.1093/jnci/djx148.
13. Kronowitz SJ, Lam C, Terefe W, *et al.* A multidisciplinary protocol for planned skin-preserving delayed breast reconstruction for patients with locally advanced breast cancer requiring postmastectomy radiation therapy: 3-year follow-up. *Plast Reconstr Surg* 2011. DOI:10.1097/PRS.0b013e3182131b8e.
14. Khajuria A, Prokopenko M, Greenfield M, Smith O, Pusic AL, Mosahebi A. A meta-analysis of clinical, patient-reported outcomes and cost of DIEP versus implant-based breast reconstruction. *Plast Reconstr Surg—Glob Open* 2019. DOI:10.1097/gox.0000000000002486.

15. Dibbs R, Trost J, Degregorio V, Izaddoost S. Free tissue breast reconstruction. *Semin Plast Surg* 2019. DOI:10.1055/s-0039-1677703.

16. Sood R, Easow JM, Konopka G, Panthaki ZJ. Latissimus dorsi flap in breast reconstruction: recent innovations in the workhorse flap. *Cancer Control* 2018. DOI:10.1177/1073274817744638.

17. American Society of Plastics Surgeons. 2014 plastic surgery statistics report. *Am Soc Plast Surg* 2014.

18. Jeevan R, Cromwell D, Browne J, van der Meulen J, Pereira J, Caddy C, *et al*. National mastectomy and breast reconstruction audit. *NHS Inf Cent* 2011.

19. Martin L, O'Donoghue JM, Horgan K, Thrush S, Johnson R, Gandhi A. Acellular dermal matrix (ADM) assisted breast reconstruction procedures: joint guidelines from the Association of Breast Surgery and the British Association of Plastic, Reconstructive and Aesthetic Surgeons. *Eur J Surg Oncol* 2013. DOI:10.1016/j.ejso.2012.12.012.

20. Jepsen C, Hallberg H, Pivodic A, Elander A, Hansson E. Complications, patient-reported outcomes, and aesthetic results in immediate breast reconstruction with a dermal sling: a systematic review and meta-analysis. *J Plast Reconstr Aesthetic Surg* 2019. DOI:10.1016/j.bjps.2018.12.046.

21. Vidya R, Berna G, Sbitany H, *et al*. Prepectoral implant-based breast reconstruction: a joint consensus guide from UK, European and USA breast and plastic reconstructive surgeons. *Ecancermedicalscience* 2019. DOI:10.3332/ecancer.2019.927.

22. Magnusson MR, Cooter RD, Rakhorst H, McGuire PA, Adams WP, Deva AK. Breast implant illness: a way forward. *Plast Reconstr Surg* 2019. DOI:10.1097/PRS.0000000000005573.

23. Lineaweaver WC. Breast implant-associated anaplastic large cell lymphoma and textured breast implants. *Ann Plast Surg* 2019. DOI:10.1097/SAP.0000000000001964.

24. Turner A, Abu-Ghname A, Davis MJ, Winocour SJ, Hanson SE, Chu CK. Fat grafting in breast reconstruction. *Semin Plast Surg* 2020. DOI:10.1055/s-0039-1700959.

25. De Decker M, De Schrijver L, Thiessen F, Tondu T, Van Goethem M, Tjalma WA. Breast cancer and fat grafting: efficacy, safety and complications—a systematic review. *Eur J Obstet Gynecol Reprod Biol* 2016. DOI:10.1016/j.ejogrb.2016.10.032.

Surgical Management of Breast Cancer– Related Lymphedema

23

Ashok BC

INTRODUCTION

Breast cancer–related lymphedema (BCRL) is a debilitating condition in which protein-rich fluid collects in the subcutaneous tissue of the upper limb following some kind of axillary intervention in the form of axillary node dissection or regional radiation for breast cancer treatment. The lymphedema can affect the upper limb on the same side and/or the breast itself in cases of breast conservation. The condition can severely affect a patient's health-related quality of life, including emotional, functional, social/family, and physical well-being. Once lymphedema sets in, it has a relentless progression unless some intervention is done. Until recently, there were not many options to treat this condition. The advent of fluorescence imaging and microsurgery has changed the way we look at and treat BCRL. This chapter briefly describes the etiology, pathology, and management of BCRL.

DEFINITION

Lymphedema manifests as progressive swelling of the upper limb, which is pitting initially but will become nonpitting later, and there might be skin changes. There may be frequent episodes of cellulitis or lymphangitis.

Four diagnostic criteria are considered to define lymphedema: A 200-mL excess as measured by perometry, 10% volume discrepancy between two limbs as measured by perometry, 2-cm change in arm circumference via tape measurement, and patient-reported symptoms of heaviness or swelling.

Risk and timing: Approximately a third of all patients who have breast surgery for cancers develop BCRL (1, 2). The risk factors are high body mass index (BMI), patients who are on taxanes (3), and patients who have axillary radiation along with axillary lymph node clearance as part of treatment. The time course of the development of BCRL is dependent on the type of treatment received. Axillary node clearance is associated with early-onset lymphedema, and axillary nodal irradiation leads to late-onset

DOI: 10.1201/9780367821982-24

lymphedema. Sentinel node biopsy is known to have a 1%–6% risk of lymphedema. The highest incidence of lymphedema is at around 12–30 months, although the risk is lifelong.

PATHOPHYSIOLOGY

There is a disequilibrium between the amount of lymph produced to the amount that is transported. Disruption of axillary lymphatics due to removal of lymph nodes might be the starting event. Added to this, there might be a reduction in the ability of the remaining lymphatics to drain the limbs effectively by the addition of radiation, and certain chemotherapeutic agents like taxanes seem to worsen lymphedema. There is a progressive accumulation of protein-rich fluid and water, leading to further structural failure of remaining lymphatics in the limb with dilatation and valve disruption and then sclerosis of lymph vessels. In later stages the proteins and glycosaminoglycans in the retained interstitial fluid stimulate adipose tissue and collagen production, which leads to skin thickening and subcutaneous soft tissue fibrosis, and the peau d'orange sign may appear. Lymphedema is associated with an increase in the risk of cellulitis due to disturbances in immune cell transport caused by a compromised lymphatic system (4). Bacterial infections like *Streptococcus* and fungal infections are common in patients with lymphedema (5).

SIGNS, SYMPTOMS, AND CLINICAL ASSESMENT

In early stages, patients may complain of slight pain, restriction of movement, fullness, heaviness, and clothing or ornaments becoming tight on the affected limbs. Swelling will be pitting in the early stages and then progress to nonpitting as time goes by. Swelling, redness, and tenderness due to lymphangitis may occur from time to time. Other skin changes include peau d'orange appearance, hyperkeratosis, and papillomatosis. Severity is measured by changes in the limb volume. Limb volume measurements can be made using a tape measure, perometer, or by water displacement. Tape girth measurements at fixed intervals and applying the frustum method to calculate limb volume give volume measurements that are simple, fast, and reproducible in a clinical setup.

INVESTIGATIONS

Investigations not only help to detect and quantify lymphedema clinically, they also determine what type of treatment can be offered to patients.

Imaging Methods

Radionuclide Lymphoscintigraphy

This not only delineates the anatomy but function as well. It involves injecting radionuclides intradermally into the limb, and the limb is scanned using a gamma camera at regular intervals. The disadvantage of lymphoscintigraphy is the use of a radioactive isotope; hence, it is contraindicated in pregnancy and breastfeeding, has poor spatial resolution, visualization of small lymphatic vessels is poor, and it takes a long time.

Near-infrared fluorescence imaging

This gives real-time visualization of the superficial lymphatics. It is used for diagnosing early lymphedema and assessing lymphatic function and the response to lymphedema therapy (6). A small quantity of Idigo cyanine green (ICG) is injected subdermally into the affected limb and scanned with an infrared camera. The result can be classified into a grade 0 subclinical or linear pattern; grade I, when mostly linear channels with a splash pattern are seen; grade II, stardust pattern areas with linear channels; grade III, stardust patterns seen in two regions; grade IV, stardust pattern in more than three regions is seen; and grade V, diffuse backflow with no normal architecture seen. Depending on the grade, treatment is offered; for example, grades I and II may be managed with lymphovenous anastomosis and grades III and IV with vascular lymph node transfer. This helps with making on-table decisions but can visualize superficial lymphatics up to only 2 cm.

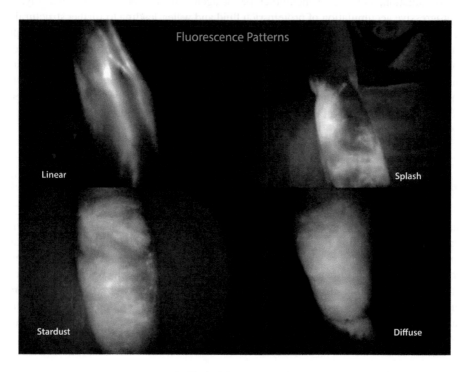

FIGURE 23.1 Different patterns of ICG fluorescence on scan.

Magnetic resonance imaging (MRI)

MRI can delineate enlarged lymph channels and fat thickness. It is useful in differentiating the liquid stage from solid stage (fibrotic and lipodystrophic) and hence helps in formulating a treatment plan. The liquid stage is amendable to lymphovenous anastomosis, vascular lymph node transfer, or liposuction, whereas the solid stage requires liposuction or an excisional procedure (7).

MANAGEMENT

There are two strategies to manage lymphedema preventively, both medical and surgical, used before edema sets in. Curative measures similar to medical or surgical measures can be used to tackle established lymphedema.

PREVENTION

Medical Prevention

In patients with risk of BRCL, preventive measures like patient education play an important role in detecting and preventing BRCL. Patients should made aware of the lifetime risk of lymphedema, early signs of lymphedema like tightness or heaviness in the limb, and lastly they should be referred to a specialist center if there are early signs of lymphedema. Manual lymphatic drainage (MLD) and compression garments in the form of stockings or short stretch bandages and upper limb/shoulder exercises are started before lymphedema sets in.

Surgical Prevention

There are three main procedures for surgical prevention.

Sentinel lymph node biopsy (*SLNB*): By doing a SLNB instead of axillary lymph node dissection (ALND), the risk of lymphedema can be reduced. First, a blue dye or ICG or radiocolloid is injected into the subdermal plane under the nipple and massaged. The first node that takes up this dye is harvested as the sentinel node. Studies have shown that this method can stage the axilla with high accuracy and has a low risk of false negativity (8).

Axillary reverse mapping (*ARM*): This was introduced by Klimberg in 2008. At the time of axillary clearance, a radiocolloid is injected into the limb subcutaneously and ICG into the breast, thereby identifying and protecting the lymphatics from the upper limb while completely removing the ones draining the breast. There are conflicting reports about the efficacy of this procedure, with some studies showing benefit (9–11) and others claiming no benefit (12, 13).

Primary lymphovenous anastomosis: At the time of axillary clearance, the severed lymphatics from the upper limb are identified using ICG fluoroscopy, and using super-microsurgical techniques the lymphatics are diverted and anastomosed to one of the tributaries of the axillary vein, thereby providing an alternate channel for limb lymphatics to drain. This is also called the lymphatic microsurgical preventive healing approach (LYMPHA) (14–16). Various studies have shown a significant benefit by adopting this procedure. The disadvantages are it adds to the cost and time of surgery. Microsurgical expertise is required, sometimes it is not possible to find suitable veins or lymphatics, and lastly some skeptics doubt the long-term efficacy of such anastomoses.

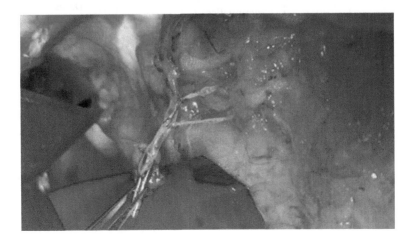

FIGURE 23.2   End-to-side anastomosis of severed lymphatics in the axilla to the lateral thoracic vein.

TREATMENT OF BCRL

There are many modalities of treatment available to treat established BCRL. The choice of procedure largely depends on the stage of the disease.

Conservative Treatment

Complete decongestive therapy (CDT) is done for patients not willing or not fit for surgical intervention. In some cases, this is done to downstage the disease so that a reconstructive procedure can be done rather than an ablative procedure like liposuction or excision. The main components of CDT are manual lymphatic drainage, compression bandaging using short stretch bandages and foams, skin care, and exercises in a three-phase protocol. CDT has been shown to decrease limb volume and improved overall quality of life (QOL) (17). However, another recent randomized controlled trial reported no significant differences in limb volume between the two groups at 6 weeks (18).

Surgical Treatment

Early stages, stage I and II, lymphovenous anastomosis is recommended. Stage III will require lymphovenous anastomosis, and stage IV may need ablative procedures like suctioning or lipodermal excision. A reasonable flowchart to manage BCRL is given in the following figure.

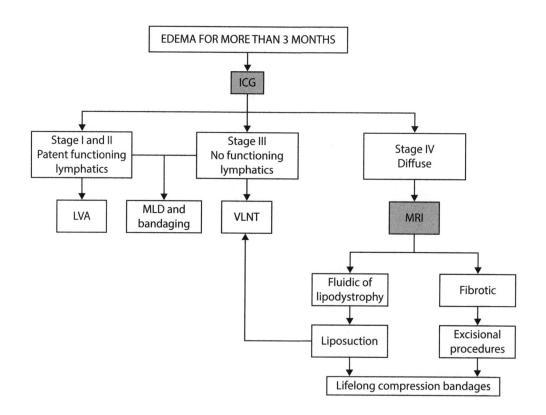

Lymphovenous Anastomosis

In stage I and II lymphedema, small linear subcutaneous lymphatics are identified using ICG scans and are anastomosed to small adjacent veins, thereby bypassing the obstruction. This anastomosis can be in an end-to-end, end-to-side, or side-to-side configuration. It can be done under local anesthesia. Studies have shown that the greater the number of anastomoses, the better the results. A systematic meta-analysis of 22 studies in patients having lymphovenous anastomosis procedures for peripheral lymphedema reveals consistent improvement and safety (19). There are concerns about long-term patency of the shunts, however.

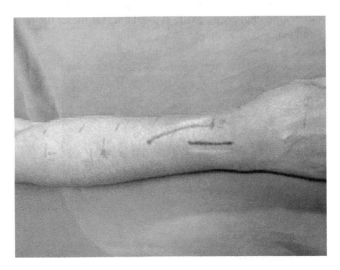

FIGURE 23.3 Multiple lymphatic channels (yellow) and adjacent veins (blue) are marked using the ICG scan and vein viewer.

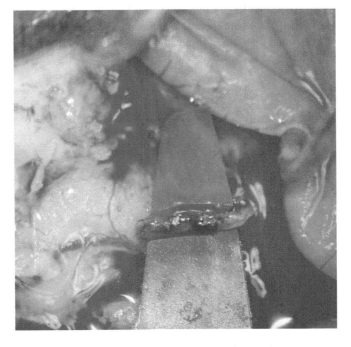

FIGURE 23.4 Lymphovenous anastomosis using 10-0 or 11-0 nylon under microscope.

Vascularized Lymph Node Transfer

Vascularized lymph node transfer (VLNT) was described by Becker. Lymph nodes, along with their blood supply, are harvested and transferred to the affected limb by the microvascular technique. VLNT is very useful in late stage II and stage III lymphedema. In these stages there are not many functioning lymphatics to perform lymphovenous anastomoses on. There are two theories on how it works: One, the nodes act like a sump, absorbing the lymph from the interstitial space and discharging it into the venous system. Second, some lymphangiogenesis occurs around the transferred tissue, which helps in reducing the edema. In reality, there might be a bit of both. Popular sites for donor nodes are the groin, right gastric, supraclavicular, submental, and opposite axilla if available. Of these, the right gastric has no risk of secondary lymphedema and hence is our choice.

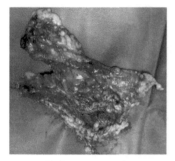 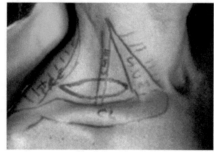 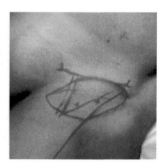

Right gastric nodes   Supraclavicular   Groin nodes

FIGURE 23.5   Donor sites of lymph nodes.

These harvested lymph nodes can be placed orthotopically, i.e., in the region where the lymph nodes were removed (axilla). Excision of all the scar tissue before transfer is necessary; otherwise, lymphatic tissue may not bridge the scar tissue and VLNT may not work. Lymph nodes can also be placed heterotopically, i.e., anywhere else on the limb where there is lymphedema, typically at the wrist or ulnar border of the forearm. The lymph nodes and their blood supply are transferred by doing microvascular anastomosis of the flap artery to limb artery and at least two veins to limb veins.

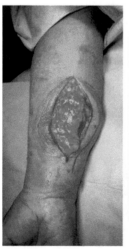 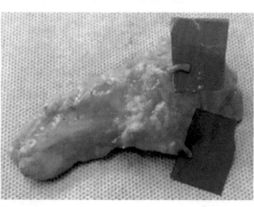 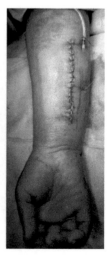

FIGURE 23.6   Lymph node transfer by microvascular transfer.

The results begin to appear in the form of wrinkling of the skin and a decrease in limb volume within a week's time. Patients need to be on compression and follow MLD protocols.

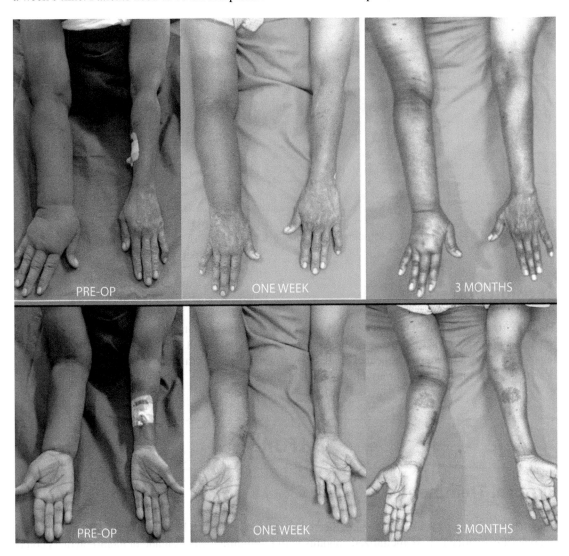

FIGURE 23.7 Postoperative picture showing almost near-normal limb volume matching the normal side.

In a series by Saaristo et al., almost all patients showed improvements after the procedure, and cure was observed in 41.6% of cases (20). They performed VLNT simultaneously during breast reconstruction in patients with lymphedema after mastectomy. Another group reported favorable outcomes after VLNT (21).

Liposuction

In patients who have nonpitting, nonfibrotic lymphedema, no functioning linear channels, and MRI proves the swelling to be fatty, liposuction under tourniquet control is an option to reduce the swelling. But this has to be followed by a strict compression regimen that is lifelong; otherwise, the edema will recur in no time (22).

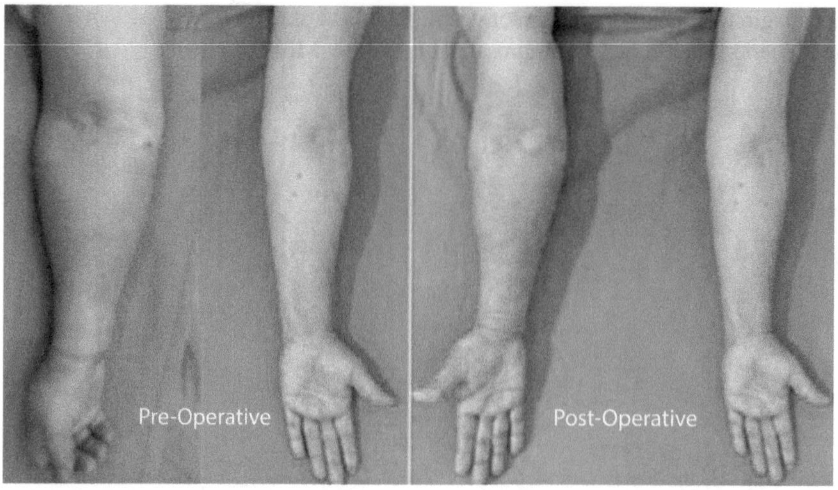

FIGURE 23.8   Preoperative and postoperative pictures after liposuction.

Excision Procedure

Though extremely rare in BCRL, in very advanced stages with skin changes, complete excision of tissues to the deep fascia with skin grafting (Charles procedure) may be useful. This is very disfiguring, takes a long time to heal, and can have repeated breakdown of suture lines or grafted areas, but the most annoying problem is weeping of grafted areas due to lymph leakage.

FUTURE

Surgical Treatment

Lymphatic reconstruction using tissue-engineered lymphatic grafts will be available in the near future for lymphedema treatment. Endothelialized conduits with intraluminal valves made of nano-polymers could be used in the future as a lymphatic graft.

BCRL affects a significant proportion of the population undergoing axillary intervention and causes a significant financial burden for both patients and the health care system. These patients require comprehensive management by a dedicated team. Today, there are both surgical and nonsurgical options available which are efficient in terms of cure and reduce and arrest the progression of the disease. Present research will bring better solutions and will improve patient evaluation and management.

REFERENCES

1. Norman SA, Localio AR, Potashnik SL, Simoes Torpey HA, Kallan MJ, Weber AL, et al. Lymphedema in breast cancer survivors: incidence, degree, time course, treatment, and symptoms. *J Clin Oncol Off J Am Soc Clin Oncol.* 2009 Jan 20;27(3):390–7.

2. McDuff SGR, Mina AI, Brunelle CL, Salama L, Warren LEG, Abouegylah M, et al. Timing of lymphedema after treatment for breast cancer: when are patients most at risk? *Int J Radiat Oncol Biol Phys*. 2019 Jan 1; 103(1):62–70.

3. Lee M-J, Beith J, Ward L, Kilbreath S. Lymphedema following taxane-based chemotherapy in women with early breast cancer. *Lymphat Res Biol*. 2014 Dec;12(4):282–8.

4. Mortimer PS, Rockson SG. New developments in clinical aspects of lymphatic disease. *J Clin Invest*. 2014 Mar;124(3):915–21.

5. Thieme Medical Publishers—Lymphedema Management. The Comprehensive Guide for Practitioners [Internet]. [cited 2022 Jan 28]. Available from: https://www.thieme.com/for-media/125-2017/1308-lymphedema-management-the-comprehensive-guide-for-practitioners

6. Sevick-Muraca EM, Kwon S, Rasmussen JC. Emerging lymphatic imaging technologies for mouse and man. *J Clin Invest*. 2014 Mar 3;124(3):905–14.

7. Sen Y, Qian Y, Koelmeyer L, Borotkanics R, Ricketts R, Mackie H, et al. Breast cancer-related lymphedema: differentiating fat from fluid using magnetic resonance imaging segmentation. *Lymphat Res Biol*. 2018 Feb;16(1):20–7.

8. Somashekhar SP, Zaveri Shabber S, Udupa Venkatesh K, Venkatachala K, Parameshwaran, Vasan Thirumalai MM. Sentinel lymph node biopsy in early breast cancer using methylene blue dye and radioactive sulphur colloid – a single institution Indian experience. *Indian J Surg*. 2008 Jun;70(3):111–9. doi: 10.1007/s12262-008-0033-9. Epub 2008 Jul 24.

9. Noguchi M. Axillary reverse mapping for breast cancer. *Breast Cancer Res Treat*. 2010 Feb;119(3):529–35.

10. Klimberg VS. A new concept toward the prevention of lymphedema: axillary reverse mapping. *J Surg Oncol*. 2008 Jun 1;97(7):563–4.

11. Toi M, Winer EP, Inamoto T, Benson JR, Forbes JF, Mitsumori M, et al. Identifying gaps in the locoregional management of early breast cancer: highlights from the Kyoto Consensus Conference. *Ann Surg Oncol*. 2011 Oct;18(10):2885–92.

12. Boneti C, Badgwell B, Robertson Y, Korourian S, Adkins L, Klimberg V. Axillary reverse mapping (ARM): initial results of phase II trial in preventing lymphedema after lymphadenectomy. *Minerva Ginecol*. 2012 Oct;64(5):421–30.

13. Tausch C, Baege A, Dietrich D, Vergin I, Heuer H, Heusler RH, et al. Can axillary reverse mapping avoid lymphedema in node positive breast cancer patients? *Eur J Surg Oncol J Eur Soc Surg Oncol*. 2013 Aug;39(8):880–6.

14. Boccardo F, Casabona F, De Cian F, Friedman D, Villa G, Bogliolo S, et al. Lymphedema microsurgical preventive healing approach: a new technique for primary prevention of arm lymphedema after mastectomy. *Ann Surg Oncol*. 2009 Mar;16(3):703–8.

15. Boccardo F, Casabona F, De Cian F, DeCian F, Friedman D, Murelli F, et al. Lymphatic microsurgical preventing healing approach (LYMPHA) for primary surgical prevention of breast cancer-related lymphedema: over 4 years follow-up. *Microsurgery*. 2014 Sep;34(6):421–4.

16. Feldman S, Bansil H, Ascherman J, Grant R, Borden B, Henderson P, et al. Single institution experience with lymphatic microsurgical preventive healing approach (LYMPHA) for the primary prevention of lymphedema. *Ann Surg Oncol*. 2015 Oct;22(10):3296–301.

17. Lasinski BB, McKillip Thrift K, Squire D, Austin MK, Smith KM, Wanchai A, et al. A systematic review of the evidence for complete decongestive therapy in the treatment of lymphedema from 2004 to 2011. *PM R*. 2012 Aug;4(8):580–601.

18. Dayes IS, Whelan TJ, Julian JA, Parpia S, Pritchard KI, D'Souza DP, et al. Randomized trial of decongestive lymphatic therapy for the treatment of lymphedema in women with breast cancer. *J Clin Oncol*. 2013 Oct 20;31(30):3758–63.

19. Rockson SG. General Overview. In: Lee B-B, Rockson SG, Bergan J, editors. *Lymphedema: A Concise Compendium of Theory and Practice [Internet]*. Cham: Springer International Publishing; 2018 [cited 2022 Jan 28]. pp. 81–5. Available from: https://doi.org/10.1007/978-3-319-52423-8_6

20. Saaristo AM, Niemi TS, Viitanen TP, Tervala TV, Hartiala P, Suominen EA. Microvascular breast reconstruction and lymph node transfer for postmastectomy lymphedema patients. *Ann Surg*. 2012 Mar;255(3):468–73.

21. Raju A, Chang DW. Vascularized lymph node transfer for treatment of lymphedema: a comprehensive literature review. *Ann Surg*. 2015 May;261(5):1013–23.

22. Executive Committee. The diagnosis and treatment of peripheral lymphedema: 2016 consensus document of the International Society of Lymphology. *Lymphology*. 2016 Dec;49(4):170–84.

CORE AREA VII: ADJUVANT AND NEOADJUVANT THERAPY

Radiation Oncology

24

Practice Guidelines

Amitabh Ray

Radiotherapy for breast cancer has a long and tumultuous history. Consensus regarding the utility of radiation in breast cancer was achieved after decades of research and meta-analyses of the large volume of data available through the same. The benefit of local radiation can be broadly divided into the three following items:

1. Curative therapy for noninvasive and invasive breast cancer as an adjuvant to surgery and systemic therapy
2. Palliative treatment for advanced or metastatic breast cancer for symptom alleviation
3. Ablative treatment in oligometastatic breast cancer to augment systemic therapy

The advances made in surgical approaches and systemic therapy are also mirrored in radiotherapy wherein shorter courses of treatment, sparing of adjacent organs at risk, maintenance of cosmesis post-radiation, and reduction of treatment volumes in selected cases have all been studied in detail and are evolving into newer options for patients in the current age. Indeed, radiation oncologists are often spoiled for choice while deciding on protocols, given the rapid advancements in the equipment hardware and software over the years. A complete discussion of all these aspects will be beyond the scope of this chapter and will only be touched upon in relevant sections.

ROLE OF RADIATION IN CURATIVE THERAPY POST-BCS IN INVASIVE BREAST CANCER

Whole-Breast Radiotherapy (WBR)

Evidence for WBR in invasive breast cancer is gleaned from the 2011 Early Breast Cancer Trialists' Collaborative Group (EBCTCG) meta-analysis of 17 randomized studies comparing postoperative

DOI: 10.1201/9780367821982-25

radiotherapy vs. none with a total of 10,801 patients with pT1–2 tumors. The majority of them (n = 7287) were node negative, 1,050 were node positive, and in 2,464 patients the nodal status was unknown (1). WBR reduced the 10-year recurrence rate (local or distant) from 35% to 19.3%, corresponding to an absolute benefit of 15.7% (p < 0.0001) for irradiated women (pN0: 15.4%, pN+: 21.2%). Moreover, WBR decreased the 15-year breast cancer death rate from 25.2% to 21.4%, corresponding to an absolute gain of 3.8% (pN0: 3.3%, pN+: 8.5%).

Post-WBR boost

The tumor bed is at highest risk for subclinical residual tumor cells and is often supplemented with an additional dose of radiation known as a tumor bed boost. In the EORTC 22881-10882 trial, a total of 5,318 patients with microscopically complete excision followed by whole-breast irradiation of 50 Gy were randomly assigned to receive either a boost dose of 16 Gy (2,661 patients) or no boost dose (2,657 patients). With a median follow-up of 10.8 years, the cumulative incidence of local recurrence was 10.2% versus 6.2% for the no boost and the boost group, respectively (P < .0001). The hazard ratio of local recurrence was 0.59 (0.46–0.76) in favor of the boost, with no statistically significant interaction per age group. The absolute risk reduction at 10 years per age group was the largest in patients ≤40 years of age: 23.9%–13.5% (P = .0014). Survival at 10 years was 82% in both arms. Radiation-related fibrosis was higher in the boost arm.

Hypofractionated whole-breast irradiation

Hypofractionated WBR schedules (39–42.9 Gy in single fractions of 2.6–3.3 Gy) have been stringently compared across continents for iso-effectiveness to normofractionation (50 Gy in single fractions of 2 Gy) in four robust trials with 7,095 patients. In these trials, 89.8% of tumors were <3 cm, 79% were node negative, 87% had small- or medium-sized breasts. The results show equivalent local control rates and cosmesis at 10 years median follow-up. However, caution needs to be exercised before selection of shorter protocols, especially in the setting of large-volume breasts or use of dose-dense chemotherapy or taxanes in systemic therapy protocols. Ultra-short protocols of 5 days (FAST FORWARD study) are still awaiting endorsement prior to universal implementation.

Radiotherapy after neoadjuvant chemotherapy and BCS/Oncoplastic surgery

The indication for radiotherapy in this setting follows the presystemic therapy stage of disease regardless of the extent of response achieved. The use of hypofractionation is usually discouraged in this subgroup of patients.

Partial breast irradiation

Accelerated partial breast irradiation (APBI) refers to radiation therapy (RT) of a smaller (partial) breast volume over a shorter time interval, covering the tumor bed with a limited margin of normal tissue. For patients at a lower risk for local recurrence, APBI can be delivered intraoperatively in a single fraction or postoperatively over 1–3 weeks by brachytherapy or external beam radiotherapy. At the present time, most regulatory authorities encourage APBI in the setting of a clinical trial where patient selection guidelines are very stringent. Outside of this, it may be considered as an option for elderly women fulfilling all of the following preconditions: Age >70 years, tumor size <2 cm, invasive ductal carcinoma, negative axillary nodes, free surgical margins, absence of EIC, and luminal A type (ER+ and PR+, G1–2, Her 2 neu negative). Meticulous and close post - therapy follow-up is essential and must be discussed with the patient prior to deciding on the protocol (3).

ROLE OF RADIOTHERAPY IN NONINVASIVE BREAST CANCER POST-CS

Among different noninvasive neoplasias of the breast, only the subgroup of pure ductal carcinoma *in situ* (DCIS) is considered for further recurrence risk reduction treatment modalities after complete excision in order to avoid a mastectomy. About half of recurrences are invasive cancers. Up to 50% of all recurrences require salvage mastectomy. Randomized clinical trials and a huge number of mostly observational studies have unanimously demonstrated that RT significantly reduces recurrence risks of ipsilateral DCIS as well as invasive breast cancer independent of patient age in all subgroups. The recommended total dose is 50 Gy administered as whole-breast irradiation (WBI) in single fractions of 1.8 or 2.0 Gy given 5 days weekly. The University of Southern California/Van Nuys Prognostic Index (USC/VNPI) is a numeric tool that quantifies five measurable prognostic factors known to be important in predicting local recurrence in conservatively treated patients with DCIS (Table 24.1). Data support excision alone for all patients scoring 4, 5, or 6 and patients who score 7 but have margin widths ≥3 mm. Excision plus radiotherapy achieves the less than 20% local recurrence threshold at 12 years for patients who score 7 and have margins <3 mm, patients who score 8 and have margins ≥3 mm, and patients who score 9 and have margins ≥5 mm. Mastectomy is required for patients who score 8 and have margins <3 mm, who score 9 and have margins <5 mm, and for all patients who score 10, 11, or 12 to keep the local recurrence rate less than 20% at 12 years.

POSTMASTECTOMY RADIOTHERAPY

The term postmastectomy radiotherapy (PMRT) describes adjuvant radiotherapy after mastectomy. Irradiation is typically delivered to the chest wall, including the regional lymphatics. Evidence from the EBCTCG meta-analysis from 2014 including 8,135 women in 22 trials in which radiotherapy included the chest wall and regional lymph nodes supports the use of radiotherapy in a defined subgroup of patients after surgery (2). Women who have had a mastectomy and axillary dissection of at least levels I and II and radiotherapy that includes the chest wall, the supraclavicular or axillary fossa (or both), and the internal mammary chain may see a reduction in the recurrence, breast cancer mortality, and overall mortality for all node-positive women. In the node-negative subgroup, radiation is indicated for primary tumor size of more than 5 cm, pT4 disease, or positive margins. Patients who receive neoadjuvant chemotherapy are considered for PMRT on the basis of prechemotherapy status regardless of the response achieved with systemic therapy. For early-stage disease, the role of radiotherapy is still investigational, and various factors including age of the patient, the Cambridge PMRT index, and biological type of breast cancer have been proposed for patient selection.

TABLE 24.1   Cambridge post mastectomy radiotherapy index

SCORE	1	2	3
Size	≤15 mm	16–40	>40
Margin	≥10 mm	1–9	<1
VN Class	Grade 1/2 without necrosis	Grade 1/2 with necrosis	Grade 3
Age	>60	40–60	<40

REGIONAL NODAL IRRADIATION (RNI) IN BREAST CANCER

The radiation of supraclavicular nodes (SCNs) and internal mammary lymph nodes (IMNs), together called RNI, has been an area of extensive debate in the radiation oncology community. In the case of four positive axillary nodes, the indication for RNI is undisputed. For patients with one to three positive nodes (pN1), data concerning the effectiveness of RNI are less certain. The MA 20 and EORTC 22922-10925 suggest *all* node-positive patients benefit from comprehensive, including SCN and IMN, without an increase in cardiovascular toxicity. It is not recommended for patients with pathologically negative axillary nodes (pN0) assessed by adequate axillary lymph node dissection (ALND) or sentinel node biopsy (SNB). The role of axillary radiation in inadequately addressed axilla is supported by data from the EORTC 10981-22023 AMAROS study where 4,806 patients who had clinically negative nodes received SNB. Patients with negative SNB did not undergo any axillary treatment (except WBI), and the 5-year rate of axillary recurrence was 0.8%. SNB was pathologically positive in 1,425 patients, who were randomized for either ALN-RT or ALND. In the ALND group, 67% had no further positive nodes, 1–3 affected nodes were found in 25%, and >4 nodes in 7.8%. The 5-year axillary recurrence rate was not significantly different: 0.43% after ALND and 1.19% after ALN-RT (5).

Role of Radiotherapy in Metastatic Breast Cancer

Radiation is a potent tool in palliation of symptoms related to the spread of cancer. Bone and brain metastases have been traditionally treated with short courses of palliative radiotherapy with appreciable symptomatic benefit. Hemostatic radiation has been useful in controlling bleeding from advanced inoperable breast cancer. Ablative radiation in the form of stereotactic brain and body radiotherapy has shown promise in phase 2 studies in improving the outcomes in oligometastatic disease when used instead of standard doses of palliative radiotherapy (4). The potential synergy of this modality with systemic therapy has stimulated a plethora of studies in this area, and the future might see a bigger role of radiation in this difficult-to-treat group of patients.

REFERENCES

1. Early Breast Cancer Trialists' Collaborative Group (EBCTCG), Darby S, McGale P, Correa C, Taylor C, Arriagada R, Clarke M, Cutter D, Davies C, Ewertz M, Godwin J, Gray R, Pierce L, Whelan T, Wang Y, Peto R. Effect of radiotherapy after breast-conserving surgery on 10-year recurrence and 15-year breast cancer death: meta-analysis of individual patient data for 10,801 women in 17 randomised trials. *Lancet.* 2011 Nov 12; 378(9804):1707–16.
2. EBCTCG (Early Breast Cancer Trialists' Collaborative Group), McGale P, Taylor C, Correa C, Cutter D, Duane F, Ewertz M, Gray R, Mannu G, Peto R, Whelan T, Wang Y, Wang Z, Darby S. Effect of radiotherapy after mastectomy and axillary surgery on 10-year recurrence and 20-year breast cancer mortality: meta-analysis of individual patient data for 8135 women in 22 randomised trials. *Lancet.* 2014 Jun 21;383(9935):2127–35. doi: 10.1016/S0140-6736(14)60488-8. Epub 2014 Mar 19. Erratum in: Lancet. 2014 Nov 22;384(9957):1848.
3. Sedlmayer F, Sautter-Bihl ML, Budach W, Dunst J, Fastner G, Feyer P, Fietkau R, Haase W, Harms W, Souchon R, Wenz F, Sauer R, Breast Cancer Expert Panel of the German Society of Radiation Oncology (DEGRO). DEGRO practical guidelines: radiotherapy of breast cancer I: radiotherapy following breast conserving therapy for invasive breast cancer. *Strahlenther Onkol.* 2013 Oct;189(10):825–33.

4. Palma DA, Olson R, Harrow S, Gaede S, Louie AV, Haasbeek C, Mulroy L, Lock M, Rodrigues GB, Yaremko BP, Schellenberg D, Ahmad B, Griffioen G, Senthi S, Swaminath A, Kopek N, Liu M, Moore K, Currie S, Bauman GS, Warner A, Senan S. Stereotactic ablative radiotherapy versus standard of care palliative treatment in patients with oligometastatic cancers (SABR-COMET): a randomised, phase 2, open-label trial. *Lancet.* 2019 May 18;393(10185):2051–2058.

5. Cardoso F, Paluch-Shimon S, Senkus E, Curigliano G, Aapro MS, André F, Barrios CH, Bergh J, Bhattacharyya GS, Biganzoli L, Boyle F, Cardoso MJ, Carey LA, Cortés J, El Saghir NS, Elzayat M, Eniu A, Fallowfield L, Francis PA, Gelmon K, Gligorov J, Haidinger R, Harbeck N, Hu X, Kaufman B, Kaur R, Kiely BE, Kim SB, Lin NU, Mertz SA, Neciosup S, Offersen BV, Ohno S, Pagani O, Prat A, Penault-Llorca F, Rugo HS, Sledge GW, Thomssen C, Vorobiof DA, Wiseman T, Xu B, Norton L, Costa A, Winer EP. 5th ESO-ESMO International Consensus guidelines for advanced breast cancer (ABC 5). *Ann Oncol.* 2020 Dec;31(12):1623–1649.

Chemotherapeutic Interventions

25

Kakali Choudhury

INTRODUCTION

Chemotherapy is an important mode of multimodal treatment of breast cancer. It uses drugs to target and kill the cancer cells. This is a systemic therapy for breast cancer and is used in different stages of breast cancer (1).

HISTORY

Breast cancer has been recognized since at least 1600 BC (2), and gradually its anatomy and surgery were invented in the 17th century onwards. The journey of chemotherapy began after the Second World War, and the first effective combination chemotherapy in breast cancer was cyclophosphamide, methotrexate, and 5FU (CMF) by Bonadonna et al. in 1976 (3). It was tested in the 1970s in the Milan trial. Their demonstration that risk of recurrence after surgery could be reduced with the addition of adjuvant chemotherapy paved the path to the modern breast conservation approach. The first anthracycline-containing regimen is cyclophosphamide and doxorubicin and is still the gold standard, which was investigated by the National Surgical Adjuvant Breast and Bowel Project (NSABP) in the 1990s (4).

TYPES OF CHEMOTHERAPY

According to the use of chemotherapy in breast cancer, it can be one of three types:

1. Adjuvant chemotherapy
2. Neoadjuvant chemotherapy
3. Palliative chemotherapy

DOI: 10.1201/9780367821982-26

Adjuvant Chemotherapy

When chemotherapy is administered after surgery in early breast cancer (stage I, II, and some III) to destroy the residual microscopic diseases in the body, it is called adjuvant chemotherapy.

The benefit of this chemotherapy depends on several factors like endocrine receptor status and subtype of tumor and also patient age and type of chemotherapy drugs used (5).

Adjuvant chemotherapy can be omitted if the tumor size is less than 2 cm, hormone receptor status is positive, grade 1, no lymphovascular invasion (LVI), and HER2-neu status is negative (6).

Adjuvant chemotherapy is strongly recommended with an increasing number of risk factors like positive nodal status, tumor more than 2 cm, estrogen receptor status negative, age less than 35 years, LVI present, grade 2 or 3, HER2-neu status positive, and Ki67 score more than 15% (6).

The Nottingham Prognostic Index (NPI) is an important scoring system to guide adjuvant therapy in breast cancer. NPI along with Allred score and Her 2 neu status help to decide the adjuvant chemotherapy in early breast cancer.

A multigene signature like the Oncotype DX score also stratifies patients according to survival benefit and recurrence risk and benefit from adjuvant chemotherapy (7).

Adjuvant chemotherapy for breast cancer has evolved over the years. The first-generation regimen is CMF (8). Then anthracyclines and taxanes were added with an increased survival benefit and reduced the mortality by about 30% (9, 10). The recommended regimens are 5flurouracil, Doxorubicin (Adriamycin) Cyclophosphamide (FAC) or 5 fluorouracil Epirubicin Cyclophosphamide (FEC) followed by Taxanes (Docetaxel/Paclitaxel) (T), Adriyamycin & Cyclophosphamide (AC) followed by T, Taxane (Docetaxel) Adriyamycin Cyclophosphamide (TAC). "Dose-dense" regimens are 2 weekly regimens of the same drugs with granulocyte colony-stimulating factor (GCSF) support and usually used for high-risk groups, such as node positive and triple negative (11, 12). The absolute benefits of adjuvant chemotherapy gained depend on the absolute risk recurrence without adjuvant chemotherapy (13, 14). NPI calculates the risk of recurrence.

The regimens are shown in Tables 25.1 and 25.2 (NCCN Guidelines Version 4.2022).

Neoadjuvant Chemotherapy

Neoadjuvant therapy is defined as the systemic therapy of breast cancer before the definitive surgical therapy.

The goal of neoadjuvant chemotherapy is to reduce the risk of distant recurrence in nonmetastatic invasive breast cancer. This preoperative therapy downstages the disease in breast and/or regional lymph nodes and also provides information regarding the response to adjuvant therapies.

Downstaging may allow less extensive surgery (like a breast conservative one instead of mastectomy), better cosmetic outcome, and fewer postoperative complications like lymphedema.

The residual invasive cancer after neoadjuvant therapy is a strong prognostic factor for the risk of recurrence, especially in triple-negative and HER2-neu–positive diseases (15).

Although originally neoadjuvant chemotherapy was indicated for locally advanced breast cancer, it is now frequently used in early operable cases to avoid mastectomy and can provide a less extensive surgery and better cosmetic outcome (16).

Hence the indications for neoadjuvant chemotherapy are as follows (17):

1. *Locally advanced breast cancer*: Stage III disease, T1–3 with N2T4 with N0-2, any T with N3 of all subtypes are candidates for neoadjuvant chemotherapy.
2. *Selected early-stage patients*: When operable tumor presents with high tumor: Breast ratio, neoadjuvant therapy is needed for breast conservation or better cosmetic outcome. It is also indicated in T2 or even T1c triple-negative or HER2-neu–positive varieties to know the response to treatment. These subgroups are associated with high rates of clinical and pathological complete

TABLE 25.1   Preoperative/Adjuvant regimen for HER2-neu–positive breast cancer

Preferred Regimens

- Paclitaxel + Trastuzumab
- TCH (Docetaxel/Carboplatin/Trastuzumab)
- TCHP (Docetaxel/Carboplatin/Trastuzumab/Pertuzumab)
- If no residual disease after preoperative therapy or no preoperative therapy:
  - Complete up to 1 year of HER2-targeted therapy with trastuzumab (category 1) ± Pertuzumab
- *If residual disease after preoperative therapy*: Ado-trastuzumab emtansine (category 1) alone
  If ado-trastuzumab emtansine discontinued for toxicity, then Trastuzumab (category 1) ± Pertuzumab
  to complete 1 year of therapy

Useful in Certain Circumstances	**Other Recommended Regimens**
- Docetaxel + Cyclophosphamide + Trastuzumab - AC followed by T + Trastuzumab (Doxorubicin/Cyclophosphamide followed by paclitaxel plus trastuzumab, various schedules) - AC followed by T + Trastuzumab + Pertuzumab (Doxorubicin/Cyclophosphamide followed by Paclitaxel + Trastuzumab + Pertuzumab, various schedules) - Neratinib (adjuvant setting only) - Paclitaxel + Trastuzumab + Pertuzumab - Ado-trastuzumab emtansine (TDM-1) (adjuvant setting only)	- AC followed by Docetaxel + Trastuzumab (Doxorubicin/Cyclophosphamide followed by Docetaxel + Trastuzumab) - AC followed by Docetaxel + Trastuzumab + Pertuzumab - (Doxorubicin/ Cyclophosphamide followed by Docetaxel + Trastuzumab + Pertuzumab)

response. Neoadjuvant treatment also guides the additional treatment after surgery if there is any residual disease.

3. *Clinically limited node-positive disease*: The patient who needs downstaging of axilla regardless of the size of primary tumor. With neoadjuvant chemotherapy, the extent of axillary dissection can be minimized, and thus the complications like lymphedema can be avoided.

4. *Patients with temporary contraindications for surgery*: Breast cancer diagnosed during pregnancy and patients requiring short-term anticoagulation like with recent deep vein thrombosis and pulmonary embolism also receive neoadjuvant chemotherapy.

After neoadjuvant chemotherapy is complete, the patient is evaluated for a response clinically and radiologically and a decision regarding surgery is made.

Palliative Chemotherapy

The goal of treatment of metastatic breast cancer is to prolong survival and improve the quality of life by reducing cancer-related symptoms. Cytotoxic chemotherapy is the standard of care in metastatic breast cancer irrespective of hormone receptor status and also along with other targeted therapies. This is called palliative chemotherapy. The survival of metastatic breast cancer patients has been improved with palliative chemotherapy, and hence they are now eligible for several lines of chemotherapy (18).

Single-agent chemotherapy is the preferred choice for palliative chemotherapy, as there is better understanding of the benefit by the drug and usually less toxicity. Combination chemotherapy can be preferred in extensive visceral disease or impending visceral crisis, but the benefit is not proven in prospective

TABLE 25.2   Preoperative/Adjuvant regimen for HER2-neu–negative breast cancer

Preferred Regimens

- Dose-dense AC (Doxorubicin/Cyclophosphamide) followed by paclitaxel every 2 weeks
- Dose-dense AC (Doxorubicin/Cyclophosphamide) followed by weekly paclitaxel
- TC (Docetaxel and cyclophosphamide)
- Olaparib, if germline *BRCA1/2* mutations
- *High-risk triple-negative breast cancer (TNBC)*: Preoperative pembrolizumab + Carboplatin + Paclitaxel, followed by preoperative Pembrolizumab + Cyclophosphamide + Doxorubicin or epirubicin, followed by adjuvant pembrolizumab
- TNBC and residual disease after preoperative therapy with taxane-, alkylator-, and anthracycline-based chemotherapy: Capecitabine

Useful in Certain Circumstances	**Other Recommended Regimens**
- Dose-dense AC (Doxorubicin/Cyclophosphamide) - AC (Doxorubicin/Cyclophosphamide) every 3 weeks (category 2B) - CMF (Cyclophosphamide/Methotrexate/Fluorouracil) AC followed by weekly paclitaxel - Capecitabine (maintenance therapy for TNBC after adjuvant chemotherapy)	AC followed by docetaxel every 3 weeks - EC (Epirubicin/Cyclophosphamide) - TAC (Docetaxel/Doxorubicin/Cyclophosphamide) Select patients with TNBC - Paclitaxel + Carboplatin (various schedules) - Docetaxel + Carboplatin (preoperative setting only)

trials. Duration of response gradually decreases with the subsequent line of chemotherapy. Chemotherapy can be withheld with adequate response and symptom relief and can be restarted after disease progression or symptom recurrence (19).

Anthracyclines and taxanes are the most effective drugs for breast cancer (20, 21). The regimen or drug selection is guided by the previous chemotherapeutic agent received, residual toxicities of previous treatment (like neuropathy or cardiac morbidity), performance status of the patient, and patient's preference. The regimens are shown in Tables 25.3 and 25.4 (NCCN Guidelines Version 4.2022).

TOXICITIES OF CHEMOTHERAPY

The chemotherapeutic agents used in breast cancer have several side effects. The side effects depend on the type and dose of the drugs used and also the duration of treatment (22). The most common effects are hair loss, nail changes, mouth sores, loss of appetite, weight changes, nausea, vomiting, diarrhea, and fatigue. Hot flashes and/or vaginal dryness due to chemotherapy-induced menopause may also occur. Hematological toxicities are also common. There is increased risk of infection due to low white blood cell (WBC) count and easy bruising or bleeding due to low platelet count. Anemia may cause fatigue (23).

Some of these side effects are now manageable by using drugs like antiemetics, steroids, GCSF, etc., and usually go away after a few weeks of completion of treatment.

Some other side effects are associated with particular drugs like cardiac toxicity with anthracyclines, nerve toxicity with taxanes, etc.

Cardiac toxicity: Anthracyclines (doxorubicin, epirubicin) can cause permanent damage like cardiomyopathy. The risk increases with higher doses and prolonged use and also with preexisting heart disease or when used with other cardiotoxic drugs like trastuzumab. This cardiac damage may appear months or years after treatment. Hence, close cardiac monitoring is needed during follow-up (24).

TABLE 25.3 Systemic therapy regimens for recurrent unresectable (local or regional) or stage IV (M1) HER2-neu–negative disease

HER2-NEGATIVE			
Preferred Regimens		**Other Recommended Regimens**	**Useful in Certain Circumstances**

• Anthracyclines
  o Doxorubicin
  o Liposomal
    doxorubicin
• Taxanes
  o Paclitaxel
• Anti-metabolites
  o Capecitabine
  o Gemcitabine
• Microtubule
  inhibitors
  o Vinorelbine
  o Eribulin
• Sacituzumab
  govitecan-hziy (for
  TNBC [category 1]
  or HR+/HER2–)
	• For HER2 IHC 1+
	  or 2+/ISH negative
	  o Fam-trastuzumab
	    deruxtecan-nxki
	    (category 1)
	• For germline
	  BRCA1/2 mutations
	  see additional
	  targeted therapy
	  options (*BINV-R*)
	• Platinum (for TNBC
	  and germline
	  BRCA1/2 mutation)
	  o Carboplatin
	  o Cisplatin
	• For PD-L1–positive
	  TNBC see additional
	  targeted therapy
	  options (*BINV-R*)
		• Cyclophosphamide
		• Docetaxel
		• Albumin-bound
		  paclitaxel
		• Epirubicin
		• Ixabepilone
			• AC (Doxorubicin/
			  Cyclophosphamide)
			• EC (Epirubicin/
			  Cyclophosphamide)
			• CMF (Cyclophosphamide/
			  Methotrexate/Fluorouracil)
			• Docetaxel/Capecitabine
			• GT (Gemcitabine/Paclitaxel)
			• Gemcitabine/Carboplatin
			• Carboplatin + Paclitaxel or
			  albumin-bound paclitaxel

Neurological toxicity: The chemotherapeutic agents like taxanes (docetaxel, paclitaxel, protein bound paclitaxel), platinum compounds (cisplatin, carboplatin), vinorelbine, eribulin, and ixabepilone can cause neurological damage in the limbs (neuropathy). These cause numbness, pain, tingling or burning sensation, sensitivity to cold or heat exposure, and weakness. These symptoms are usually not persistent but sometimes may cause permanent damage. These can be treated by medications.

Hand-foot syndrome: This toxicity is mostly related to capecitabine and liposomal doxorubicin. The palms and soles have redness, tingling, and numbness and then they may be swollen, painful, with blisters and peeling of the skin. There is no specific treatment of hand-foot syndrome, and it is usually cured after changing or stopping the drug.

Second malignancy: This is a very rare but serious long-term toxicity. The drugs like doxorubicin may cause myelodysplastic syndrome (MDS) or acute leukemias.

Menstrual changes and fertility: Premature menopause and infertility may occur due to the effect of chemotherapy. Hence, a prior gynecological consultation should be done to deal with these problems.

CONCLUSION

Chemotherapy is one of the important systemic therapies in the management of breast cancer in almost every stage and irrespective of type. Although newer modalities of treatment are coming like targeted therapy, CDK inhibitors, PARP inhibitors, and newer techniques in surgery and radiotherapy, still chemotherapy is the mainstay of treatment to increase survival in breast cancer. Newer molecules are coming with higher efficacy and lesser toxicities to improve survival as well as quality of life.

TABLE 25.4 Systemic therapy regimens for recurrent unresectable (local or regional) or stage IV (M1) HER2-neu–positive disease

HER2-POSITIVE			
Setting	**Regimen**	**NCCN Category of Preference**	**NCCN Category of Evidence**
First line	Pertuzumab + Trastuzumab + Docetaxel	Preferred regimen	1
	Pertuzumab + Trastuzumab + Paclitaxel	Preferred regimen	2A
Second line	Fam-trastuzumab deruxtecan-nxki	Preferred regimen	1
	Ado-trastuzumab emtansine (T-DM1)	Other recommended regimen	2A
Third line and beyond (optimal sequence is not known)	Tucatinib + Trastuzumab + Capecitabine	Other recommended regimen	1
	Trastuzumab + Docetaxel or Vinorelbine	Other recommended regimen	2A
	Trastuzumab + Paclitaxel ± Carboplatin	Other recommended regimen	2A
	Capecitabine + Trastuzumab or lapatinib	Other recommended regimen	2A
	Trastuzumab + Lapatinib (without cytotoxic therapy)	Other recommended regimen	2A
	Trastuzumab + Other agents	Other recommended regimen	2A
	Neratinib + Capecitabine	Other recommended regimen	2A
	Margetuximab-cmkb + Chemotherapy (capecitabine, eribulin, gemcitabine, or vinorelbine)	Other recommended regimen	2A

REFERENCES

1. DeSantis C, Siegel R, Bandi P, Jemal A. (2011). Breast cancer statistics, 2011. *CA Cancer J Clin* 61:409–418. [PubMed]
2. Smith E. (2006). *The Edwin Smith surgical papyrus: hieroglyphic transliteration, translation and commentary VI*. Breasted JH (ed). Kissinger Publishing: Montana. [Google Scholar]
3. Bonadonna G, Brusamolino E, Valagussa P, Rossi A, Brugnatelli L, Brambilla C, De Lena M, et al. (1976). Combination chemotherapy as an adjuvant treatment in operable breast cancer. *N Engl J Med* 294:405–410.
4. Fisher B, Brown AM, Dimitrov NV, et al. (1990). Two months of doxorubicin- cyclophosphamide with or without reinduction therapy compared with 6 months of cyclophosphamide, methotrexate and 5 fluorouracil therapy in positive node breast cancer patients with tamoxifen non responsive tumors: results from the Nation Surgical Adjuvant Breast and Bowel Project B-15. *J Clin Oncol* 8:1483–1496.
5. NIH Consensus Conference. (1991). Treatment of early stage breast cancer. *J Am Med Assoc* 265:391–395.

6. NICE. (2014). Early and locally advanced breast cancer. Diagnosis and treatment. NICE clinical guideline 80. London: National Institute for Health and Care Excellence.
7. NICE. (2013). Gene expression profiling and expanded immunohistochemistry tests for guiding adjuvant chemotherapy decisions in early breast cancer management: MamaPrint, Oncotype DX, IHC4 and MammoStrat. NICE Diagnostics Guidance 10. London: National Institute for Health and Care Excellence.
8. Earl HM, Hiller L, Dunn JA, et al. (2012). Adjuvant Epiribicin followed by Cyclophosphamide, Methotrexate and Fluracil (CMF) vs CMF in early breast cancer: results with over 7 years median follow up from the randomazied NEAT/BR9601 trials. *Br J Cancer* 107:1257–1267.
9. Martin M, Pienkowski T, Kissin M, et al. (2005). Adjuvant docetaxel for node positive breast cancer. *N Engl J Med* 352:2302–2313.
10. Jones S, Homes FA, et al. (2009). Docetaxel with cyclophosphamide is associated with an overall survival benefit compared with doxorubicin and cyclophosphamide: 7 year follow up of US Oncology Research Trial 9735. *J Clin Once* 27:1177–1183.
11. Citron ML, Berry DA, et al. (2003). Randomizied trial of dose deans versus conventionally scheduled and sequential versus concurrent combination chemotherapy as post operative adjuvant treatment of node positive primary breast cancer: first report of Intergroup Trial C9741/Cancer and Leukemia Group B Trial 9741. *J Clin Once* 21:1431–1439.
12. French Adjuvant Study Group. (2001). Benefit of a high dose epirubicin regimen in adjuvant chemotherapy for node positive breast cancer patients with poor prognostic factors: 5 year follow up results of French Adjuvant Study Group 05 randomised trial. *J Clin Oncol* 19:602–611.
13. EBCTCG. (2012). Comparisions between different polychemotherapy regimens for early breast cancer: meta-analyses of long term outcome among 100000 women in 123 randomised trials. *Lancet* 379:432–444.
14. EBCTCG. (2005). Effects of chemotherapy and hormonal therapy for early breast cancer on recurrence and 15 year survival: an overview of the randomised trials. *Lancet* 365:1687–1717.
15. Von Minckwitz G, Untch M, Blohmer J, et al. (2012). Definition and Impact of pathological complete response on prognosis after neoadjuvant chemotherapy in various intrinsic breast cancer subtypes. *J Clin Oncol* 30:1796–1804.
16. Hanrahan EO, Hennessy BT, Valero V. (2005). Neoadjuvant chemotherapy for breast cancer: an overview and review of recent clinical trials. *Exp Opin Pharmacother* 6:1477–1491.
17. Goldhirsch A, Gelber RD, et al. (2013). Personalising the treatment of women with early breast cancer: highlights of the St Gallen International Expert Consensus on the Primary Therapy of Early Breast Cancer 2013. *Ann Oncol* 24:2206–2223.
18. Geels P, Eisenhauer E, Bezjak A, et al. (2000). Palliative effect of chemotherapy: objective tumor response is associated with symptom improvement in patients with metastatic breast cancer. *J Clin Oncol* 18(12):2395–2405.
19. Cardoso F, Costa A, Senkus E, et al. (2017). 3rd ESO-ESMO International Consensus Guidelines for Advanced Breast Cancer (ABC 3). *Ann Oncol* 28(1):16–33.
20. Marty M, Cognetti F, Maraninchi D, et al. (2005). Randomized phase II trial of the efficacy and safety of trastuzumab combined with docetaxel in patients with human epidermal growth factor receptor 2-positive metastatic breast cancer administered as first-line treatment: the M77001 Study Group. *J Clin Oncol* 23(19):4265–4274.
21. Slamon DJ, Leyland-Jones B, Shak S, et al. (2001). Use of chemotherapy plus a monoclonal antibody against HER2 for metastatic breast cancer that overexpresses HER2. *N Engl J Med* 344(11):783–792.
22. Russo S, Cinausero M., et al. (2014). Factors affecting patient'sperception of anti-cancer treatments side effects: an observational study. Expert. Open. Drug Say 13(2):139–150.
23. Leonard RC, Howell A. (2000). A systematic review of docetaxel, paclitaxel and vinorelbine in the treatment of advanced breast cancer. *Adv Breast Cancer* 2:1–3.
24. O'Shaughnessy J, Miles D, Vukelja S, et al. (2002). Superior survival with Capecitabine plus Docetaxel combination chemotherapy anthracyclin pretreated patients with advanced breast cancer: phase III trial results. *J Clin Oncol* 20:2812–2823.
25. Russo S, Cinausero M, et al. (2014). Factors affecting patient'sperception of anti-cancer treatments side effects: an observational study. *Expert Open Drug Say* 13(2):139–150.
26. Muss HB, Berry DA, Cirrincione C, et al. (2007). Toxicity of older and younger patients treated with adjuvant chemotherapy for node-positive breast cancer: the Cancer and Leukemia Group B Experience. *J Clin Oncol* 25:3699–3704.
27. Curigliano G, Cardinale D, Suter T, et al. (2012). Cardiovascular toxicity induced by chemotherapy, targeted agents and radiotherapy: ESMO Clinical Practice Guidelines. *Ann Oncol* 23(Suppl. 7):vii155–vii166. [PubMed] [Google Scholar] Guidelines for cardiotoxicity in oncology.

Molecular Targets and Immunotherapy 26

Joydeep Ghosh

INTRODUCTION

The treatment of breast cancer has come a long way from the times of chemotherapy, to hormonal therapies, to finding drivers like human epidermal growth factor receptor 2 (HER2) and targeting them, to molecular targets and immunotherapies (1, 2). With every prominent discovery, there has been a significant leap in the outcomes of patients. Today we are standing at a time point, and from here, treatment decisions are going to be made purely based on targeted therapies and immunotherapy. There is a possibility that with better outcomes, the role of nonspecific cytotoxic regimens might become redundant. In this chapter, we shall discuss the updates in molecular and targeted therapies. We shall divide it into the curative setting and metastatic setting and discuss each one concerning molecular targets and immune blockade.

NEOADJUVANT AND ADJUVANT SETTINGS

Anti–HER2 Blockade

Trastuzumab, which is an HER2 blocker, was found to be effective in multiple randomized trials, initially in the metastatic setting and followed by the adjuvant and neoadjuvant settings (3–5). In the neoadjuvant and adjuvant settings, the latest Early Breast Cancer Trialists Collaborative Group (EBCTCG) meta-analysis involving 13,864 patients has shown that trastuzumab used in early breast cancer significantly reduces risks of breast cancer recurrence (response rate 0.66, 95% confidence interval [CI] 0.62–0.71; $p < 0.0001$) and death from breast cancer (0.67, 0.61–0.73; $p < 0.0001$) (6). Initially, single HER2 blockade was found to be effective in improving the pathological complete response (pCR) rates as well as the event-free survival for patients treated with neoadjuvant chemotherapy (7). Then came the era of dual HER2 blockade with the use of a pertuzumab and trastuzumab combination, which significantly improved the response rates and proportion of pCR (8). The pCR rates with double HER2 blockade ranges from 45% to 60% depending on various chemotherapy backbones (9). Strategies have also introduced trastuzumab emtansine (TDM1) in the neoadjuvant setting, which has led to inferior pCR rates (10).

DOI: 10.1201/9780367821982-27

Hormone Receptor–Positive Cancer

Breast cancer is no longer a "one size fits all" disease. It has been subclassified based on immunohistochemistry and endocrine receptor expression to luminal A, B HER amplified, and basal types (11). Out of these, luminal A has the best prognosis and the most endocrine-responsive tumor. With the advent of molecular signature assessments, various risk prediction tools have paved the way for personalized therapy in the adjuvant setting. Oncotype DX is once such widely used platform which tested the role of chemotherapy in the adjuvant setting for an intermediate-risk group. It was shown that patients with an intermediate risk have no benefits with the addition of chemotherapy to adjuvant endocrine therapy in small node-negative tumors. Endocrine therapy was noninferior to chemoendocrine therapy in the analysis of invasive disease-free survival (hazard ratio for invasive disease recurrence, second primary cancer, or death [endocrine vs. chemoendocrine therapy], 1.08; 95% CI 0.94–1.24; P = 0.26) (12). The other molecular-based platforms for risk stratification are Mammaprint, PAM 50, and EndoPredict (13–15). In recent times, there have been studies in the neoadjuvant space for endocrine therapy. Strategies have used neoadjuvant tamoxifen as well as aromatase inhibitors. An ideal patient would be operable breast cancer in an elderly lady with a strong hormone receptor positivity and low Ki65 score. This is the subset that benefits the most from neoadjuvant endocrine therapy (NAET). In the GEICAM trial, exemestane for 24 weeks was compared to standard chemotherapy of anthracyclines and taxanes. The response rate was 66% with chemotherapy and 40% with NAET (16). In the NEOCENT trial, similarly, the response rate was 55% with chemotherapy and 59% with NAET (17).

Cyclin-dependent kinase (CDK4/6) has established its role as the primary treatment of metastatic hormone receptor–positive breast cancer. It is now being tested in the neoadjuvant setting. In the PALLET trial, palbociclib was combined with letrozole (PA) as neoadjuvant therapy and compared to letrozole alone. Although PA enhanced the suppression of malignant cell proliferation (Ki67), it did not increase the clinical response rate over 14 weeks (18). In another study, exemestane was combined with letrozole and compared to 5-fluorouracil, epiurubicin and cyclophosphamide (FEC) chemotherapy. It showed that neoadjuvant everolimus plus letrozole may achieve a better ultrasound response with fewer toxicities compared to chemotherapy (19).

Triple-Negative Breast Cancer (TNBC)

Of all the molecular aberrations driving research in breast cancer therapy, a major chunk of them are happening in TNBC. This is largely because TNBC has a varied molecular abnormality, and we do not have well-defined targets, unlike hormone receptor–positive or HER2 positive.

A major breakthrough was the incorporation of BReast CAncer gene (*BRCA*) 1 and 2 gene testing. A recent trial (OlympiAD) randomized patients who were BRCA 1/2 positive and HER2 negative after curative intent surgery, chemotherapy, and radiotherapy to a PARP inhibitor (olaparib) versus placebo for 1 year. The 3-year invasive disease-free survival was 85.9% in the olaparib group and 77.1% in the placebo group (95% CI, 4.5–13.0; hazard ratio [HR] for invasive disease or death, 0.58; 99.5% CI, 0.41–0.82; P < 0.001) (20). This trial included both hormone receptor–positive and –negative populations.

The GeparOla trial brought olaparib into the neoadjuvant setting, in combination with paclitaxel for patients with homologous recombinant deficiency. The pCR rate with paclitaxel and olaparib was 55.1% versus 48.6% (90% CI 34.3–63.2%) (21). Another trial utilizing veliparib in combination with the taxane platinum concluded that there is no significant increase in the pCR rate with the addition of veliparib (22).

Immunotherapy, just like with other cancers, has also been tested in the neoadjuvant setting for breast cancer. In the KEYNOTE-522 trial, triple-negative early breast cancer patients were randomized to pembrolizumab plus chemotherapy versus chemotherapy alone. For those who received pembrolizumab, they were given the same in the adjuvant phase for nine cycles. The primary endpoint of pCR was 64.8% (95% CI, 59.9–69.5) in the pembrolizumab-chemotherapy group and 51.2% (95% CI, 44.1–58.3) in the placebo-chemotherapy group (95% CI, 5.4–21.8; P < 0.001) (23). Neoadjuvant treatment with atezolizumab in combination with nab-paclitaxel and anthracycline-based chemotherapy significantly improved pathological complete response rates: 58% versus 41% (95% CI 6–27; one-sided p = 0.0044 [significance boundary 0.0184]) (24).

METASTATIC SETTING

The impact of research with molecular targets has had a greater impact on treatment decisions in the metastatic setting than the curative setting. This can also be looked at as a stage in the drug development and testing, where it is usually first tested in a metastatic setting, followed by a curative setting. Since the treatment approaches vary significantly among the three common breast cancer types, we shall discuss each of them separately.

HER2-Positive Breast Cancer

The first-line treatment gold standard regimen is the combination of taxane with pertuzumab and trastuzumab as per the CLEOPATRA trial, leading to a median overall survival (OS) of 56 months versus 41 months with taxane trastuzumab alone (25). In the second line, TDM1 is the standard of care now, with the EMILIA trial showing the significant benefit of improved OS of 30.9 months vs. 25.1 months (HR, 0.68; 95% CI, 0.55–0.85; P < 0.001), compared to lapatinib with capecitabine (26). Also in the third line, the best strategy remains TDM1, with the TH3RESA trial showing improved survival of 22 months versus 15.8 months with chemotherapy of physicians' choice (HR 0.68 [95% CI 0.54–0.85]; p = 0.0007) (27). Another antibody-drug conjugate, trastuzumab deruxtecan (TDX1), has been found to be effective in not just HER2-positive but also HER2-low tumors. In a phase 2 study with TDX1 in previously treated HER2-positive metastatic breast cancer (MBC), the median response duration was 14.8 months (95% CI, 13.8–16.9), and the median duration of progression-free survival was 16.4 months (95% CI, 12.7 to not reached) (28).

Oral tyrosine kinase inhibitors (TKIs) have also been proven to be beneficial in this set of patients. A newer TKI, tucatinib, has shown significant improvement in both visceral and central nervous system (CNS) metastasis, compared to trastuzumab and capecitabine in the HER2CLIMB trial (29, 30).

The new drug margetuximab shares HER2 specificity with trastuzumab but incorporates an engineered Fc region to increase immune activation. Margetuximab improved primary progression-free survival (PFS) (5.8 versus 4.9 months) over trastuzumab (HR, 0.76; 95% CI, 0.59–0.98; P = .03); in the SOFIA trial (31). Overall, the role of anti-HER2 blockade is emerging fast and is expected to make the role of chemotherapy redundant.

Hormone Receptor–Positive Breast Cancer

With the advent of CDK4/6 inhibitors, the treatment has been revolutionized with three molecules, namely palbociclib, ribociclib, and abemaciclib. In the first line, all of them nearly doubled the PFS compared to aromatase inhibitor alone (32–34). In addition, ribociclib has shown to be beneficial in premenopausal patients, also improving both PFS and OS (33).

Preclinical studies have established the role of PIK3CA in the development of resistance to standard first-line treatment. Based on the same, the SOLAR1 trial demonstrated significant improvement in PFS of alpelisib with fulvestrant in the second line for those with PIK3CA mutant (11.0 months [95% CI, 7.5–14.5] in the alpelisib-fulvestrant group, as compared with 5.7 months (95% CI, 3.7–7.4) with fulvestrant alone (35). Presently, there are insufficient data to recommend routine testing for *ESR1* mutations to guide therapy for HR-positive, HER2-negative MBC.

Triple-Negative Breast Cancer

Due to the wide variety of possible driver mutations in TNBC, there has been significant development with various molecules. The targeted approach in TNBC revolved around *BRCA* positivity, androgen receptor targeting, and immunotherapy. We shall discuss each one of them next.

BRCA1/2

The prevalence of *BRCA* 1 and 2 has varied from 5% to 15% based on various registry studies (36, 37). So, strategies to inhibit cell growth with PARP inhibitors have been tested in two trials. The EMBRACA study showed the median PFS was significantly longer with talazoparib, compared to chemotherapy (8.6 months vs. 5.6 months, the HR for disease progression or death, 0.54; 95% CI, 0.41–0.71; P < 0.001) (38). Also, in the OlympiAD study, the median PFS was significantly longer in the olaparib group compared to chemotherapy (7.0 months vs. 4.2 months; HR, 0.58; 95% CI, 0.43–0.80; P < 0.001) (39).

Androgen receptor blockade

In patients who have androgen receptor (AR) receptor positivity, enzalutamide led to a clinical benefit rate at 16 weeks of 25% (95% CI, 17%–33%) (40).

Immune checkpoint inhibitors

TNBC has multiple subtypes, one of which is rich in T-cell infiltrates. So, they are supposed to respond to immune checkpoint inhibitors. Paclitaxel was combined with atezolizumab in the treatment of first-line therapy for metastatic TNBC; however, it did not lead to any improvement in the PFS (41). Also, pembrolizumab was tested in combination with chemotherapy, and it showed an improvement in the median PFS from 5.6 to 9.7 months (HR for progression or death, 0.65, 95% CI 0.49–0.86; one-sided p = 0.0012 [primary objective met]) (42).

Antibody-drug conjugates have also been proven to be beneficial in TNBC. In one study, sacituzumab govitecan improved the progression free survival (PFS) from 1.7 months to 5.6 months compared to chemotherapy alone (HR for disease progression or death, 0.41; 95% CI, 0.32–0.52; P < 0.001). There was also an improvement in the OS (43).

Targeting the PI3K/Akt/mTOR pathway is also being investigated as one of the treatment strategies. Ipatasertib with paclitaxel improved the PFS compared to taxane alone (44). Trials with capivasertib are on the way.

Inhibition of vascular endothelial growth factor (VEGF) with bevacizumab has also been used as a target. In the TANIA trial, PFS was significantly longer for those patients treated with bevacizumab plus chemotherapy than for those with chemotherapy alone (median: 6.3 months [95% CI 5.4–7.2] vs 4.2 months [3.9–4.7], respectively, stratified HR 0.75 [95% CI 0.61–0.93] (45). A subgroup analysis of the RIBBON II trial showed that for TNBC, there is a role of improvement of PFS with the addition of bevacizumab with chemotherapy in the second line, but it did not achieve any survival benefit (46).

Trials are underway looking at the epigenetic pathway modification, DNA methyltransferase (DNMT) inhibition, and histone deacetylase (HDAC) inhibition as well as inhibition of the cell cycle (47–50).

CONCLUSION

There has been a major leap in recent times in terms of strategies to treat breast cancer with more precise molecular targets. It is beyond the capacity of this chapter to discuss every aspect in detail. We have tried to highlight the most clinically relevant areas. Overall, it's great progress and is going to change how we treat breast cancer in a big way.

REFERENCES

1. Larionov AA (2018) Current therapies for human epidermal growth factor receptor 2-positive metastatic breast cancer patients. *Front Oncol* 8:89
2. Ades F, Tryfonidis K, Zardavas D (2017) The past and future of breast cancer treatment-from the papyrus to individualised treatment approaches. *Ecancermedicalscience* 11:746
3. Kast K, Schoffer O, Link T, et al (2017) Trastuzumab and survival of patients with metastatic breast cancer. *Arch Gynecol Obstet* 296:303–312
4. Takada M, Toi M (2020) Neoadjuvant treatment for HER2-positive breast cancer. *Chin Clin Oncol* 9:32
5. Cameron D, Piccart-Gebhart MJ, Gelber RD, et al (2017) 11 years' follow-up of trastuzumab after adjuvant chemotherapy in HER2-positive early breast cancer: final analysis of the HERceptin Adjuvant (HERA) trial. *Lancet* 389:1195–1205
6. Early Breast Cancer Trialists' Collaborative group (EBCTCG) (2021) Trastuzumab for early-stage, HER2-positive breast cancer: a meta-analysis of 13 864 women in seven randomised trials. *Lancet Oncol* 22:1139–1150
7. Gianni L, Eiermann W, Semiglazov V, et al (2010) Neoadjuvant chemotherapy with trastuzumab followed by adjuvant trastuzumab versus neoadjuvant chemotherapy alone, in patients with HER2-positive locally advanced breast cancer (the NOAH trial): a randomised controlled superiority trial with a parallel HER2-negative cohort. *Lancet* 375:377–384
8. Gianni L, Pienkowski T, Im Y-H, et al (2012) Efficacy and safety of neoadjuvant pertuzumab and trastuzumab in women with locally advanced, inflammatory, or early HER2-positive breast cancer (NeoSphere): a randomised multicentre, open-label, phase 2 trial. *Lancet Oncol* 13:25–32
9. Choi JH, Jeon CW, Kim YO, Jung S (2020) Pathological complete response to neoadjuvant trastuzumab and pertuzumab therapy is related to human epidermal growth factor receptor 2 (HER2) amplification level in HER2-amplified breast cancer. *Medicine* 99:e23053
10. Hurvitz SA, Martin M, Symmans WF, et al (2018) Neoadjuvant trastuzumab, pertuzumab, and chemotherapy versus trastuzumab emtansine plus pertuzumab in patients with HER2-positive breast cancer (KRISTINE): a randomised, open-label, multicentre, phase 3 trial. *Lancet Oncol* 19:115–126
11. (2021) Molecular Subtypes of Breast Cancer. https://www.breastcancer.org/symptoms/types/molecular-subtypes. Accessed 11 Dec 2021
12. Sparano JA, Gray RJ, Makower DF, et al (2018) Adjuvant chemotherapy guided by a 21-gene expression assay in breast cancer. *N Engl J Med* 379:111–121
13. Brandão M, Pondé N, Piccart-Gebhart M (2019) Mammaprint™: a comprehensive review. *Future Oncol* 15:207–224
14. Pu M, Messer K, Davies SR, et al (2020) Research-based PAM50 signature and long-term breast cancer survival. *Breast Cancer Res Treat* 179:197–206
15. Almstedt K, Mendoza S, Otto M, et al (2020) EndoPredict® in early hormone receptor-positive, HER2-negative breast cancer. *Breast Cancer Res Treat* 182:137–146
16. Alba E, Calvo L, Albanell J, et al (2012) Chemotherapy (CT) and hormonotherapy (HT) as neoadjuvant treatment in luminal breast cancer patients: results from the GEICAM/2006-03, a multicenter, randomized, phase-II study. *Ann Oncol* 23:3069–3074
17. Palmieri C, Cleator S, Kilburn LS, et al (2014) NEOCENT: a randomised feasibility and translational study comparing neoadjuvant endocrine therapy with chemotherapy in ER-rich postmenopausal primary breast cancer. *Breast Cancer Res Treat* 148:581–590
18. Johnston S, Puhalla S, Wheatley D, et al (2019) Randomized phase II study evaluating Palbociclib in addition to letrozole as neoadjuvant therapy in estrogen receptor-positive early breast cancer: PALLET trial. *J Clin Oncol* 37:178–189
19. Wu W, Chen J, Deng H, et al (2021) Neoadjuvant everolimus plus letrozole versus fluorouracil, epirubicin and cyclophosphamide for ER-positive, HER2-negative breast cancer: a randomized pilot trial. *BMC Cancer* 21:862
20. Tutt ANJ, Garber JE, Kaufman B, et al (2021) Adjuvant Olaparib for patients with BRCA1- or BRCA2-mutated breast cancer. *N Engl J Med* 384:2394–2405
21. Fasching PA, Link T, Hauke J, et al (2021) Neoadjuvant paclitaxel/Olaparib in comparison to paclitaxel/carboplatinum in patients with HER2-negative breast cancer and homologous recombination deficiency (GeparOLA study). *Ann Oncol* 32:49–57

22. Loibl S, O'Shaughnessy J, Untch M, et al (2018) Addition of the PARP inhibitor veliparib plus carboplatin or carboplatin alone to standard neoadjuvant chemotherapy in triple-negative breast cancer (BrighTNess): a randomised, phase 3 trial. *Lancet Oncol* 19:497–509

23. Schmid P, Cortes J, Pusztai L, et al (2020) Pembrolizumab for early triple-negative breast cancer. *N Engl J Med* 382:810–821

24. Mittendorf EA, Zhang H, Barrios CH, et al (2020) Neoadjuvant atezolizumab in combination with sequential nab-paclitaxel and anthracycline-based chemotherapy versus placebo and chemotherapy in patients with early-stage triple-negative breast cancer (IMpassion031): a randomised, double-blind, phase 3 trial. *Lancet* 396:1090–1100

25. Swain SM, Baselga J, Kim S-B, et al (2015) Pertuzumab, trastuzumab, and docetaxel in HER2-positive metastatic breast cancer. *N Engl J Med* 372:724–734

26. Verma S, Miles D, Gianni L, et al (2012) Trastuzumab emtansine for HER2-positive advanced breast cancer. *N Engl J Med* 367:1783–1791

27. Krop IE, Kim S-B, Martin AG, LoRusso PM, Ferrero J-M, Badovinac-Crnjevic T, Hoersch S, Smitt M, Wildiers H (2017) Trastuzumab emtansine versus treatment of physician's choice in patients with previously treated HER2-positive metastatic breast cancer (TH3RESA): final overall survival results from a randomised open-label phase 3 trial. *Lancet Oncol* 18:743–754

28. Modi S, Saura C, Yamashita T, et al (2020) Trastuzumab deruxtecan in previously treated HER2-positive breast cancer. *N Engl J Med* 382:610–621

29. Murthy RK, Loi S, Okines A, et al (2020) Tucatinib, trastuzumab, and capecitabine for HER2-positive metastatic breast cancer. *N Engl J Med* 382:597–609

30. Lin NU, Borges V, Anders C, et al (2020) Intracranial efficacy and survival with tucatinib plus trastuzumab and capecitabine for previously treated HER2-positive breast cancer with brain metastases in the HER2CLIMB trial. *J Clin Oncol* 38:2610–2619

31. Rugo HS, Im S-A, Cardoso F, et al (2021) Efficacy of Margetuximab vs Trastuzumab in patients with pretreated ERBB2-positive advanced breast cancer: a phase 3 randomized clinical trial. *JAMA Oncol* 7:573–584

32. Finn RS, Martin M, Rugo HS, et al (2016) Palbociclib and letrozole in advanced breast cancer. *N Engl J Med* 375:1925–1936

33. Hortobagyi GN, Stemmer SM, Burris HA, et al (2016) Ribociclib as first-line therapy for HR-positive, advanced breast cancer. *N Engl J Med* 375:1738–1748

34. Sledge GW Jr, Toi M, Neven P, et al (2017) MONARCH 2: Abemaciclib in combination with fulvestrant in women with HR+/HER2- advanced breast cancer who had progressed while receiving endocrine therapy. *J Clin Oncol* 35:2875–2884

35. André F, Ciruelos E, Rubovszky G, et al (2019) Alpelisib for PIK3CA-mutated, hormone receptor-positive advanced breast cancer. *N Engl J Med* 380:1929–1940

36. Sharma P, Klemp JR, Kimler BF, et al (2014) Germline BRCA mutation evaluation in a prospective triple-negative breast cancer registry: implications for hereditary breast and/or ovarian cancer syndrome testing. *Breast Cancer Res Treat* 145:707–714

37. Couch FJ, Hart SN, Sharma P, et al (2015) Inherited mutations in 17 breast cancer susceptibility genes among a large triple-negative breast cancer cohort unselected for family history of breast cancer. *J Clin Oncol* 33:304–311

38. Litton JK, Rugo HS, Ettl J, et al (2018) Talazoparib in patients with advanced breast cancer and a germline BRCA mutation. *N Engl J Med* 379:753–763

39. Robson M, Im S-A, Senkus E, et al (2017) Olaparib for metastatic breast cancer in patients with a germline BRCA mutation. *N Engl J Med* 377:523–533

40. Traina TA, Miller K, Yardley DA, et al (2018) Enzalutamide for the treatment of androgen receptor-expressing triple-negative breast cancer. *J Clin Oncol* 36:884–890

41. Miles D, Gligorov J, André F, et al (2021) Primary results from IMpassion131, a double-blind, placebo-controlled, randomised phase III trial of first-line paclitaxel with or without atezolizumab for unresectable locally advanced/metastatic triple-negative breast cancer. *Ann Oncol* 32:994–1004

42. Cortes J, Cescon DW, Rugo HS, et al (2020) Pembrolizumab plus chemotherapy versus placebo plus chemotherapy for previously untreated locally recurrent inoperable or metastatic triple-negative breast cancer (KEYNOTE-355): a randomised, placebo-controlled, double-blind, phase 3 clinical trial. *Lancet* 396:1817–1828

43. Bardia A, Hurvitz SA, Tolaney SM, et al (2021) Sacituzumab govitecan in metastatic triple-negative breast cancer. *N Engl J Med* 384:1529–1541

44. Kim S-B, Dent R, Im S-A, et al (2017) Ipatasertib plus paclitaxel versus placebo plus paclitaxel as first-line therapy for metastatic triple-negative breast cancer (LOTUS): a multicentre, randomised, double-blind, placebo-controlled, phase 2 trial. *Lancet Oncol* 18:1360–1372

45. von Minckwitz G, Puglisi F, Cortes J, et al (2014) Bevacizumab plus chemotherapy versus chemotherapy alone as second-line treatment for patients with HER2-negative locally recurrent or metastatic breast cancer after first-line treatment with bevacizumab plus chemotherapy (TANIA): an open-label, randomised phase 3 trial. *Lancet Oncol* 15:1269–1278

46. Brufsky A, Valero V, Tiangco B, Dakhil S, Brize A, Rugo HS, Rivera R, Duenne A, Bousfoul N, Yardley DA (2012) Second-line bevacizumab-containing therapy in patients with triple-negative breast cancer: subgroup analysis of the RIBBON-2 trial. *Breast Cancer Res Treat* 133:1067–1075

47. Miranda Furtado CL, Dos Santos Luciano MC, Silva Santos RD, Furtado GP, Moraes MO, Pessoa C (2019) Epidrugs: targeting epigenetic marks in cancer treatment. *Epigenetics* 14:1164–1176

48. Muvarak NE, Chowdhury K, Xia L, et al (2016) Enhancing the cytotoxic effects of PARP inhibitors with DNA demethylating agents - a potential therapy for cancer. *Cancer Cell* 30:637–650

49. Sulaiman A, McGarry S, Lam KM, et al (2018) Co-inhibition of mTORC1, HDAC and ESR1α retards the growth of triple-negative breast cancer and suppresses cancer stem cells. *Cell Death Dis* 9:815

50. Teo ZL, Versaci S, Dushyanthen S, et al (2017) Combined CDK4/6 and PI3Kα inhibition is synergistic and immunogenic in triple-negative breast cancer. *Cancer Res* 77:6340–6352

CORE AREA VIII: MISCELLANEOUS

Special Issues in Breast Tumors

27

27A *Phyllodes Tumor*

Diptendra Kumar Sarkar and Srija Basu

The nomenclature of phyllodes is derived from the word "leaf." It is because of the typical shape of these tumors which mimics a leaf.

Phyllodes tumors account for 1% of breast neoplasms.

SURGICAL PATHOLOGY

A phyllodes tumor is characterized by microscopic leaf-like projections from its wall. Thus, enucleation is often associated with multicentric recurrences. A phyllodes tumor can be, depending on the biological behavior, subclassified into:

1. Benign
2. Borderline
3. Malignant

TUMOR CHARACTERISTICS	BENIGN	BORDERLINE	MALIGNANT
Stromal proliferation	Minimal	Moderate	Severe Nonvisualization of duct at 40×
Mitosis/10 hpf	0–4	5–9	≥10
Margin	Well circumscribed with pushy margin	Microscopic perilesional invasion	Infiltrative margin
Stromal atypia (Pleomorphism)	+	++	++++

DOI: 10.1201/9780367821982-28

PRESENTATION

Phyllodes tumor usually presents in the mid-30s with a painless progressive lump in the breast. Often they may grow very rapidly to attain a large size almost encroaching the whole breast. On clinical examination a large mass with a bosselated (lobulated) surface is palpable. Often the overlying skin contains dilated veins (caused due to increased size of the mass). Skin involvement is a rarity. Axillary lymph nodes are usually not palpable.

DIAGNOSIS

Triple assessment is the cornerstone of diagnosis. Mammography shows a mass in the breast with a smooth surface without any microcalcification. High-resolution ultrasonography (HRUSG) shows lesions in the breast with a smooth lobulated surface. The surrounding halo is present. The anteroposterior diameter is usually less than the transverse diameter. Characteristically there are intralesional clefts. Core biopsy is confirmatory. Histopathological examination (HPE) can differentiate between fibroadenoma and phyllodes tumor. In case of a malignant phyllodes tumor, CT of the thorax may be done to exclude pulmonary metastasis.

TREATMENT

Wide local excision is the treatment of choice. As a phyllodes tumor has leaf-like microscopic extensions, enucleation is not recommended. In large lesions with volume loss, oncoplasty may be required to attain symmetry. In some cases with large lesions occupying the whole of the breast or in patients with recurrent malignant phyllodes tumors, simple mastectomy with or without reconstruction may be needed. Axillary lymph node dissection is not recommended in phyllodes tumors. Historically, radiation therapy (RT) has had a little role in the management of phyllodes tumors. Weak evidence (retrospective review) shows improved local control with RT. Adjuvant CT is associated with marginally improved survival, but the evidence is weak. Phyllodes tumor is associated with 25%–30% local recurrence, and thus strong clinic-radiological follow-up is recommended.

Special Issues in Breast Tumors

27

27B Sarcoma Tumor

Diptendra Kumar Sarkar and Srija Basu

Sarcomas of the breast are a rare and varied group of mesenchymal-derived neoplasias. The incidence of primary breast sarcomas varies between 0.5% and 3% of malignant tumors of the breast (1). They account for less than 5% of all sarcomas (2).

ETIOLOGY

Breast sarcomas may be primary or secondary. Primary breast sarcomas arise from the mesenchymal tissues of the breast. The risk factors are largely unknown. Like other soft tissue sarcomas, some genetic conditions are associated with a higher risk for breast sarcomas. These include Li–Fraumeni syndrome, familial adenomatous polyposis, and neurofibromatosis type 1 (3–5). Breast sarcomas are associated with a *TP53* mutation. There are environmental exposures that have been suggested as risk factors for breast sarcomas, like exposure to arsenic compounds, vinyl chloride, and alkylators (6).

The overall most common type of breast sarcoma is secondary breast sarcoma, especially secondary angiosarcoma. Secondary breast sarcomas occur following external beam radiation therapy for the breast or other intrathoracic malignancies. The most common antecedent malignancies in radiation-induced sarcomas are breast carcinoma and non-Hodgkin's lymphoma (2).

CLINICAL PRESENTATION

Breast sarcomas commonly occur in the fifth to sixth decade but are also found in the premenopausal age group. The clinical presentation includes a unilateral large, firm, mobile, and painless breast mass, which usually grows faster compared with epithelial breast cancer. Breast sarcomas usually lack other features such as nipple discharge or skin retraction. Sarcomas of the breast frequently metastasize hematogenously to the lungs, bone marrow, and liver. Lymphatic spread is rare, but more commonly seen in certain soft tissue sarcomas (STS) histological subtypes (i.e., angiosarcoma, epithelioid sarcoma).

DOI: 10.1201/9780367821982-29

INVESTIGATIONS AND DIAGNOSIS

Triple assessment is the mainstay of diagnosis.

The mammographic appearance of a breast sarcoma usually manifests as a dense, nonspiculated mass without microcalcifications. Sonographically, breast sarcomas appear homogeneously hypoechoic without shadowing as in sarcomas of other sites, a PET/CT scan may be helpful in diagnosing local, recurrent, regional, and distant disease; however, it is not specific, and its role in breast sarcoma has not yet been proven.

Core needle biopsy is an optimal procedure of choice. As is the case in all other primary STS sites, breast sarcomas comprise a diverse array of histological subtypes. The major primary breast sarcomas include angiosarcoma, malignant fibrous histiocytoma, and stromal sarcoma as the most common histological subtypes.

Metastatic workup should include a chest CT scan due to the propensity of these tumors to metastasize to the lungs. Patients diagnosed with myxoid/round cell liposarcoma should undergo an additional abdominal/pelvic CT since these tumors tend to spread to fat-bearing areas in the retroperitoneum. The role of PET/CT in the metastatic workup of breast sarcoma is inconclusive.

TREATMENT

Surgery

Surgery remains the mainstay of treatment, with some role for adjuvant chemotherapy and radiotherapy. Surgery may be in the form of wide local excision or mastectomy. Several studies have found both to be comparable to each other in terms of local recurrence and survival (7–9). For larger tumors or high tumor-to-breast ratios, the overall cosmesis is often better with a mastectomy and reconstruction than with a wide excision. Deep-seated tumors that are near or involve the chest wall may require en bloc resection of the chest wall. Negative (R0) margins of resection are strongly associated with a better outcome (7, 10–12). Most surgeons consider a minimum of a 1-cm tumor-free margin to be adequate.

Angiosarcomas, however, are extremely aggressive and recur within 1 year of surgery (13). Angiosarcomas often have infiltrative cutaneous disease that extends beyond the tumor, and recurrences are often seen at the margins of the prior operation. Thus special attention should be given to ensuring the skin margin is clear; margins of 3 cm have been proposed (14). Hence, several surgeons prefer a mastectomy rather than breast conservation surgery for this histology. Moreover, given the high risk of recurrence with this histology, reconstruction should be delayed.

Axillary nodal dissection

Breast sarcomas generally spread by local infiltration and by the hematogenous route. Lymph nodal spread is rare, and prophylactic nodal dissection is not indicated. For patients with clinically suspicious nodes, ultrasound-guided fine needle aspiration of enlarged nodes is advisable. When lymph node metastases are detected in a patient with a breast sarcoma, the pathology should be reassessed, as it may be metaplastic carcinoma or carcinosarcoma (14). Lymph node dissection should only be performed if the histological subtype is carcinosarcoma (15, 16). Sentinel nodal assay has not been studied, but since nodal spread is rare, it is not advisable.

Adjuvant Radiation Therapy

Primary breast sarcomas

The benefits of adjuvant radiation therapy (RT) for primary breast sarcomas is controversial. Data from several studies are conflicting regarding benefits of adjuvant RT in primary breast sarcoma. Adjuvant RT is usually not used for most breast sarcomas where wide margins (>1 cm) are achieved. If margins are close, then a reresection is recommended to obtain wider margins. In cases of high-grade breast sarcomas and positive margins in whom resection is not feasible, adjuvant RT may be tried. However, RT can't replace inadequate surgery, and re-excision is recommended wherever feasible.

For large, deep tumors where close or positive margins are expected, preoperative (neoadjuvant) RT may be indicated in an attempt to increase resectability (17).

Radiotherapy-associated breast sarcomas

Adjuvant RT for radiation-associated breast sarcomas is undefined, and in the background of prior RT to the same area, the potential adverse effects of a high cumulative RT dose need to be considered. However, particularly for therapy-related angiosarcomas, the concern for late side effects must be counterbalanced by the high recurrence rates of surgery alone.

Reirradiation, often with a hypofractionated dose, has been used in the neoadjuvant or adjuvant setting in some patients with favorable outcomes (18, 19). Thus, treatment must be individualized according to patient and tumor characteristics.

Adjuvant Chemotherapy

As with adjuvant RT, the role of adjuvant chemotherapy for breast sarcoma is undefined. Adjuvant chemotherapy is not recommended routinely after resection of a breast sarcoma. The use of adjuvant chemotherapy must be individualized, taking into account the patient's performance status, comorbid factors, tumor size, and histologic subtype.

There are no trials specifically addressing the benefit of adjuvant chemotherapy for breast sarcomas. A retrospective analysis suggested improved disease-free survival for patients who received adjuvant chemotherapy (20), while another study found reduced recurrence rates (21). Few studies report no benefit (22).

Chemotherapy as adjuvant therapy is hence considered only for specific cases. Adjuvant chemotherapy is a reasonable option for patients with high-risk or recurrent sarcomas, and because of their worse outcome, for angiosarcomas. These include patients with high-grade breast sarcomas that are >5 cm in size or have nodal involvement. Considering the relatively poor prognosis of angiosarcomas in patients even with a tumor size from 3 to 5 cm, adjuvant chemotherapy is reasonable but only after assessing the risk-to-benefit ratio. When adjuvant or neoadjuvant chemotherapy is chosen, the combination of doxorubicin plus ifosfamide is used. However, in a patient with a treatment-related angiosarcoma who has received prior anthracycline-based chemotherapy, a taxane-containing regimen is considered.

Role of Neoadjuvant Therapy

Neoadjuvant rather than adjuvant therapy may be useful in the setting of a large or recurrent initially unresectable or borderline resectable high-grade tumor. Decisions about neoadjuvant therapy should be made on a case-by-case basis with a multidisciplinary group of sarcoma experts. Preoperative (neoadjuvant) RT may be preferred over chemotherapy given the risk of progression on chemotherapy. Given the importance of R0 surgical margins for local control and survival, neoadjuvant therapy may increase the likelihood of successful surgical resection for large high-grade breast sarcomas.

POST-TREATMENT SURVEILLANCE

The recommended follow-up scheme is as follows:

- For patients with stage I disease, history and physical examination at 3- to 6-monthly intervals for the first 2 years and yearly thereafter. Periodic imaging of the primary site is also indicated.
- For patients with stage II or III disease, history and physical examination and chest imaging at 3- to 6-monthly intervals for 2 or 3 years, then every 6 months for the next 2 years, then annually.
- For patients at higher risk of local recurrence, such as those with positive margins or in whom the primary tumor site is not easily examined, MRI is preferred over CT scanning.

RECURRENT AND METASTATIC DISEASE

- *Locally recurrent disease*: In most breast sarcoma recurrences are common, and surgery may be potentially curative (10, 11).
- *Metastatic disease*: Palliative chemotherapy can offer some benefits in patients with metastatic breast sarcoma. In rare cases, potentially curative metastectomy may be feasible in patients with isolated limited pulmonary metastases (23).

PROGNOSIS

Five-year disease-free survival rates for breast sarcomas range from 44% to 66%, and 5-year overall survival rates are between 49% and 67% (7, 8, 11, 24–27).

The prognosis for breast sarcomas is highly dependent upon histologic grade and tumor size. Positive surgical margins increase the risk for local recurrence and death.

Histologic subtype does not influence prognosis with the exception of angiosarcoma.

Radiation-associated sarcomas are reported to have a worse clinical outcome than sporadic breast sarcomas.

REFERENCES

1. Surov A, Holzhausen HJ, Ruschke K, Spielmann RP. Primary breast sarcoma: prevalence, clinical signs, and radiological features. *Acta Radiol [Internet]*. 2011 Jul [cited 2022 Aug 7];52(6):597–601. Available from: http://journals.sagepub.com/doi/10.1258/ar.2011.100468
2. Duncan MA, Lautner MA. Sarcomas of the breast. *Surg Clin North Am [Internet]*. 2018 Aug [cited 2022 Aug 7];98(4):869–76. Available from: https://linkinghub.elsevier.com/retrieve/pii/S0039610918300434
3. Malkin D, Li FP, Strong LC, Fraumeni JF, Nelson CE, Kim DH, et al. Germ line p53 mutations in a familial syndrome of breast cancer, sarcomas, and other neoplasms. *Science*. 1990 Nov 30;250(4985):1233–8.
4. Birch JM, Alston RD, McNally RJ, Evans DG, Kelsey AM, Harris M, et al. Relative frequency and morphology of cancers in carriers of germline TP53 mutations. *Oncogene*. 2001 Aug 2;20(34):4621–8.

5. Lim SZ, Ong KW, Tan BKT, Selvarajan S, Tan PH. Sarcoma of the breast: an update on a rare entity. *J Clin Pathol [Internet]*. 2016 May [cited 2022 Sep 19];69(5):373–81. Available from: http://jcp.bmj.com/lookup/doi/10.1136/jclinpath-2015-203545

6. Lahat G, Lazar A, Lev D. Sarcoma epidemiology and etiology: potential environmental and genetic factors. *Surg Clin North Am [Internet]*. 2008 Jun [cited 2022 Sep 19];88(3):451–81. Available from: https://linkinghub.elsevier.com/retrieve/pii/S0039610908000388

7. Confavreux C, Lurkin A, Mitton N, Blondet R, Saba C, Ranchère D, et al. Sarcomas and malignant phyllodes tumours of the breast – a retrospective study. *Eur J Cancer [Internet]*. 2006 Nov [cited 2022 Sep 25]; 42(16):2715–21. Available from: https://linkinghub.elsevier.com/retrieve/pii/S0959804906007283

8. Fields RC, Aft RL, Gillanders WE, Eberlein TJ, Margenthaler JA. Treatment and outcomes of patients with primary breast sarcoma. *Am J Surg*. 2008 Oct;196(4):559–61.

9. North JH, McPhee M, Arredondo M, Edge SB. Sarcoma of the breast: implications of the extent of local therapy. *Am Surg*. 1998 Nov;64(11):1059–61.

10. Pandey M, Mathew A, Abraham EK, Rajan B. Primary sarcoma of the breast. *J Surg Oncol [Internet]*. 2004 Sep 1 [cited 2022 Sep 25];87(3):121–5. Available from: https://onlinelibrary.wiley.com/doi/10.1002/jso.20110

11. Zelek L, Llombart-Cussac A, Terrier P, Pivot X, Guinebretiere JM, Le Pechoux C, et al. Prognostic factors in primary breast sarcomas: a series of patients with long-term follow-up. *JCO [Internet]*. 2003 Jul 1 [cited 2022 Sep 25];21(13):2583–8. Available from: https://ascopubs.org/doi/10.1200/JCO.2003.06.080

12. Shabahang M, Franceschi D, Sundaram M, Castillo MH, Moffat FL, Frank DS, et al. Surgical management of primary breast sarcoma. *Am Surg*. 2002 Aug;68(8):673–7; discussion 677.

13. Monroe AT, Feigenberg SJ, Mendenhall NP. Angiosarcoma after breast-conserving therapy. *Cancer*. 2003 Apr 15;97(8):1832–40.

14. Al-Benna S, Poggemann K, Steinau HU, Steinstraesser L. Diagnosis and management of primary breast sarcoma. *Breast Cancer Res Treat [Internet]*. 2010 Aug [cited 2022 Sep 25];122(3):619–26. Available from: http://link.springer.com/10.1007/s10549-010-0915-y

15. An analysis of 78 breast sarcoma patients without distant metastases at presentation. PubMed [Internet]. [cited 2022 Sep 25]. Available from: https://pubmed.ncbi.nlm.nih.gov/10661345/

16. Sarcoma and Cystosarcoma phyllodes tumors of the breast – a retrospective review of 58 cases. PubMed [Internet]. [cited 2022 Sep 25]. Available from: https://pubmed.ncbi.nlm.nih.gov/8185030/

17. Breast sarcoma: Treatment [Internet]. [cited 2022 Sep 25]. Available from: https://medilib.ir/uptodate/show/83132#rid14

18. Palta M, Morris CG, Grobmyer SR, Copeland EM, Mendenhall NP. Angiosarcoma after breast-conserving therapy: long-term outcomes with hyperfractionated radiotherapy. *Cancer*. 2010 Apr 15;116(8):1872–8.

19. Feigenberg SJ, Mendenhall NP, Reith JD, Ward JR, Copeland EM. Angiosarcoma after breast-conserving therapy: experience with hyperfractionated radiotherapy. *Int J Radiat Oncol Biol Phys*. 2002 Mar 1;52(3):620–6.

20. Gutman H, Pollock RE, Ross MI, Benjamin RS, Johnston DA, Janjan NA, et al. Sarcoma of the breast: implications for extent of therapy. The M. D. Anderson experience. *Surgery*. 1994 Sep;116(3):505–9.

21. Torres KE, Ravi V, Kin K, Yi M, Guadagnolo BA, May CD, et al. Long-term outcomes in patients with radiation-associated angiosarcomas of the breast following surgery and radiotherapy for breast cancer. *Ann Surg Oncol*. 2013 Apr;20(4):1267–74.

22. Lagrange JL, Ramaioli A, Chateau MC, Marchal C, Resbeut M, Richaud P, et al. Sarcoma after radiation therapy: retrospective multiinstitutional study of 80 histologically confirmed cases. Radiation Therapist and Pathologist Groups of the Fédération Nationale des Centres de Lutte Contre le Cancer. *Radiology*. 2000 Jul;216(1):197–205.

23. Lahat G, Dhuka AR, Lahat S, Smith KD, Pollock RE, Hunt KK, et al. Outcome of locally recurrent and metastatic angiosarcoma. *Ann Surg Oncol*. 2009 Sep;16(9):2502–9.

24. McGowan TS, Cummings BJ, O'Sullivan B, Catton CN, Miller N, Panzarella T. An analysis of 78 breast sarcoma patients without distant metastases at presentation. *Int J Radiat Oncol Biol Phys*. 2000 Jan 15;46(2):383–90.

25. Terrier P, Terrier-Lacombe MJ, Mouriesse H, Friedman S, Spielmann M, Contesso G. Primary breast sarcoma: a review of 33 cases with immunohistochemistry and prognostic factors. *Breast Cancer Res Treat*. 1989 Jan;13(1):39–48.

26. Adem C, Reynolds C, Ingle JN, Nascimento AG. Primary breast sarcoma: clinicopathologic series from the Mayo Clinic and review of the literature. *Br J Cancer*. 2004 Jul 19;91(2):237–41.

27. Ciatto S, Bonardi R, Cataliotti L, Cardona G. Sarcomas of the breast: a multicenter series of 70 cases. *Neoplasma*. 1992;39(6):375–9.

Breast Cancer in Developing Countries **28**

Issues and Solutions

Diptendra Kumar Sarkar

Working guidelines for patients with suspected breast carcinoma include the following.

> *Evaluation*: Triple assessment.
> *History and clinical breast examination (CBE), must include*:

1. Upper inner quadrant
2. Lower inner quadrant
3. Lower outer quadrant
4. Upper outer quadrant
5. Nipple–areola complex
6. Axillary extension of breast
7. Axilla
8. Ipsilateral arm
9. Neck
10. Opposite breast

Radiology

1. *High-resolution ultrasonography (HRUSG) of both breast and axilla*: This is available across all areas and is strongly recommended in all age groups. Below 35 years, it is the standard of care. In BI-RADS III lesions and complex cystic lesions, elastography may be helpful.
2. *Mammogram of both breasts*: It is recommended above the age of 35 years. However, USG correlation is strongly recommended in all cases. Nonavailability of mammogram technology should not be a deterrent to management of breast lumps
3. MRI is routinely not recommended, which is used in special circumstances such as:
   a. Evaluation of the breast following prosthesis placement.
   b. In inconclusive situations.
   c. Post-radiation recurrences.
   d. To assess multifocality/multicentricity (in special situations).
   e. Response to neoadjuvant systemic therapy (NST).
   f. Young females with hereditary ovarian and breast cancer (HOBC).

DOI: 10.1201/9780367821982-30

Core biopsy

This is the standard of care. In palpable (clinical) solid lesions (HRUSG), nonguided biopsy can be performed. In impalpable or complex lesions, radiology-guided biopsies are preferred to reduce false-negative results. Fine needle aspiration cytology (FNAC) is used to assess axillary lymph nodes. Immunohistochemistry (IHC) should be performed in all cases of breast cancer. Estrogen receptor (ER), progesterone receptor (PR), HER2-neu, and Ki67 status should be performed in cases of invasive duct carcinomas.

Staging of breast cancer

1. *Early breast cancer (EBC)*: It is not essential to evaluate for systemic metastasis in EBC. Liver function test is the only investigation recommended in the absence of any symptoms. In patients with systemic symptoms or in whom post-surgery high-volume axillary disease is noted, systemic evaluation is needed.
2. *Locally advanced breast cancer (LABC)*: All LABCs should have CT thorax, CT abdomen and pelvis, and bone scan done. In some centers, whole-body PET-CT scan is done. Other systemic evaluation is based on specific symptoms

Genetic testing: BRCA testing is recommended in women with triple-negative breast cancer (TNBC) less than 60 years.

Treatment guidelines

1. *EBC*: Surgery is preferred in most cases as first-line treatment. However, in TNBC and HER2-neu–enriched cancers, NST may be chosen as first-line therapy for lesions more than 3 cm in size. In patients opting for breast conservation surgery (BCS), an unacceptable tumor-to-breast ratio may be a factor in selecting up-front NST.
   a. BCS is the standard of care in unicentric EBC. Frozen section for margin evaluation is not mandatory. The walls and the cavity should be clipped for future localization and radiotherapy. Proper orientation of the specimen should be done for pathological evaluation. A 1-cm macroscopic and negative inked margin microscopically is considered an R0 resection. Mastectomy should be considered in patients who are contraindicated for BCS. Cavity shaving should be offered to patients with multifocal or diffuse positive margins. In unifocal positivity, radiotherapy may be offered. Repeated (twice) positive margins should mandate mastectomy.
   b. Sentinel lymph node biopsy (SLNB) using a dual tracer is the standard of care for N0 axilla. Isosulfan blue or methylene blue, technninium-99m sulfur colloid, and indocyanine green are the three most commonly used dyes for SLNB. Lower nodal sampling can also be used instead of SLNB in resource-constrained centers. In most centers, positive SLNB is an indication for axillary lymph node dissection (ALND). In selected cases, a conservative approach (non-ALND) can be followed. Facilities for targeted axillary dissection are unavailable in most mid/low socioeconomic countries and should be planned only after a proper learning curve is achieved.
   c. Adjuvant therapy after surgery: In all patients with BCS, radiotherapy (RT)   becomes mandatory. In patients who underwent mastectomy-based surgery, RT is indicated if there are more than four nodes or there is perinodal extension. The choice of adjuvant therapy depends on risk categorization. Traditional prognostic (tumor size, nodal status, grade, ER status) and predictive markers, online software, and molecular signatures may be used to choose the appropriate adjuvant therapy.

2. *LABC*: NST is the standard of care followed by surgery and RT with or without endocrine manipulation.

    a. *NST*: Before initiation of NST, one must consider placing a marker at the center of the lesion if BCS is planned. In the case of luminal cancers, three to four cycles of chemotherapy are given and the lesion is assessed (BCS or mastectomy) for surgery. Following surgery, adjuvant therapy is continued. In case the lesion is still inoperable, further NST is given. In the case of TNBC, NST is completed before proceeding to surgery. In HER2-enriched lesions, NST (dual blockade with trastuzumab and pertuzumab) is given for up to six cycles to achieve a complete pathological response. Neoadjuvant endocrine therapy is used in elderly females who otherwise are not good candidates for chemotherapy.

    b. *Surgery*: In T4b lesions (except a small subset of patients with minimal skin involvement where extreme oncoplasty may work), mastectomy remains the procedure of choice. In T3 lesions breast conservation may be done with or without OPS. ALND or targeted axillary dissection is the standard of care for post-NST axilla.

    c. *RT*: RT is an integral form of treatment in LABC.

    d. *Endocrine manipulation*: Depends on status of hormone receptors.

3. *Metastatic breast cancer*:

    a. *Surgery*: Surgery of primary tumors is done in the case of fungating or ulcerative lesions for better palliation or for oligometastatic disease (fewer than four metastases).

    b. *Systemic therapy*: Depends on the biological subtype, presenting symptom, and performance status of the patient.

      • *Chemotherapy*: Anthracyclines, taxanes, platinum, capecitabine, cyclophosphamide, methotrexate, and others. Sequential single agents are preferred over combinations.

      • *Hormone therapy*: Ovarian suppression is indicated in premenopausal metastatic breast cancer (MBC). It can be surgical (bilateral oophorectomy) or RT (ovarian radiation) or medical (gonadotropin-releasing hormone [GnRH] analogues). In others, tamoxifen, aromatase inhibitors, fulvestrant, megestrol acetate, CD 4/6 inhibitors, and everolimus may be used.

      • *HER2-targeted therapy*: Trastuzumab, lapatinib, pertuzumab, and trastuzumab-emtansine.

      • *RT*: It is used to reduce pain in bone metastasis. It is also routinely used for brain metastasis.

      • *Bone-targeted therapy*: All patients with bone metastasis should receive a bone-modifying agent (zoledronic acid) at 4- to 22-week intervals.

Breast cancer screening—Global strategies

1. *High economy*: Mammography-based screening is recommended.

2. *Mid/Low economy*: Clinical breast examination done by trained health workers (nonmedical) done at 2- to 5-yearly intervals is found to be appropriate. It is also recommended to promote breast self-examinations among females through community health workers as a mode of breast cancer awareness.

Breast Cancer Survivorship

29

Diptendra Kumar Sarkar

INTRODUCTION

The word "survivorship" has a wide meaning, and it is difficult to define it in a sentence. The perspective is different in different individuals. However, it encompasses the "journey" of an individual from "diagnosis" of breast cancer (BC) to her "lifelong" issues related to the "new normal" after being diagnosed and treated for BC.

A survivorship care plan (SCP) includes

1. Documenting details of management
2. Detecting recurrences (structured follow-up plan)
3. Detecting additional cancers
4. Lifestyle modifications to lower recurrences
5. Short-term efforts to address the physical and psychological issues related to treatment
6. Long-term efforts to address the physical and psychological issues related to treatment
7. Financial issues in a survivor
8. Role of caregivers

DOCUMENTATION

As time progresses, most patients fail to remember the details of treatment provided and the issues that arose out of it. The American Society of Clinical Oncology (ASCO) recommends the following information be collected:

- *Background information*: Family history, genetic counseling, hereditary or predisposing factors, and genetic test results
- *Diagnosis*: Cancer type (HPE)/Subtype (immunohistochemistry [IHC])/location(quadrant)/ Date of diagnosis
- *Stage of diagnosis*

DOI: 10.1201/9780367821982-31

- *Surgery*: Date/Surgical procedure
- *Systemic therapy*: No/Yes (CT/MTT/endocrine/immunotherapy/others)
- *Radiation therapy*
- *Side effects* that continued after completing treatment
- *Follow-up*: Need for ongoing adjuvant therapy (yes/no). Schedule of follow-up visits

DETECTING RECURRENCE

The classical model for follow-up includes 3-monthly follow-ups for 2 years followed by 6-monthly follow-up for 3 years.

- *Clinical examination of breast, axilla, and neck and other systemic evaluations.*
- *Mammogram/High-resolution ultrasonography (HRUSG)*: Done at 6 and 12 months after breast-conserving therapy (BCT) and subsequently yearly.
- *Pelvic examination/Transvaginal USG*: Recommended yearly in individuals who are on tamoxifen.
- *Bone mineral density*: It is recommended in individuals who are on an aromatase inhibitor.
- *USG abdomen/CT abdomen/Chest X-ray [CXR]/CT thorax/Bone scan or PET-CT scan*: These tests are not routinely recommended in asymptomatic survivors. Evaluation is indicated only if a patient shows specific symptoms of metastasis.
- *Serum cancer markers*: Not recommended routinely.

DETECTING ADDITIONAL CANCERS

Apart from the recurrence of BC, many individuals may develop a second primary tumor in their lifetime. While some cancers are linked to hereditary genetic mutations, others may develop sporadic cancers. The sporadic cancers can again be truly sporadic or may be linked to side effects of treatment rendered to the patients.

- *Hereditary predispositions*: Opposite breast, ovary and fallopian tubes, colon, pancreas, prostate (male), and others
- *Treatment related*: Radiation-induced (lung, sarcomas, leukemias, and myelodysplastic syndrome [MDS]), chemotherapy (leukemia and MDS), and tamoxifen related (endometrial cancers)
- *Truly unrelated sporadic cancers*

Patients should be made aware of symptoms of other cancers and should be evaluated clinically or with investigations if the need arises.

LIFESTYLE MODIFICATIONS TO LOWER RECURRENCE

A large proportion of cancer survivors look at cancer as an event to make positive lifestyle modifications. It impacts post-therapy life immensely. The survivors are more prone to certain illnesses because of the treatment of cancer.

- *Healthy diet*: Chemotherapy changes the dietary habit of many patients. Consulting dietitians about modifying the diet during treatment has a good impact on lifestyle. Continuing a healthy diet regimen after completion of treatment improves quality of life (QOL) and reduces recurrence (by reducing obesity).

- *Regular exercise*: 150 minutes of exercise per week has shown cancer recurrence to be reduced by up to 30%. Moderate aerobic exercise (walking) and resistance training have been shown to be very effective. It is recommended to start slowly and increase the performance over months. Apart from reducing recurrence, exercise also has shown to have a positive impact on QOL and mental health.
- *Managing stress*: Stress reduction after cancer treatment is pivotal. Engaging in survivorship groups (peer) and social engagements is helpful. In extreme cases psychological support is beneficial.
- *Reducing smoking and alcohol use*: Both of these substances are linked to recurrences, second primary, and other noncancerous diseases.

Short-term efforts to address the physical and psychological issues related to treatment are as follows:

1. *Diagnosis*: The mental trauma is sudden, and therefore stress is high. Dealing with acute mental stress requires extreme empathetic care. Discussion with a specialized nurse counselor and survivor group is helpful. A road map of treatment (discussed in multiple meetings) is also beneficial.
2. *Surgery*: The team must discuss the options for surgical treatment (including the pros and cons) and help the patient in appropriate decision making. In developing countries, the decision of choosing a mastectomy is often guided by family members and nonoriented physicians. Patients also tend to choose mastectomy for mythical "safety." However, many decisions have long-term impact, and many regret later taking the instant impulsive decisions. The patient must also be put into a program of early physiotherapy to reduce lymphedema and disability of the arm, shoulder, and hand.
3. *Systemic therapy*: All patients undergoing chemotherapy/molecular targets and other therapies develop distressing side effects. While some are reversible, some might have long-term impacts on health. Appropriate counseling and follow-up are essential.

Long-term side effects of treatment include the following:

1. *Attention, memory, and thinking problems*: Many patients develop issues related to thinking, concentration, attention deficit, and memory deficits. These are grouped together into a nomenclature called "cancer-related cognitive impairment." Loosely it is called "chemofog" or "chemobrain."
2. *Emotional lability*: Many survivors develop emotional lability and posttraumatic stress disorders. Discussion and counseling by social workers, survivor groups, and survivorship nurses are helpful. Clinical psychologists also are helpful. Psychiatric help is reserved for extreme cases.
3. *Cancer-related fatigue*: This is also a common problem that needs to be addressed in survivorship programs.
4. *Bones and joints*: Patients receiving steroids or aromatase inhibitors are prone to the development of osteoporosis. Periodic bone mineral density (BMD) is indicated to assess the deterioration of bone health.
5. *Gastrointestinal (GI) side effects*: Radiation and/or systemic chemotherapy may induce dysphagia, indigestion, and chronic diarrhea. Appropriate dietary changes and supportive care are needed.
6. *Pulmonary side effects*: Chemotherapy and radiation therapy induce pulmonary parenchymal damage and fibrosis. All patients with breathlessness on exertion should be evaluated (apart from excluding metastasis) by radiology and pulmonary function test.

7. *Cardiac side effects*: Molecular targets, radiotherapy, and chemotherapy produce cardiac side effects. While most are short-term and reversible (from conduction defects to myocardial ischemia), a minority may develop long-term cardiomyopathy. This coupled with increasing age adds to cardiac comorbidity in a subset of patients.

8. *Peripheral neuropathy (PN)*: Paranesthesia, reduced deep reflexes, and weakness are common after chemotherapy. Vincristine, taxanes, and cisplatin are common agents responsible for PN. The side effect is cumulative and is partially reversible after discontinuation of CT.

9. *Endocrine side effects*: Sexual function after treatment is least addressed. There are multiple factors which influence sexual health. Psychological effects of the disease and treatment is one of the key factors. Body image alterations, chronic physical and mental issues, effects of medications (reduced libido, vaginal dryness, premature menopause, dyspareunia, and difficulty in achieving orgasm), and the role of partners play a complex role in reviving pretreatment sexual health.

10. *Lymphedema and disability of the arm, shoulder, and hand (DASH)*: Axillary surgery combined with radiation is associated with a high incidence of lymphedema. Early initiation of active and passive physiotherapy and active exercises are the key to reducing these complications. Prophylactic lymphovenous bypass and secondary lymphovenous bypass (for established progressive lymphedema) is used in select cases.

FINANCIAL ISSUES IN A SURVIVOR

Treatment of BC is very expensive. While some countries rely on insured health structures, others offer assured health for their citizens. But prolonged treatment leads to a delayed return to work for many patents. This issue also needs to be addressed.

ROLE OF CAREGIVERS

Caregivers play a major role in the physical and mental recovery of a patient. Though the approach is individualized in most cases, appropriate counseling of caregivers has been shown to have a major impact in survivorship programs.

Recent Trials in Surgical Management of Breast Cancer

30

Sanjit Kumar Agrawal and Rosina Ahmed

INTRODUCTION

Through well-designed clinical and translational trials, breast cancer research has made significant contributions to patients' survival and quality of life. The treatment is more personalized now as per the biology of breast cancer and treatment responses. We are in the era of de-escalation of invasive therapies in early breast cancer (EBC) and escalation in a minority of advanced breast cancer patients. The last decade has added many new promising molecular agents for metastatic breast cancer treatment.

The methodology, population, intervention, and results of recent practice-changing breast cancer surgical trials are summarized in this chapter. Additionally, some of the ongoing trials, which are likely to impact the practice, are detailed in brief.

PRIMARY BREAST SURGERY

Locoregional breast cancer treatment includes surgery and radiotherapy (RT) in appropriately selected patients. Primary breast surgery has slowly evolved from radical mastectomy to breast conservation surgery (BCS). The first de-escalation effort for less extensive surgery was made by the NSABP B04 randomized controlled trial (RCT), which compared radical mastectomy with less extensive surgery and reported no difference in overall survival (OS) in 25 years of follow-up (1). NSABP B-06, an RCT comparing lumpectomy + axillary lymph node dissection (ALND) with or without breast irradiation with modified radical mastectomy in EBC patients reported no difference in OS between the two groups in 20 years of follow-up. However, RT significantly decreased local recurrence in the lumpectomy group (14.3% with RT vs 39.2% without RT) (2). Similar results published by the Veronesi et al. and EBCTG meta-analysis have established the safety of BCS with RT compared to mastectomy in EBC patients (3, 4). Additionally, recently, population-based registry studies indicate superior survival with breast conservation than with mastectomy (5, 6). A Swedish prospective cohort study of 48,986 EBC patients has reported inferior OS

DOI: 10.1201/9780367821982-32

with mastectomy with or without RT (Mx-RT [hazard ratio] (HR), 1.79; 95% confidence interval [CI] 1.66–1.92, Mx + RT [HR, 1.24; 95% CI, 1.13–1.37]) than BCS + RT (6). With neoadjuvant chemotherapy and a pathological complete response in 50%–70% of triple-negative and HER2-positive breast cancer patients, the trend is slowly evolving towards no breast surgery in excellent responders (7). Vacuum-assisted biopsy (VAB) around the marker clips was compared with breast surgery with an accuracy of 98% (95% CI, 87%–100%), a false-negative rate of 5% (95% CI, 0%–24%), and a negative predictive value of 95% (95% CI, 75%–100%) in detecting residual breast cancer (8). An ongoing multicenter clinical trial (NCT02945579) of 50 patients with the omission of breast surgery in triple-negative breast cancer (TNBC) and HER2-positive patients demonstrated that image-guided VAB shows no residual tumor with ipsilateral breast tumour recurrence (IBTR) as a primary outcome; however, the final results are still pending and may put forward the concept of no breast surgery in eligible patients (9).

AXILLARY STAGING

The importance of axillary staging was established by Fisher et al. by the NSABP 04 RCT. The trial's long-term results have shown that ALND was associated with better local control, with no effect on OS (1). ALND was the only tool for axillary staging in the majority of breast cancer patients until 2000 throughout most of the world. Sentinel lymph node biopsy (SLNB) was introduced in the early 20th century to overcome the ALND procedure complications like shoulder stiffness and lymphedema. SLNB has been proven noninferior to ALND for axillary staging in clinically node-negative EBC patients with similar disease-free survival (DFS), OS, and axillary recurrence rates with a significant decrease in lymphedema rate (10, 11).

Until 2010, ALND was the standard of care for all breast cancer patients with a metastatic sentinel lymph node (SLN) for axillary staging in EBC. The universal role of ALND in breast cancer, as mentioned earlier, in patients with metastatic SLNs was challenged by the published results of three well-designed RCTs (Z0011, IBCSG -23, and AMAROS) between 2010 and 2020. The landmark RCT Z0011 included EBC patients undergoing BCS with tumor size <5 cm and up to two metastatic SLNs (ALND in the standard arm and no axillary surgery in the experimental arm. The 10-year survival outcomes reported no difference between the two arms in terms of OS (83.6% vs 86.3%, noninferiority p = 0.02), DFS (78.2% vs 80.2%, p = 0.32), and locoregional relapse-free survival (81.2% vs 83%, p = 0.41) (12). The IBCSG 23-01 study randomized EBC patients (both BCS and mastectomy) with one or more micrometastatic (≤2 mm) sentinel nodes into ALND vs no axillary surgery. The 9.3-year median follow-up results showed no difference in DFS between the two arms and established the noninferiority of no axillary surgery with ALND (13). The AMAROS RCT included EBC patients (both BCS and mastectomy) with metastatic SLNs (no restriction for the number of positive SLNs) and assigned patients into ALND vs axillary RT. The 10-year axillary recurrence rate was 1.82% in the axillary RT arm compared to 0.93% in the ALND arm (p = NS) (14).

The feasibility and accuracy of the SLNB procedure in node-positive patients who were rendered node-negative post–neoadjuvant chemotherapy (NACT) were evaluated by three validation studies (ACOSOG Z1071, SENTINA, and SNFNAC) (15–17). Validation of ALND followed the SLNB to define the false-negative rate (FNR) of the SLNB procedure in the post-NACT setting. The overall FNR was more than 10% in all three studies. The FNR was <10% when >2 SLNs were removed; immunohistochemistry (IHC) was used in the frozen section examination and considered ITC a positive SLN. Targeted axillary dissection is an emerging procedure in this setting with the removal of both the SLN and clipped node (metastatic node clipped before chemotherapy) to reduce the FNR of SLNB alone. The reported FNR was 10.1% with SLNB only, 4.2% with clipped node removal, and 1.4% with both SLNB + clipped node removal in the MD Anderson study (18).

The ongoing trials SOUND, INSEMA, and EUBREAST 01 further the feasibility of SLNB vs observation only in EBC patients. Both SOUND and INSEMA RCTs comparing SLNB vs observation in the selected group of EBC patients have finished their enrollment (19). The EUBREAST 01 is a single-arm prospective phase 2 trial focused on the post-NACT setting. In this study, no axillary SLNB will be done in CT1-3No TNBC and HER2 +ve BC patients with pathological complete response (pCR) in the breast post-NACT (20).

PREOPERATIVE CHEMOTHERAPY, ENDOCRINE THERAPY, AND RESPONSE-GUIDED ADJUVANT TREATMENT

In the last 25 years, there has been a gradual evolution in the indications for preoperative systemic treatment. In early trials, neoadjuvant therapy was most commonly given for inoperable diseases, and not all patients had surgery following their systemic treatment. However, two major trials, NSABP B-18 and B-27, established the overall equivalence of DFS and OS in patients who had chemotherapy in the neoadjuvant and adjuvant settings (21). These trials also provided evidence that patients with a pCR after chemotherapy may have better survival outcomes. These results led to the use of pCR as the basis for a response-guided approach to subsequent therapy and laid the foundation for further studies examining the safety of conservative approaches to breast and axilla surgery in this scenario, the relationship between pCR and outcome in different breast cancer subtypes, and whether further therapy could improve outcome in a patient who had residual disease after chemotherapy.

First-Line Treatment – Surgery or Chemotherapy?

An EBCTCG meta-analysis (2017) included data from 10 major studies and found similar distant recurrence and breast cancer mortality in neoadjuvant and adjuvant chemotherapy patients (22). Patients who had breast conservation after NACT had an increased relative risk of local recurrence at 15 years of 1.37 (95% CI 1.11–1.64) compared to patients having up-front surgery. The highest risk of local recurrence following breast conservation was in the first 4 years, with little difference beyond 10 years. The study recommended careful tumor localization, detailed pathological assessment of margins, and appropriate radiotherapy to mitigate the increased risk of local recurrence following NACT.

pCR as a Prognostic Tool

The importance of breast cancer subtypes and pCR in predicting survival was established in a meta-analysis of almost 12,000 patients from 12 major NACT trials (23). Locoregional recurrence (LRR) varied from 4.2% for a low-grade luminal subtype to 12.2% for triple-negative and 14.8% for HER2-enriched tumors. In addition, the risk of LRR differed with the extent of residual disease in the breast. The LRR was 6.2% in pCR patients, 6.7% (1.6 times higher) with residual disease in the breast alone, and 11.8% (2.7 times higher) with residual disease in the breast and the axillary lymph nodes. pCR was associated with improved event-free survival and overall survival in two subgroups: Triple-negative (HR for EFS: 0.24, 95% CI 0.18–0.33; for OS: 0.16, 0.11–0.25) and HER2 overexpressed who received trastuzumab (HR for EFS: 0.15, 0.09–0.27; for OS: 0.08, 0.03, 0.22).

Once pCR was recognized as a prognostic tool, different approaches attempted to increase the pCR rate, particularly in high-risk patient groups. Dose-dense regimens reduce the interval between chemotherapy cycles with a significantly higher pCR rate (13.5% vs 9.2%) (24). In a different approach in HER2-positive patients, dual HER2 blockade in the APHINITY trial resulted in a higher pCR rate and an estimated improvement in 6-year invasive DFS (IDFS) (HR 0.81 [95% CI, 0.66–1.00], $P = .045$) compared to single-agent trastuzumab only (25).

Response-Guided Adjuvant Therapy

In patients with high-risk breast cancer subtypes, studies have been designed to evaluate the result of additional therapy in the adjuvant setting for patients who did not achieve pCR after NACT.

- The CREATE-X trial showed that adding adjuvant capecitabine in triple-negative patients with residual disease following NACT could improve 5-year DFS (74.1% compared to 67.6%) (26).
- Patients with HER2-enriched breast cancer typically receive trastuzumab for 1 year. In the KATHERINE trial, patients with residual disease following trastuzumab and NACT were randomized to a change in maintenance HER2-targeted therapy from trastuzumab to T-DM1 for 3 years with DFS improvement from 77.0% to 88.3% (27).
- Patients with *BRCA* gene mutations and HER2-negative breast cancer were studied in the OlympiA trial. In these patients, adding 1 year of adjuvant olaparib improved the 3-year DFS from 80.4% to 87.5% (28).

Neoadjuvant Endocrine Therapy

Low-grade endocrine receptor–positive tumors may be relatively chemoresistant, with poor response to NACT. For these patients, neoadjuvant endocrine therapy has been studied in several trials, mostly restricted to postmenopausal women. PROACT and IMPACT compared the response to tamoxifen and aromatase inhibitors (AIs), and Z1031 found an equivalent response to three different AIs (29). Biomarkers, including Ki67, and scoring systems such as the preoperative endocrine prognostic index (PEPI) have attempted to identify the optimal duration of endocrine therapy to define which patients will benefit from the addition of chemotherapy in the adjuvant setting. In other studies, novel agents have been studied in combination with neoadjuvant endocrine therapy in selected settings (PIK-3 inhibitors in LORELEI, CDK 4/6 inhibitors in neoMONARCH and CORALLEEN).

GERMLINE MUTATION CARRIERS

There are very few randomised trials in this group of patients. However, a meta-analysis provides evidence that the outcome of treatment is similar in patients with or without germline mutations. (30)

Breast Cancer Treatment Options in Germline Mutation Carriers

1. *Surgery*: A meta-analysis published in 2014 found that gene-mutated patients with BCS had similar outcomes in distant recurrence, breast cancer–related death, and OS (31). In terms of recurrence, there was a significantly higher risk of contralateral breast cancer (relative risk [RR] 3.56, 95% CI 2.50–5.08). The evidence for higher ipsilateral recurrence was not significant overall, although studies with longer-term follow-up over 7 years showed some increased RR. Overall, the review concluded that breast conservation was safe and the results could be further improved with appropriate adjuvant therapy, including chemotherapy, tamoxifen, and oophorectomy.
2. *Systemic therapy*: Evidence from several studies has evaluated the addition of platinum compounds to standard first-line chemotherapy in gene-mutated individuals. Still, the results are mixed, with no clear recommendation for platinum in the neoadjuvant setting (32). The OlympiA trial provided evidence of improved DFS at 3 years following 1 year of adjuvant olaparib (see the section on response-guided adjuvant therapy earlier).

Risk-Reducing Surgery in Mutation Carriers Affected with Breast Cancer

1. Contralateral prophylactic mastectomy reduced the risk of new contralateral breast cancer but did not confer a survival benefit. The risk reduction was 90% in patients who had cotralateral risk reducing mastectomy (CRRM) alone and 95% in those who additionally had risk-reducing bilateral salpingo-oophorectomy (BSO) (33).
2. Although the appropriate timing for such an intervention is unclear, there is evidence that this option is increasingly offered to patients (34).
3. Risk-reducing salpingo-oophorectomy protects against ovarian cancer. However, earlier studies supported a new breast cancer risk reduction by up to 50%. Recent reviews that address biases in the older evidence suggest that the benefit may be much more limited, particularly in premenopausal women (35).

Risk-Reducing Surgery in Unaffected Mutation Carriers

1. Bilateral risk-reducing mastectomy effectively reduces both incidence and death from breast cancer (33).
2. Risk-reducing BSO reduces the risk of ovarian cancer by 80% and all-cause mortality by 68% in female *BRCA1/2* carriers (36).

METASTATIC BREAST CANCER (MBC)

The role of surgery in MBC is reserved mainly for the palliative role only. Three seminal RCTS (TMH Mumbai trial, MF07-01, and ECOG 2018) studied the association of surgery with OS in MBC. The TMH, Mumbai (NCT 0019377) study reported a median OS of 19.2 months in the surgical group vs 20.5 months in the nonsurgical group (HR = 1.04. P = 0.79) (37). The MF07-01 trial showed no survival benefit of surgery at 3 years of follow-up; however, the post hoc analysis has shown some survival benefit with surgery (OS 46 months in surgery vs 37 months in the nonsurgical group [HR = 0.66, P = 0.005]). In addition, the unplanned subgroup analysis has shown survival benefits in patients with solitary bone metastasis (HR 0.47, CI 0.23–0.98, p = 0.04) (38). The ECOG 2018 trial reported no survival benefit of surgery in MBC with a 3-year OS of 68.4% in surgery + systemic treatment vs 67.9% in systemic therapy only arm (HR = 1.09, 90% CI: 0.80, 1.49) (39).

The role of surgery in oligometastatic disease is debatable. The ongoing phase 2R/3 trial of standard-of-care therapy with or without stereotactic body radiotherapy (SBRT) and/or surgical ablation for newly oligometastatic breast cancer (NRG-BR002) has included MBC patients with <2 metastases in CT/PET CT with progression-free survival (PFS) as a primary outcome (40). The NRG BR002 trial results will provide the level 1 evidence of locoregional treatment in oligometastatic breast cancer.

REFERENCES

1. Fisher B, Jeong JH, Anderson S, Bryant J, Fisher ER, Wolmark N. Twenty-five-year follow-up of a randomized trial comparing radical mastectomy, total mastectomy, and total mastectomy followed by Irradiation. *N Engl J Med*. 2002 Aug 22;347(8):567–75.

2. Fisher B, Anderson S, Bryant J, Margolese RG, Deutsch M, Fisher ER, et al. Twenty-year follow-up of a randomized trial comparing total mastectomy, lumpectomy, and lumpectomy plus irradiation for the treatment of invasive breast cancer. *N Engl J Med.* 2002 Oct 17;347(16):1233–41.

3. Veronesi U, Saccozzi R, Del Vecchio M, Banfi A, Clemente C, De Lena M, et al. Comparing radical mastectomy with quadrantectomy, axillary dissection, and radiotherapy in patients with small cancers of the breast. *N Engl J Med.* 1981 Jul 2;305(1):6–11.

4. Early Breast Cancer Trialists' Collaborative Group. Favourable and unfavourable effects on long-term survival of radiotherapy for early breast cancer: an overview of the randomised trials. *Lancet.* 2000 May 20;355(9217):1757–70.

5. Christiansen P, Carstensen SL, Ejlertsen B, Kroman N, Offersen B, Bodilsen A, et al. Breast conserving surgery versus mastectomy: overall and relative surviva l – a population based study by the Danish Breast Cancer Cooperative Group (DBCG). *Acta Oncol Stockh Swed.* 2018 Jan;57(1):19–25.

6. de Boniface J, Szulkin R, Johansson ALV. Survival after breast conservation vs mastectomy adjusted for comorbidity and socioeconomic status: a Swedish national 6-year follow-up of 48 986 women. *JAMA Surg.* 2021 Jul 1;156(7):628–37.

7. Heil J, Pfob A, Morrow M. De-escalation of breast and axillary surgery in exceptional responders to neoadjuvant systemic treatment. *Lancet Oncol.* 2021 Apr 1;22(4):435–6.

8. Kuerer HM, Rauch GM, Krishnamurthy S, Adrada BE, Caudle AS, DeSnyder SM, et al. A clinical feasibility trial for identification of exceptional responders in whom breast cancer surgery can be eliminated following neoadjuvant systemic therapy. *Ann Surg.* 2018 May;267(5):946–51.

9. Eliminating Surgery or Radiotherapy After Systemic Therapy in Treating Patients with HER2 Positive or Triple Negative Breast Cancer – Tabular View. ClinicalTrials.gov [Internet]. [cited 2022 Jan 17]. Available from: https://clinicaltrials.gov/ct2/show/record/NCT02945579

10. Krag DN, Anderson SJ, Julian TB, Brown AM, Harlow SP, Costantino JP, et al. Sentinel-lymph-node resection compared with conventional axillary-lymph-node dissection in clinically node-negative patients with breast cancer: overall survival findings from the NSABP B-32 randomised phase 3 trial. *Lancet Oncol.* 2010 Oct;11(10):927–33.

11. Mansel RE, Fallowfield L, Kissin M, Goyal A, Newcombe RG, Dixon JM, et al. Randomized multicenter trial of sentinel node biopsy versus standard axillary treatment in operable breast cancer: the ALMANAC Trial. *J Natl Cancer Inst.* 2006 May 3;98(9):599–609.

12. Giuliano AE, Ballman KV, McCall L, Beitsch PD, Brennan MB, Kelemen PR, et al. Effect of axillary dissection vs no axillary dissection on 10-year overall survival among women with invasive breast cancer and sentinel node metastasis: the ACOSOG Z0011 (Alliance) randomized clinical trial. *JAMA.* 2017 Sep 12;318(10):918–26.

13. Galimberti V, Cole BF, Viale G, Veronesi P, Vicini E, Intra M, et al. Axillary dissection versus no axillary dissection in patients with breast cancer and sentinel-node micrometastases (IBCSG 23-01): 10-year follow-up of a randomised, controlled phase 3 trial. *Lancet Oncol.* 2018 Oct;19(10):1385–93.

14. Rutgers E, Donker M, Poncet C, Straver M, Meijnen P, van de Velde C, et al. Abstract GS4-01: radiotherapy or surgery of the axilla after a positive sentinel node in breast cancer patients: 10 year follow up results of the EORTC AMAROS trial (EORTC 10981/22023). *Cancer Res.* 2019 Feb 15;79(4_Supplement):GS4–01.

15. Boughey JC, Suman VJ, Mittendorf EA, Ahrendt GM, Wilke LG, Taback B, et al. Sentinel lymph node surgery after neoadjuvant chemotherapy in patients with node-positive breast cancer: the ACOSOG Z1071 (Alliance) clinical trial. *JAMA.* 2013 Oct 9;310(14):1455–61.

16. Kuehn T, Bauerfeind I, Fehm T, Fleige B, Hausschild M, Helms G, et al. Sentinel-lymph-node biopsy in patients with breast cancer before and after neoadjuvant chemotherapy (SENTINA): a prospective, multicentre cohort study. *Lancet Oncol.* 2013 Jun;14(7):609–18.

17. Boileau JF, Poirier B, Basik M, Holloway CMB, Gaboury L, Sideris L, et al. Sentinel node biopsy after neoadjuvant chemotherapy in biopsy-proven node-positive breast cancer: the SN FNAC study. *J Clin Oncol Off J Am Soc Clin Oncol.* 2015 Jan 20;33(3):258–64.

18. Caudle AS, Yang WT, Krishnamurthy S, Mittendorf EA, Black DM, Gilcrease MZ, et al. Improved axillary evaluation following neoadjuvant therapy for patients with node-positive breast cancer using selective evaluation of clipped nodes: implementation of targeted axillary dissection. *J Clin Oncol.* 2016 Apr 1;34(10):1072–8.

19. Simons JM, Smidt ML. De-escalation of axillary management in early stage breast cancer. *Ann Breast Surg [Internet].* 2020 Mar 25 [cited 2022 May 29];4(0). Available from: https://abs.amegroups.com/article/view/5713

20. Reimer T, Glass A, Botteri E, Loibl S, D. Gentilini O. Avoiding axillary sentinel lymph node biopsy after neoadjuvant systemic therapy in breast cancer: rationale for the prospective, multicentric EUBREAST-01 trial. *Cancers.* 2020 Dec 9;12(12):3698.

21. Rastogi P, Anderson SJ, Bear HD, Geyer CE, Kahlenberg MS, Robidoux A, et al. Preoperative chemotherapy: updates of National Surgical Adjuvant Breast and Bowel Project Protocols B-18 and B-27. *J Clin Oncol.* 2008 Feb 10;26(5):778–85.
22. Early Breast Cancer Trialists' Collaborative Group (EBCTCG). Long-term outcomes for neoadjuvant versus adjuvant chemotherapy in early breast cancer: meta-analysis of individual patient data from ten randomised trials. *Lancet Oncol.* 2018 Jan;19(1):27–39.
23. Cortazar P, Zhang L, Untch M, Mehta K, Costantino JP, Wolmark N, et al. Pathological complete response and long-term clinical benefit in breast cancer: the CTNeoBC pooled analysis. *Lancet.* 2014 Jul 12; 384(9938):164–72.
24. Petrelli F, Coinu A, Lonati V, Cabiddu M, Ghilardi M, Borgonovo K, et al. Neoadjuvant dose-dense chemotherapy for locally advanced breast cancer: a meta-analysis of published studies. *Anticancer Drugs.* 2016 Aug;27(7):702–8.
25. Piccart M, Procter M, Fumagalli D, de Azambuja E, Clark E, Ewer MS, et al. Adjuvant pertuzumab and trastuzumab in early HER2-positive breast cancer in the APHINITY trial: 6 years' follow-up. *J Clin Oncol.* 2021 May;39(13):1448–57.
26. Masuda N, Lee SJ, Ohtani S, Im YH, Lee ES, Yokota I, et al. Adjuvant capecitabine for breast cancer after preoperative chemotherapy. *N Engl J Med.* 2017 Jun 1;376(22):2147–59.
27. von Minckwitz G, Huang CS, Mano MS, Loibl S, Mamounas EP, Untch M, et al. Trastuzumab emtansine for residual invasive HER2-positive breast cancer. *N Engl J Med.* 2019 Feb 14;380(7):617–28.
28. Tutt ANJ, Garber JE, Kaufman B, Viale G, Fumagalli D, Rastogi P, et al. Adjuvant olaparib for patients with BRCA1- or BRCA2-mutated breast cancer. *N Engl J Med.* 2021 Jun 24;384(25):2394–405.
29. Barchiesi G, Mazzotta M, Krasniqi E, Pizzuti L, Marinelli D, Capomolla E, et al. Neoadjuvant endocrine therapy in breast cancer: current knowledge and future perspectives. *Int J Mol Sci.* 2020 May 16; 21(10):3528.
30. van den Broek AJ, Schmidt MK, van't Veer LJ, Tollenaar RAEM, van Leeuwen FE. Worse breast cancer prognosis of BRCA1/BRCA2 mutation carriers: what's the evidence? A systematic review with meta-analysis. *PLoS ONE.* 2015;10(3):e0120189.
31. Valachis A, Nearchou AD, Lind P. Surgical management of breast cancer in BRCA-mutation carriers: a systematic review and meta-analysis. *Breast Cancer Res Treat.* 2014 Apr;144(3):443–55.
32. Mylavarapu S, Das A, Roy M. Role of BRCA mutations in the modulation of response to platinum therapy. *Front Oncol.* 2018 Feb 5;8:16.
33. Carbine NE, Lostumbo L, Wallace J, Ko H. Risk-reducing mastectomy for the prevention of primary breast cancer. *Cochrane Database Syst Rev.* 2018 Apr 5;4:CD002748.
34. Scheepens JCC, Veer L van 't, Esserman L, Belkora J, Mukhtar RA. Contralateral prophylactic mastectomy: a narrative review of the evidence and acceptability. *Breast.* 2021 Apr 1;56:61–9.
35. Conduit C, Milne RL, Friedlander ML, Phillips KA. Bilateral salpingo-oophorectomy and breast cancer risk for BRCA1 and BRCA2 mutation carriers: assessing the evidence. *Cancer Prev Res Phila Pa.* 2021 Nov;14(11):983–94.
36. Marchetti C, De Felice F, Palaia I, Perniola G, Musella A, Musio D, et al. Risk-reducing salpingo-oophorectomy: a meta-analysis on impact on ovarian cancer risk and all cause mortality in BRCA 1 and BRCA 2 mutation carriers. *BMC Womens Health.* 2014 Dec 12;14(1):150.
37. Badwe R, Hawaldar R, Nair N, Kaushik R, Parmar V, Siddique S, et al. Locoregional treatment versus no treatment of the primary tumour in metastatic breast cancer: an open-label randomised controlled trial. *Lancet Oncol.* 2015 Oct;16(13):1380–8.
38. Soran A, Ozmen V, Ozbas S, Karanlik H, Muslumanoglu M, Igci A, et al. Randomized trial comparing resection of primary tumor with no surgery in stage IV breast cancer at presentation: protocol MF07-01. *Ann Surg Oncol.* 2018 Oct;25(11):3141–9.
39. Khan SA, Zhao F, Solin LJ, Goldstein LJ, Cella D, Basik M, et al. A randomized phase III trial of systemic therapy plus early local therapy versus systemic therapy alone in women with de novo stage IV breast cancer: a trial of the ECOG-ACRIN Research Group (E2108). *J Clin Oncol.* 2020 Jun 20;38(18_suppl): LBA2–LBA2.
40. Chmura SJ, Winter KA, Al-Hallaq HA, Borges VF, Jaskowiak NT, Matuszak M, et al. NRG-BR002: a phase IIR/III trial of standard of care therapy with or without stereotactic body radiotherapy (SBRT) and/ or surgical ablation for newly oligometastatic breast cancer (NCT02364557). *J Clin Oncol.* 2019 May 20; 37(15_suppl):TPS1117–TPS1117.

Index

Page numbers in *italics* and **bold** refer to figures and tables, respectively.

9780367609696